Praise for *The XX Brain*

"An empowering guide giving women the destiny."

—David Perlmutter, MD, #1 N
author of *Grain Brain*

"*The XX Brain* is a must-read for every woman who wants to protect her brain. Dr. Mosconi presents invaluable information and practical solutions to be—and stay—your best."

—Louann Brizendine, MD, *New York Times* bestselling
author of *The Female Brain*

"Women over 35 need to know that perimenopause is a dramatic transition state not just in terms of mood, sex drive, and hot flashes—but in terms of brain health and function. Lisa Mosconi is the leading authority on the female brain as it navigates hormonal upheaval, and she is here to close our knowledge gap. I give her extraordinary new book my highest recommendation."

—Sara Gottfried, MD, *New York Times* bestselling
author of *The Hormone Cure*

"Women's brains have unique risk factors for dementia that until now have been ignored by science. Lisa Mosconi's pathbreaking work changes this paradigm to show women how they specifically can protect and enhance brain function throughout life. Essential reading!"

—Max Lugavere, *New York Times* bestselling
author of *Genius Foods*

"This is a groundbreaking, must-read book, right on target with what I have found about women's brains. As we age it is critical for us to act aggressively in promoting not just our health but our brain health through lifestyle. I highly recommend it."

—Anna Cabeca, DO, author of *The Hormone Fix*

"*The XX Brain* is an exciting and empowering read for all women. Dr. Mosconi provides actionable advice to protect your brain and thrive throughout your lifetime! I highly recommend making your brain a priority now and taking charge before the inevitable hormonal shifts of perimenopause. In this book, Dr. Mosconi will show you how."

—JOLENE BRIGHTEN, ND, AUTHOR OF *BEYOND THE PILL*

"This extraordinary book gives women cutting-edge, research-based advice on what they particularly need to know to keep their brains functioning at maximum capacity. Highly recommended!"

—JJ VIRGIN, *NEW YORK TIMES* BESTSELLING
AUTHOR OF *THE VIRGIN DIET*

"In her new book, *The XX Brain*, [Dr. Mosconi] explains the differences between the female and male brains and explores the different ways the brain affects women's health. She offers practical tips on how to optimize brain health and discusses the unique risks women have for developing Alzheimer's disease and actions they can take to help prevent it."

—*THE WALL STREET JOURNAL*

"In *The XX Brain*, Mosconi makes a compelling argument: Brain health is women's health."

—GOOP

"*The XX Brain*: I'm buying this for every woman I love in my life."

—MANDY MOORE

THE XX BRAIN

The Groundbreaking Science
Empowering Women to Maximize Cognitive
Health and Prevent Alzheimer's Disease

LISA MOSCONI, PhD

Foreword by Maria Shriver

Avery / an imprint of Penguin Random House / New York

AVERY

an imprint of Penguin Random House LLC
penguinrandomhouse.com

First trade paperback edition 2022
Copyright © 2020 by Lisa Mosconi

Most Avery books are available at special quantity discounts for bulk purchase
for sales promotions, premiums, fund-raising, and educational needs. Special
books or book excerpts also can be created to fit specific needs. For details, write
SpecialMarkets@penguinrandomhouse.com.

The Library of Congress has cataloged
the hardcover edition of this book as follows:

Names: Mosconi, Lisa, author.
Title: The XX brain: the groundbreaking science empowering women to maximize
cognitive health and prevent Alzheimer's disease / Lisa Mosconi, PhD.
Description: New York: Avery, an imprint of Penguin Random House LLC,
[2020] | Includes bibliographical references and index.
Identifiers: LCCN 2019038997 (print) | LCCN 2019038998 (ebook) |
ISBN 9780593083116 (hardcover) | ISBN 9780593083123 (epub)
Subjects: LCSH: Alzheimer's disease—Prevention. | Alzheimer's
disease—Psychological aspects. | Women—Health and hygiene.
Classification: LCC RC523.2 .M68 2020 (print) |
LCC RC523.2 (ebook) | DDC 616.8/311—dc23
LC record available at https://lccn.loc.gov/2019038997
LC ebook record available at https://lccn.loc.gov/2019038998

ISBN (paperback) 9780593542132

Printed in the United States of America
3rd Printing

To the women of the world, and the brains
that make them who they are

CONTENTS

FOREWORD

I AM A DAUGHTER OF Alzheimer's disease.

My father, Sargent Shriver, was diagnosed with Alzheimer's in 2003. In 2011, he passed away from the disease. He'd been blessed with a particularly sharp mind, a beautifully tuned instrument that often left us awed and inspired. It was stunningly painful to watch this walking encyclopedia of a man go from knowing what seemed to be so much about so many things to being unable to recognize what a spoon or a fork was or remember my name—let alone being able to recall his own.

It was my father struggling with Alzheimer's, and later my mother suffering from a stroke (a strong risk factor for dementia), that propelled me to make it my mission to help find a cure for this devastating illness.

For over fifteen years, I have been on the front lines of the fight against Alzheimer's. As an activist and as a journalist, I work to raise awareness of this disease and to find ways to protect the precious future of America's minds. I've testified before Congress, founded the Women's Alzheimer's Movement, produced the award-winning *Alzheimer's Project* with HBO, written a bestselling children's book on Alzheimer's to start a conversation across generations, and executive-produced the Oscar-winning film *Still Alice*, the story of a woman beset with dementia.

In 2010, in collaboration with the Alzheimer's Association, I published *The Shriver Report: A Woman's Nation Takes on Alzheimer's*, in which we reported publicly for the first time that two-thirds of all those who end up with Alzheimer's are women. This startling fact prompted me to make women the top priority of my Alzheimer's advocacy.

Think about it. Every sixty-five seconds another person develops Alzheimer's disease; and of these newcomers, roughly two-thirds will be women—and we still don't know why. For a woman over sixty, the risk of developing Alzheimer's is twice that of developing breast cancer. With risks this steep, why isn't anyone and everyone talking about this crisis?

It is also women who make up two-thirds of the 40 million unpaid

American caregivers—17 million of them attending to dementia patients alone. Perhaps not surprisingly, comparable figures are found the world over. These caregivers are women who simultaneously work inside or outside their homes (or both). While juggling a life that often includes caring for young children, women take on the arduous task of caring for loved ones suffering from dementia, too. The latter is an enormously strenuous job in and of itself. With their own health risks already at stake, how are these women expected to take adequate care of themselves while coping with the daily physical burden, stress, and grief to which they are exposed—day in, day out, year after year?

Addressing these questions has been at the heart of my work at the Women's Alzheimer's Movement, or WAM. One of the most critical missions at WAM is to educate women about their risk for developing this devastating disease—and, perhaps even more important, to empower them with the information they need to take charge of their lives, health, and families by learning to care for their brain throughout their lives. We also fund women-based Alzheimer's research and are now developing ways to put that research to practical use. Our goal is to help establish medical centers of excellence, designed for people, especially women, to find the doctors and expertise they need to learn how to delay or prevent Alzheimer's disease. We know that there are distinct pathways to developing the disease in women that differ from those in men, and that there are specific junctures in a woman's medical journey that may increase her risk for developing the disease. So why not learn as much as we can about a woman's brain and its connection to her overall health so we can offer interventions, thereby delaying, if not preventing, the onset of Alzheimer's?

The book you have before you, *The XX Brain*, does nothing less than lead the way.

Dr. Lisa Mosconi has devoted her entire career to studying this very issue. She, too, has a story impacted by Alzheimer's. Lisa's grandmother was one of four children; she had two younger sisters and a brother. All three sisters would die of Alzheimer's while their brother was spared. As Lisa's grandmother became too ill to function, Lisa's mother took on the grueling role of primary caregiver and, along with it, the heartbreak, stress, and exhaustion that comes with shouldering such a task. Lisa witnessed firsthand how Alzheimer's appeared to selectively target the women around her, while seeing the brunt of the caregiving also fall to the women of the household. The myriadfold impact this had on her life drove her to search for the answers you'll find in this book.

Dedicating her life's work to this mission, Lisa now offers a means by which women can protect themselves from dementia, whether that means caring for others or suffering from the disease ourselves.

As you're about to read in the pages ahead, the medical profession has long accepted a gender disparity when it comes to brain health—one that was explained away by the fact that women tend to live longer than men. But now we know that other things are going on as well.

While most scientists in the field were focused on the hallmark plaques and tangles that Alzheimer's is known for, Lisa sensed a link between metabolic health and the increased Alzheimer's prevalence in women. She followed her gut, suspecting that our hormones might play a key role in rendering women more vulnerable to the disease. Thanks to Lisa and other like-minded scientists dissatisfied with the status quo, a movement began that was determined to take a closer look at how sex hormones, and the very XX chromosomes that inspired the title of this book, have unique impacts on our health as women. As it turns out, along with Alzheimer's, other conditions such as depression, stress-related illnesses, autoimmune diseases, and inflammation all affect women differently, and often more dramatically, than they do men.

I met Lisa when I went to get a cognitive baseline test from a leading expert in the Alzheimer's prevention field, Dr. Richard Isaacson. Richard started an Alzheimer's prevention program at Weill Cornell and New York–Presbyterian Hospital, an idea way ahead of its time. WAM has been supporting his efforts since 2016, as he looks for the scientific evidence to prove a link between lifestyle interventions and an improvement in cognitive function, including reducing one's risk for

Alzheimer's. In 2017, Richard introduced me to the new scientist he had just lured over from another hospital to work alongside him as associate director of the clinic, knowing that I would be interested in the work she was pursuing, given its focus on women. Lisa had just published the first study to show that women's brains become more vulnerable to Alzheimer's in the years leading up to and after menopause, and much of her work since has been on looking at the connection between younger women's hormones and the impact on their brains. She is one of the reasons we now know that women need to start thinking about brain health not after menopause but decades before. Her innovative work led us to invite her to join the WAM Scientific Advisory Council; and starting in 2018, we also began funding one of her research projects.

When I was interviewing her on the *Today* show, Lisa said something that struck me to my core: "Eight hundred and fifty million women all around the world have just entered, or are about to enter, menopause." Let me repeat: *Eight hundred and fifty million women.* She continued, "As if hot flashes, insomnia, and weight gain weren't enough, for some women, menopause may well be the beginning of a lifelong battle with dementia."

Clearly, we need a solution.

As a society, we're not sufficiently aware of how hormonal and health issues especially relevant to women—certain medications, pregnancy, perimenopause, even lack of sleep—affect our *brains*. Most of the prescription drugs women take have been tested only on men. Most of the doctors that women my age are used to seeing are male. Unless he's your gynecologist, he's not talking to you about hormones. He's not talking to you about menopause. No one's talking to you about perimenopause.

This uniquely female physiology both merits and demands wonder, respect, and research in ways we are only just beginning to adequately address. Perhaps this crisis, precipitated by an Alzheimer's epidemic that hits women so relentlessly from every angle, might at the same time trigger a revolution in women's health care—one that has been such a long time coming.

It is in this very spirit that Dr. Mosconi comes to the rescue.

Lisa's work has been pivotal in discovering that a woman's brain is more sensitive to hormonal fluctuations, as well as to specific medical and lifestyle risk factors, than a man's. In *The XX Brain*, Lisa meticulously guides us in the ways we can both nourish and protect ourselves, body and mind, to ensure our brains remain resilient throughout our lives—before, during, and after menopause. She will teach you to be your own detective in understanding and testing for your own risks, prime you in the process of crafting a health plan, and then supply you with the keys to optimize all therapeutic options available to you. Her results are personalized and targeted, offering a robust, customized program that harnesses cutting-edge discoveries to your best advantage. As a scientist, she knows better than to offer a quick-fix, magic-bullet approach. Rather, she asks you to be an active participant in your health care.

Taking care of our brains must begin early. It takes perseverance. It takes discipline. But the payoffs are *for life*.

Among the most exciting developments in the area of brain health is the news of how lifestyle modifications can be tailored to the repair, rejuvenation, and longevity of the brain. Where drugs continue to fail, women, in particular, have shown markedly responsive results to gender-targeted medical and lifestyle adjustments. Lisa has been at the forefront of these advances from their start.

This knowledge is crucial, as Alzheimer's is a disease that begins in the brain twenty to thirty years before any symptoms emerge. Although viable improvements have been shown at every age, intervening as far ahead of time as possible is key to prevention. How we live today impacts each of our tomorrows. Even if your health has not been a priority before, you can begin to make changes now that can quite literally *save the day*.

Personally, I've been following many of the brain-health recommendations included in this book. I have changed my diet, but not as much as I probably should. I do sleep. I'm trying to focus on trying to reduce my stress. I've always exercised, but I try to do it differently. I try to cut down on toxic situations. I try to walk out in nature and shut off the technology. I have a spiritual life, which is a big part of my being. I try to stay socially engaged. I try to learn new things. I'm actually learning to play poker.

As it did for me, I hope that *The XX Brain* will get you all fired up to blaze a trail with the wisdom Lisa will place at your fingertips. As women, we have every right to demand evidence-based, scientifically sound information about what we as mothers, wives, sisters, daughters, and granddaughters can do *right now* to reduce any risk we might have while optimizing our cognitive health. It is high time we equip ourselves with the knowledge of how to access help for our loved ones in need, while arming ourselves with the awareness and tools necessary to secure our own physical and mental well-being.

Lisa and I share this common passion. We are devoted to educating women to prioritize brain health in much the same way that we're encouraging a more vigilant approach to valuing ourselves and our bodies as a whole. We want to inspire you to advocate for women's health, to stay curious while you educate yourself, to speak up and reach out for the answers to supply what you need to thrive in good health.

I wish I'd had this book in my twenties. I wish someone had spoken to me after each of my four children was born about the changes I might expect to my cognitive health during and after pregnancy. I wish someone had counseled me in my forties about the changes that would occur not just to my body but also to my brain over the next decade. I didn't get this information earlier, but I am grateful this book now exists for my daughters and the generations of women I hope will learn how to care for their brains—and lower their risk for developing Alzheimer's and other dementias.

I often say that your mind is your greatest asset. It's going to be with you for your entire lifetime, so the time to start taking care of it is *now*. And while we all should start caring for our brains when we're young, the fact is that no matter what our age, it's never too late to start, including today. I hope with Lisa's help you'll be inspired to do so, and enjoy the journey of being introduced to your brain!

Maria Shriver

RECLAIMING WOMEN'S HEALTH

ALL OVER THE WORLD, WOMEN'S EQUALITY, which has come so far since the days of American suffragettes and Women's Lib, is being re-evaluated in real time. Between #MeToo on the one hand and "lean in" on the other, between the increasing demand on women to contribute equally to the workforce and to the household despite the persistent gap in wages, questions come up every day about how equal, or how different, women are. At the same time, there are headline conversations about what it even means to be female to begin with.

I started writing this book in the aftermath of #MeToo, a movement that was born of a new recognition of the various ways women are outright abused and assaulted. But there are deeper shades of nuance in this movement, ones that speak instead to how women are more subtly undermined—not assaulted, but neglected, dismissed, and at times sabotaged.

On a global scale, women are derailed financially by consistently and universally being paid less than men. They are minimized legally, even considered a form of property in many ways and in many parts of the world. They are hindered intellectually, as women make up two-thirds of the 774 million illiterate adults on the planet, figures that haven't budged in twenty years. Such disparities are being brought to light all over, though it's yet to be seen whether any change will result from more voices or louder speech.

But for all the discussions about the many ways women are treated differently from men, one topic that remains woefully neglected is the one that is closest to my heart: the notion of gender disparity around health and wellness.

As surely as women's social, financial, and physical security remain inequitable, women's health is in deep jeopardy. Women were promised we could "have it all." We've discovered that means "doing it all" instead. And not only do we now get to do it all, but we do so for lower pay and less recognition, and not at all surprisingly, at the expense of our health. We are trained and encouraged to see how many balls we can keep in the air at any given time, and to apply our deepest determination to keep them there, *just so.*

We tend to hold ourselves to very high standards as we navigate this awkward obstacle course, many of us severely overtaxing our bodies and minds in the process. As we juggle madly, society pushes us to do so without breaking a sweat, with broad smiles on our faces, and all the while keeping an eye on the mirror to make sure we "look good" in the process. On the long list of societal, cultural, and familial demands on women, our being healthy just doesn't seem to make the cut. It doesn't take a scientist to point out that there is something askew here.

But it does take a scientist to denounce the way that women are also overlooked *medically*, where our needs too often go unrecognized, misattributed, or unaddressed. This is in large part due to the fact that the field of medicine has been historically male dominated, which led to the fundamental model for most medical research being not a person, but a *man*. For a number of reasons, which we'll discuss shortly, medical interventions have been largely tested with, dosed for, and modeled based on their effects on men.

This is not the source of a conspiracy theory, but rather an acknowledgment of the compound effects of assumptions made over centuries, which have led to our teaching and practicing "bikini medicine." For those of you not familiar with the term: Historically, medical professionals believed that the only thing that set women apart from men were those body parts that lie beneath the small triangles of a bikini—namely, our reproductive organs. Setting these "parts" aside, as if one could, meant that most doctors would diagnose and treat both sexes in the exact same way. This biased approach remains just as prevalent and deeply destructive in the hard sciences as it is in many other aspects of culture at large.

Given the worldview derived from that model, the very notion of women's health is problematic. If you ask doctors to look at a female patient through the lens of "women's health," they will likely run a mammogram or collect cells from the cervix to examine them for cancer. Doing blood tests for estrogen and other hormones is just as common a practice. In other words, women's health is confined to the health of our reproductive organs. Let's be clear that all these procedures have indeed changed and bettered the lives of millions of women around the world. However, these same lines of research, inquiry, and intervention are a direct consequence of a reductive understanding of *what a woman is*.

BRAIN HEALTH IS WOMEN'S HEALTH

From where I sit, as the director of the Women's Brain Initiative at Weill Cornell Medical College and associate director of the first Alzheimer's Prevention Clinic in the United States, I scan the press every day for a headline that's never yet appeared. It's for the unwritten story about distinguishing women's health outcomes in one part of the body that no bikini will ever cover: the brain.

Women's brain health is one of the most underrepresented and unspoken concerns, one that is constantly glossed over as a result of the male-based medical paradigm. Somehow, in the landscape of things that we're told a woman should be concerned with, her brain has seldom been one of them. Further, very few doctors have the knowledge or framework to address the many ways that brain health plays out differently in women than in men.

In my work, I also rely on those aforementioned women's health tests to better understand and help our patients. But when I think about women's health, I reach for brain imaging techniques like magnetic resonance imaging (MRI) and positron emission tomography (PET) to see what's happening inside our patients' heads. Because this is where some of the truly momentous dynamics of women's health are taking place. Far more than our breasts and tubes, our brains are under the greatest threat.

If that sounds hyperbolic, here are the statistics that most people aren't familiar with:

- Women are twice as likely to have anxiety and depression as men.

- Women are over three times more likely than men to be diagnosed with an autoimmune disorder, including those that attack the brain, like multiple sclerosis.

- Women are up to four times more likely to suffer from migraines and headaches than men.

- Women are more prone than men to developing meningiomas, the most common brain tumors.

- Strokes kill more women than men.

But looking further through a neuroscientist's lens, we can see an even more consequential danger in our collective and individual futures. There is a silent and looming epidemic brewing that is going to impact women greatly—one that most people are completely unaware of.

Alzheimer's Sets Its Sights

Alzheimer's disease haunts the twenty-first century. In most regions of the world, there isn't a person alive who doesn't have a personal story about how the disease has touched someone they care for, whether it be a parent or grandparent, a beloved relative, or a close friend. Beyond the pain of these personal stories, a broader collective narrative has emerged.

Of all the challenges to brain aging, nothing compares to the unprecedented scale of Alzheimer's disease, which has become the most common form of dementia, currently affecting 5.7 million people in the United States alone. With rates increasing at their current clip, the disease will almost triple by 2050. That means that, by then, 15 million Americans will be suffering from Alzheimer's. For context, that number is equal to the populations of New York, Chicago, and Los Angeles combined. On a global scale, Alzheimer's patients will number somewhere between the populations of Russia and Mexico!

Bottom line: we are facing nothing less than an Alzheimer's epidemic.

At the same time, we have yet to be made aware of the fact that these numbers do not tell a story of equality when it comes to the victims of this epidemic. Not many people know that Alzheimer's has its own epidemiology, with a deeply outsize representation among a selective part of the population. Alzheimer's has, in fact, set its sights predominantly on women. To provide the most blunt and startling statistic: today, *two out of every three Alzheimer's patients are women.*

Today, Alzheimer's is as real a threat to women's health as breast cancer is. Women in their sixties are about twice as likely to develop Alzheimer's over the rest of their lives as they are to develop breast cancer. And yet breast cancer is clearly identified as a women's health issue, while Alzheimer's is not. One of the most startling facts about the disease is that a forty-five-year-old woman has a one in five chance of developing Alzheimer's during her remaining life, while a man of the same age has only a one in ten chance. This is no dismissal of the suffering that men with Alzheimer's will experience. But we need to confront the reality that, at the end of the day, many more women end their lives suffering from the disease. And this is only the first blow in a one-two punch.

The second blow is that, when it comes to providing caregiving throughout this continuing crisis, it is women once more who will bear the bulk of the burden. As it is mostly women who will find themselves, inadvertently or not, drafted into full-time caregiving roles. Currently, there are 10 million American women providing unpaid health care and assistance to loved ones with dementia, all simultaneously shouldering the steep emotional and financial tolls that accompany that crushing task.

It is time to come to terms with these numbers—not only to confront the large-scale epidemic, but also to finally acknowledge, investigate, and react to the very targeted crisis ahead in women's health. In recent years, scientists like myself have grown more and more eager to uncover what it is about women's brains that make us susceptible to Alzheimer's as well as to a host of other medical conditions that affect the brain. Why is this happening? Can we stop it from happening? Our investigations have raised an entire range of thought-provoking existential and scientific questions, not the least of which is: How is it possible we haven't figured this out yet?

To Change the Future, Confront the Mistakes of the Past

Certain medical conditions have affected the genders differently over the history of humankind. How we came to understand (and misunderstand) those conditions relative to women's health is a much shorter history. It's important to point out again that this wasn't a deliberate attempt to undermine women's health, but neither was it a thoughtful process about how certain decisions would affect us.

In the 1950s and early '60s, it was fairly common to prescribe a drug called thalidomide for the treatment of nausea in pregnant women. A few years later, it became evident that what was once thought to be an innocuous treatment had resulted in severe birth defects in thousands of children. This prompted the United States Food and Drug Administration (FDA) to prohibit use of the drug. They also recommended that women of childbearing age be excluded from all exploratory clinical trials until evidence of safety and effectiveness had become available, to avoid risks to the fetus. That cautionary stance was, however, misinterpreted and applied to all types of trials, which effectively disqualified women of any age from puberty through menopause from participating in medical research. As a result, women were no longer informing medical research either.

On top of that, animal studies focused on males, too, since menstrual cycles were thought to make female animals too "unpredictable" to study. So for decades, research was overwhelmingly conducted on male cells, male mice, and male patients, which in turn supplied medical practice with data that didn't apply (or applied inconsistently) to half of the population. "Normal" meant "male."

Eventually, the AIDS epidemic of the 1980s brought the first real challenge to "protectionist" policies preventing women's participation in research. Activists fought diligently to convince the FDA to give patients access to experimental drugs that could potentially treat AIDS. This slow and hard-won victory mobilized thousands of women to demand their fair share of access. At the same time, a dramatic increase in medical school enrollment among women during the 1970s resulted in an emerging group of medical professionals willing and able to question the status quo policies that were hobbling women's health care. With women taking strong roles in Congress then as well, and professional females now active in the health-care field, and women's advocacy groups on alert, a united front began to form that demanded attention to these oversights. Why had women's health care been confined to ob-gyn practices? How could women's health needs be relegated to little more than an often-ignored maternal leave and child-care services?

The uproar that followed led to the Government Accountability Office (a congressional watchdog that keeps an eye on federal spending) publishing, in the 1990s, a provocative report arguing that women were not adequately included in clinical trials. After all, some of the largest studies at the time, such as the Physicians' Health Study and the Multiple Risk Factor Intervention Trial (known by the ironic acronym MR. FIT), were 100 percent male-only trials. The report was so persuasive that it prompted the National Institutes of Health to create the Office of Research on Women's Health. Just a couple of years later, the Revitalization Act was launched, requiring that women be considered as participants in research on human subjects.

Today, we scientists are required by law to recruit both men and women for our research. However, rather than looking at each gender's effects separately, most studies end up lumping them together. Then, by applying careful statistical manipulation to the data collected, any important indicators of gender differentials are often removed. We ought to be careful about trusting such findings. Far from being caused by intellectual laziness or shortsightedness, this practice is often due to a bottom-line lack of funding. In order to look at men and women independently, studies would need twice the number of patients, twice the time, and twice the money. Many scientists have no other option than to keep removing gender from the equation, suppressing its undeniable impact on study outcomes. As a result, what doctors know about preventing, diagnosing, and treating disease continues to this day to be pulled from male-biased or "gender-less" studies.

The Consequences for Women

This persistence in considering men and women as biologically identical is particularly frustrating considering that gender-specific genetic and hormonal factors have an enormous impact on one's response to a drug, as well as on its efficacy.

For starters, we have long known that women metabolize drugs differently than men do and often require different doses. However, dosages are rarely adjusted by sex, which results in women having almost double the chance of an adverse drug reaction than men. Pointing to this effect, there are reports noting that eight out of the ten prescription drugs removed from the market between 1997 and 2000 posed greater health risks for women than for men. Another stunning example of this trend is revealed in the too often untold story behind flibanserin, the first "female Viagra." When the drug was evaluated for side effects, the studies were conducted on twenty-three men and only two women!

America's most popular sleep drug, zolpidem (better known as Ambien), is yet another case of how these biases are often permitted to reach dangerous conclusions before consideration is shown to gender differences in medicine. In 2012, it became clear that men and women taking the exact same dose of Ambien exhibited dramatically different reactions. Women on the drug were more likely to be found the next morning sleepwalking, sleep-eating, and even sleep-driving, leading to drug-specific reports of car accidents. Why? As it turns out, women reach maximum blood levels of Ambien at much lower doses than men. Finally, the medical community called for a reexamination of the drug's indications, which led to the FDA cutting the previously recommended dose for women by a whopping half! But for the previous twenty years or so, millions of women had been overmedicated and subsequently compromised while on Ambien, simply by following instructions that ignored a woman's specific criteria. As if all this weren't enough, high cumulative doses of Ambien have recently been linked to a greater risk of dementia.

This begs the question of how many other examples exist of female gender-related oversights in the field of medicine. The more we study, the more we are finding instances, such as spectacular discrepancies in our ability to simply diagnose women correctly. In fact, in addition to being prescribed drugs to the point of overdosing, women are also more likely to be misdiagnosed, or to have their symptoms go unrecognized as a result of doctors being informed (or rather, misinformed) by a process based on faulty data.

The field of cardiology has produced some of the best-known examples of medicine gone wrong with regard to female patients. Tragically, women are seven times more likely to be misdiagnosed and discharged mid–heart attack than men. The problem is that doctors fail to recognize women's symptoms, as they can differ widely from men's while also being generally more subtle. Evidently, only one in eight female patients report feeling the so-called Hollywood heart attack (with chest-clutching and crushing pain radiating down the left arm), which, as it turns out, is a typical male symptom. Rather, over 70 percent of women show flu-like symptoms, such as shortness of breath, a cold sweat, or nausea, along with pain in the back, jaw, or stomach—all of which can occur without any chest pain.

What other symptoms are we missing when we diagnose a woman as if she were a man? How many of us have already been misdiagnosed and continue to be misdiagnosed? Perhaps as a compounding result of the issues mentioned above, it is unfortunately very common for women to have their health concerns downplayed or dismissed. To add insult to injury, women are more likely than men to be told their pain is psychosomatic, hypochondriac, or influenced by emotional distress. More often than not, a woman in pain will walk out of the doctor's office with a prescription for antidepressants instead of painkillers.

The Bottom Line, and Where It Leads Us

In medicine, the simple fact is that we don't do as good a job of taking care of women as we do men. A woman often ends up having to prove she is as sick as a man, or has to mirror male symptoms, to receive the same level of care. This concept has become so obvious in medical practice that it led to the coining of a concept called "the Yentl syndrome." The term derives from the 1983 film *Yentl*, starring Barbra Streisand, in which her character pretends to be a Jewish man in order to gain access to schooling to become a rabbi. The Yentl syndrome is bringing our attention to an age-old and ongoing struggle: men have long had the majority of advantages, privileges, and access, while women have had to fight for the same.

As this is present in all aspects of our health care, it is no surprise then that it is equally true when it comes to the health of our brains. Women are falling prey to Alzheimer's, but also to depression, migraines, and a number of other conditions that affect the brain. Yet modern medicine is largely unprepared to help them.

Fortunately, scientists have come to the rescue. In recent years, an incredible amount of work has been done both to denounce and to investigate the gender disparity in brain health. With this book, my mission is to take this work past the rigors and paywalls of peer-reviewed research, and to give a wider voice to the "forgotten gender."

Since university, I have focused on developing tools and strategies to optimize cognitive health, while at the same time warding off Alzheimer's, particularly in women. The passion that has shaped my career was born in great part from having seen the devastating effects of Alzheimer's on my own family. Witnessing my grandmother's bitter downward spiral into dementia propelled me to devote my entire career to researching any and all possibilities of detecting the disease ahead of time. When both of my grandmother's younger sisters developed Alzheimer's, too, while their brother did not, my determination grew stronger still. I now find myself keeping a close watch on my mom for any warning signs, though I feel reassured as she carefully attends to a healthy diet and practices her yoga headstands at age seventy-six. As a middle-aged woman, I am concerned about my own risk. As a mother, I want to make sure my daughter has answers, options, and solutions.

As a scientist, I have dedicated my entire career to helping make preventative medical care to maintain cognitive function an integral part of every woman's medical requirements, as commonplace as regular mammograms, Pap tests, and colonoscopies. Together, let us literally turn the page toward a tomorrow in which there is a dedicated equality of assessment and treatment in health care, our brains included, providing true hope for all.

Caring for the XX Brain

The XX Brain confronts the unspoken crisis in women's health by revealing how the two powerful X chromosomes that distinguish women from men not only impact our reproductive organs but, due to their interactions with the rest of our genetic makeup, environment, and lifestyle, also influence each and every aspect of our health—our brain first and foremost.

As women, we experience gaps in income, power, and representation, but we also face a gap in knowledge about our health, collectively and individually. It's time to rectify this and to address our unique symptoms and concerns as related to our brains and to our bodies as a whole. We all want our cognitive life span to match our life span—we can't wait until signs of cognitive decline appear. We must be proactive now.

My goal with this book is to arm each reader with strategies that will give the female brain precisely what it needs, not just to power through any pitfalls, but to thrive. These recommendations have emerged from my many years of clinical research and interactions with both women and men at different levels of cognitive fitness. Some had perfect memories and impressive attention spans. Others would sometimes forget names and details, and worry that their memory was no longer as good as it used to be. Others still were already suffering from cognitive deterioration or dementia. After observing the potential vulnerabilities in women, and which factors set women's brains apart from men's, I've devised a specific program to maximize women's cognitive power and provide the practices necessary to maintain this self-care over the course of a lifetime.

The strategies I will outline are designed to enhance mental acuity, memory, and cognitive skills, as well as to reduce the risk of Alzheimer's, specifically in women. I will also address many common conditions affecting women of all ages, from depression and anxiety to stress and insomnia, along with medical conditions such as hormonal imbalances, diabetes, obesity, and heart disease, as these all deeply impact our brain health, too. These practices are essential for any woman who wishes to maximize her cognitive health, no matter her age.

Luckily, it is never too late to take care of yourself. No matter when you start, the benefits are scientifically undeniable. By virtue of sharpening our personal choices, we can free ourselves from the expense and side effects of "magic pill" medications, from meekly accepting our supposed genetic "luck of the draw," and from succumbing to invasive treatments or surgeries.

This specialized prevention program requires three basic steps:

1. Understanding when and why the female brain risks damage as we age.
2. Carefully testing our own risk factors.
3. Applying this knowledge in our daily lives as we make the choice to protect our brains, our bodies, and our very precious vitality from such damage.

To this end, the book is divided into three parts:

Part 1. Take In: The Research Behind the Practice provides the foundational elements needed to understand how the female brain works and its challenges, threats, and opportunities for optimization. Here I share firsthand accounts of discoveries made through my own research combined with my personal experiences both as a scientist and as a woman.

Part 2. Take Action: Get Tested outlines the key diagnostic procedures needed to optimize brain health and attend to disease prevention in women, with a particular focus on the screening process. We will take into consideration that no two women are alike—and so identifying the root causes of your own risks and symptoms is key to devising the best treatment plan for *you*. What do you need to know to take care of yourself more efficiently? Which tests are truly valuable, and what exactly do they measure? How do you define your "baseline"? What are your personal risk factors, and how can you work collaboratively with your doctor to address these risks?

Part 3. Take Charge: Optimize Your Brain Health, Minimize Your Risks provides evidence-based recommendations designed to manage risk while improving and protecting cognitive performance in women. We will tackle the wide host of symptoms commonly reported by women over thirty, including fatigue, insomnia, mood swings, and stress. Among these symptoms is forgetfulness, an issue we will carefully examine. We will also look at the bodily transformations that can lead to weight gain, insulin resistance, and a higher risk of heart disease, with a particular focus on hormonal declines and the onset of menopause. In doing so, we will sidestep the all too often confusing and conflicting health news online and arm ourselves instead with the latest proven studies on lifestyle medicine, including medical care, dietary choices and supplements that are scientifically valid, and the exercise, sleep, and stress-reduction solutions that work.

Understanding when a woman first becomes vulnerable allows us to determine when she needs to start making changes and which of these changes are the most effective in reducing risk and maintaining cognitive function. This is a road map for you to follow, one that sets your compass in the direction of optimal and lifelong brain health, and away from brain diseases like Alzheimer's. Whether your goal is to boost your brainpower for the long haul, feel calmer and happier, have more energy or improve your sleep, minimize memory lapses or cut your risk of dementia altogether, I am confident that taking these simple brain-enhancing steps will help your brain be at its very best for all your years to come.

As a reader, you might be a man who also cares about women—perhaps your mother, or your partner, or your daughter—or maybe you're just genuinely interested in the other half of the population. Thank you, truly, for caring. Although this book is unapologetically for women and about women, in truth, our goals of advancing women's health care will never become reality without men's help. This isn't about women against men, without men, or instead of men. On the contrary, it's about understanding women in a broader context. Every woman's brain needs the right food, sleep, and exercise, but it's no new discovery that it also needs the empathy, love, and support of the men (and other women) around it.

PART 1

TAKE IN: THE RESEARCH BEHIND THE PRACTICE

CHAPTER 1

THE INNER WORKINGS OF THE FEMALE BRAIN

JOHN GRAY'S BESTSELLER *Men Are from Mars, Women Are from Venus*, in which he coined that now-famous metaphor, speaks to pop science's long-term fascination with the psychological differences between men and women. There's no shortage of comedy routines that enjoy poking fun at this infamous battle of the sexes. If we were so inclined, we could hop on the bandwagon, imagining a female brain that consisted of zones such as the must-have-chocolate-now node, the gossip gland, or the busy kids-and-marriage center. Of course, our male counterparts would possess their own set of similarly satirized areas, including a pair of power tool glands, a quick-firing lame excuse lobe, and the ever-defiant "getting lost and not admitting it" region.

The origins of behavioral differences between men and women have been a topic of conversation since ancient history. However, the idea that the brain could be the principal means by which males and females behave differently is strikingly modern, having only been accepted as a true determining factor in the 1960s. Before then, people were convinced that our genitals themselves were at the crux of the matter. Then in 1992, scientists made a very powerful discovery: Our so-called sex hormones, such as estrogen and testosterone, influence not only sexual behavior but brain function as well. In other words, the hormones inextricably involved with our sexuality turn out to be just as crucial in the overall functioning of our minds.

Although our gender and its hormones don't offer a universal explanation for our health or behavior, gender differences in the brain manifest themselves in many fascinating and often overlooked ways. This is in part due to the fact that hormones are made by our DNA, and as we know, our DNA is different depending on our sex. However, not many people know that the X chromosome is actually much larger than the relatively tiny Y chromosome, containing a lofty 1,098 genes as compared with the Y chromosome's 78. This means that a woman, wielding her double X, possesses over 1,000 more genes than a man, many of which are critical for both hormonal production and brain activity.

X MARKS THE SPOT: THE ESTROGEN-DRIVEN BRAIN

All women are intuitively aware of the constant conversation between their brains and their hormones, and many of us find ourselves attributing our moods to them. Actually, our female hormones do have strong, deep effects on the brain that go far beyond the typical attributes of PMS and the variety of other ups and downs associated with our cycles.

Hormones are powerful chemicals involved in almost every process in the body and brain, including cellular metabolism, tissue growth, and recovery from injury. By doing so, hormones keep our brains acute, energized, and youthful. At the same time, they keep our bones strong, our gut active, and our sex life potent. They also affect our weight, immune function, and even how we turn food into fuel. Thanks to their all-encompassing roles, our hormones influence every aspect of our physiology, and subsequently, our health—physical and mental. When your hormones are out of whack, you feel it everywhere, from your joints to your thoughts. Depending on whether they are in balance or going awry, we'll experience changes not only in a number of bodily functions but also in our cognitive power, mood, and mental alertness, right down to how we think, talk, feel, and remember.

While all hormones are important in this regard, most of the research points to 17ß-estradiol, more commonly known as "estrogen," as a major, if not the major, hormonal driver of women's brain health.

Estrogen is a "master regulator" in the female brain, serving many roles that actually have nothing to do with reproduction, but rather everything to do with energy. Estrogen is key in the regulation of energy production and overall balance of various brain functions (homeostasis). This is particularly important in keeping brain cells healthy and active, as well as fostering brain activity in regions responsible for memory, attention, and planning .

Importantly, estrogen is also a neuro-protective hormone, playing a crucial defensive role in the brain by boosting the immune system, thereby shielding neurons from harm. And not only does it protect our nerve cells, but estrogen also encourages the formation of new connections between those cells. A well-connected brain is in turn more resilient and adaptable. Moreover, estrogen just so happens to be "nature's Prozac," too. Its levels influence the brain's production of gamma-aminobutyric acid (GABA), a chemical that soothes the nervous system, thanks to its calming properties, while also promoting the release of endorphins, the body's natural painkillers. Finally, our hormones all contribute to blood flow and circulation in the brain, which is crucial to ensuring the brain has an adequate supply of oxygen and nutrients.

All these effects start taking place inside our brains from the very moment of conception, during the development of the embryo in the womb. Over time, circulating hormones play an important role in the sexual differentiation of the brain. Androgens (male hormones like testosterone) produce a "male" brain, while a lack of those androgens, with a subsequent increase in estrogens (female hormones) in their place, produce a "female" brain.

Though these differences are subtle, if you were to closely inspect the brains of men and women, as I so often do for my work, you might notice them. For example, depending on which type of hormone is more abundant in your brain (estrogen in women, testosterone in men), you may be making more or less of certain neurotransmitters, the chemical messengers that the brain uses for signaling, communication, and information processing. Generally, men's brains produce more serotonin, the "feel good" neurotransmitter involved in mood, sleep, and even appetite. Women produce more dopamine instead—a brain chemical responsible for one's drive and reward-motivated behavior.

Even more intriguing is the fact that some parts of our brains are "sexually dimorphic," which means they are built a bit differently from each other depending on gender. For instance, the fact that men and women don't see things in the same way turns out to be as literal an observation as it is a figurative one. Deep within the visual cortex, the part of the brain that is responsible for processing visual information, we find one good example of why men and women don't always see eye to eye. While men possess more M cells, those cells responsible for movement detection, women have more P cells, the cells in charge of detecting objects and shapes. (Could this explain women's superior ability to find things in the fridge?)

Moving on to our ears, women also generally hear better than men, in part because we have 11 percent more neurons in the primary auditory cortex, the part of the brain that decodes sound. Additionally, although men have generally bigger brains by virtue of having generally bigger bodies, women have thicker cerebral cortices that seem better interconnected. In particular, in women's brains, the hippocampus (the memory center of the brain) and the amygdala (the emotional center of the brain) are more tightly connected to the frontal cortex, which is in charge of abstract thinking, planning, and reasoning.

As a result, gender differences in brain connectivity are particularly pronounced in the limbic system, the part of the brain that includes the hippocampus and amygdala mentioned above, and that resonates with the experiences of love and affection, thereby responding to the innumerable factors involved in having a family. This part of the brain is responsible for generating the motivations and emotions that govern parental instincts, everything from nursing children to protecting them, not to mention the impulse to engage and play with them. If you have children, perhaps you have tiptoed into your children's rooms at night to check their breathing, or to deposit a kiss on their foreheads before being able to sleep yourself. Or maybe you have found yourself smiling at the thought of reading your children their favorite bedtime story, in spite of the fact that you've probably read that very same tale over a hundred times already. Those are all signs of the limbic lobe in action. Men have it too, but women possess its qualities in spades. Suddenly some familiar cultural stereotypes don't seem quite so strange, do they?

It is important to point out that although male and female brains are to some extent wired differently and exhibit some biochemical differences, this doesn't have a big effect on behavior. To be perfectly clear, there is nothing in our biology to justify the gender gap in equality, wages, or opportunities. There is also no scientific basis for a "gendered brain." Blue versus pink, Barbie versus Lego, businessman versus secretary—these are all social constructs that have nothing to do with how our brains are built or operate. Unfortunately, though, results from scientific studies have all too often been manipulated to imply that one gender, the male gender, is better or more intellectually advanced than the other. You may have caught wind of the idea that "brilliance in math is a male phenomenon," a bias that disregards the fact that men have had access to higher education for significantly longer than women—not to mention that there are plenty of brilliant female mathematicians in spite of these obstacles: Ada Lovelace, Emmy Noether, and Katherine Johnson, to name but a few. The truth of the matter is that men and women are equally intellectually capable, though we may arrive at our results by way of somewhat different neural routes.

All that said, from a raw biological perspective, men and women are different to some degree. Such diversity produces gender-specific health risks and vulnerabilities. In particular, closer to my research and more urgent to consider, a growing body of literature shows that male and female brains age differently, in part because of changes in hormonal quantity and quality.

Our brains go through a series of hormonal transitions throughout our lives as we progress from childhood to puberty, and eventually on to loss of fertility and the onset of menopause. While puberty is accompanied by an explosion of hormonal power, the loss of fertility in women can be more of a blow than anticipated. If you consider estrogen as fuel for the brain, rather than for babies, the magnitude of the change becomes a lot clearer.

IT IS, INDEED, "ALL IN YOUR HEAD"

As mentioned at the beginning of this book, my colleagues and I have been focused on brain health with specific regard to what happens as women age. By "age," I don't mean achieving "senior" status. I mean any woman who is past adolescence. Over the years, we have performed several brain imaging studies on healthy women aged twenty-one to eighty and compared them with studies of healthy men of the same age. We measured multiple factors, starting with how the brain was processing glucose, its principal source of fuel. We scanned for Alzheimer's plaques, and also checked for brain atrophy and any evidence of stroke or vascular issues. We then followed many of these patients over time, some of them for a couple of years, others for as long as fifteen to twenty years.

When we are taking stock of the differences that confront men and women, there is one glaring distinction during the crucial period of midlife: women are in the process of navigating menopause, while men are not. As we proceeded, our work revealed a variety of findings, the most striking of which by far was that the delicate decline of women's fertility, with the arrival of menopause, affects our brains big-time. It turns out that menopause affects much more than a woman's fertility. For most women, hormonal changes trigger a host of well-known menopausal symptoms, such as hot flashes, night sweats, disturbed sleep, depression, and memory lapses. Although these symptoms are typically associated with our ovaries, in reality they originate somewhere else entirely: inside the brain itself. The ebb in hormones, a hallmark of menopause, causes the loss of a key protective element in the female brain. In fact, diminishing hormones are known to accelerate the aging process. Throughout the body, as we get older, hormones that build muscle and bone are on the decline, while those that break down tissue increase. The result is that our cells experience more wear and tear with less access to repair. The skin gets more wrinkly, the hair turns more dry, bones become more frail. Unfortunately, the same can happen inside our brains, weakening our neurons and making our brains more vulnerable to aging and disease.

For most women, these changes manifest themselves as bothersome hot flashes and mood swings. But for some women, hormonal changes potentially diminish the brain's ability to resist diseases like Alzheimer's.

This is quite evident when we look at the brain scans shown in the figure below. The scan to the left shows brain "metabolism," or activity levels, in a woman with no signs of menopause, a stage known as pre-menopause. The scan to the right shows brain activity in a post-menopausal woman instead. The gray scale reflects brain activity, with lighter gray indicating more activity, and darker gray indicating lower activity. The scan of the post-menopausal woman looks darker overall, which means that her brain has substantially lower brain metabolism than the pre-menopausal woman's brain to the left. This isn't just an isolated case. This is what the "average" brain looked like after menopause. In some women, these reductions were quite marked, with over 30 percent reduced brain activity. Alarmingly, similar findings were discovered in women at the perimenopausal (almost menopausal) stage, who also showed marked reductions. Men of the same age, on the other hand, showed minimal changes, and in many cases, none.

FIGURE 1. MENOPAUSE: BRAIN ACTIVITY BEFORE AND AFTER

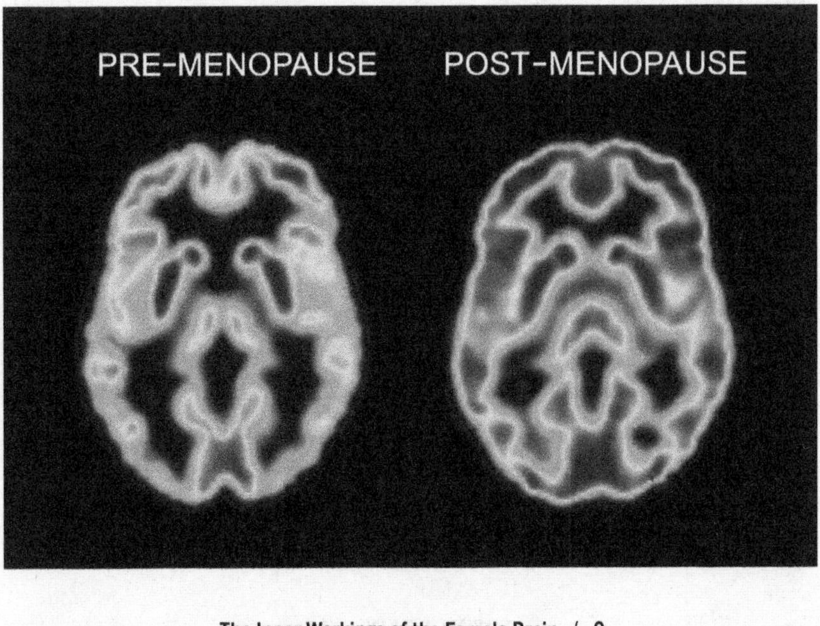

PRE-MENOPAUSE   POST-MENOPAUSE

Of greater concern, some women transitioning to menopause also showed an increased accumulation of amyloid plaques, a major hallmark of Alzheimer's disease. Additionally, these women showed progressive metabolic decline as well as shrinkage of the memory centers of the brain. These findings are a big red flag, because a similar pattern of brain changes is often found in patients in the earliest stages of Alzheimer's.

The timing also points to an increased risk of future Alzheimer's. One of the most shocking findings that scientists stumbled upon is that Alzheimer's begins in the brain decades before the first symptom. Specifically, Alzheimer's starts with negative changes to the brain beginning in midlife, in our forties and fifties . . . not in old age. For some, this might come as a great surprise, so let me clarify. We've always associated Alzheimer's with the elderly because that's when the disease has finally wreaked enough havoc for cognitive symptoms to consistently appear. In actuality, the disease launches its attack many years prior.

In some way, Alzheimer's is like a stock market crash. It doesn't come out of nowhere—it appears at the end of a long sequence of interrelated economic factors that ultimately produce the crash. Likewise, Alzheimer's isn't like you suddenly caught a cold. Just like heart disease or even cancer, these conditions don't bubble up overnight. Rather, Alzheimer's is the result of a number of genetic, medical, and lifestyle events that have been happening along the way. Their effects end up impacting the brain most in midlife, with symptoms that appear as we get older—a process that seems to start earlier in some women's brains, during the transition to menopause.

So if you've ever been told by a well-meaning doctor that the symptoms you have are all in your head, here's your proof that all you've been experiencing is scientifically valid and viable. Most important, it also allows us to finally do something about it! To clarify: Menopause doesn't "cause" Alzheimer's. As an event, menopause is more like a trigger in which the superpower of estrogen and its companion hormones is revoked, and the brain has to find new ways to perform efficiently. It is then, when the brain is busy adjusting, that the risk goes up for other issues to become actual medical problems. For many women, the brain shifts associated with menopause generate forgetfulness, memory lapses, even cognitive slippage. Others find themselves experiencing unprecedented mood swings, anxiety, and depressive symptoms. For others still, these changes can potentially lead to Alzheimer's making an appearance. As disturbing as this sounds, perhaps this is one of the vital clues that will allow us to figure out why Alzheimer's hits women harder than men.

BEYOND ALZHEIMER'S: THE "ESTROGEN HYPOTHESIS"

The impact of hormonal changes on women's brains is not limited to the threat or consequences of Alzheimer's. The role of hormones in women's brain health, with estrogen leading the charge, has been gaining increasing recognition in various medical fields, leading to important and sometimes frightening discoveries.

The field of psychiatry has unraveled perhaps one of the most extreme examples, providing evidence that fluctuations in hormonal levels during menopause might trigger a previously unrecognized form of schizophrenia. Historically, schizophrenia was regarded as a disorder of the young, affecting mostly males. In more recent years, scientists identified a demonstrable "second peak" of first-onset schizophrenia after age forty-five (or more specifically in the years leading up to menopause), affecting predominantly females.

Recognition of this new form of schizophrenia highlighted a deeply embedded bias in the way doctors had thought about the disease for centuries, overlooking the many middle-aged women who came to them for help. Records from the late nineteenth century abound with cases of American women suffering from late-onset schizophrenia who were instead labeled "insane from suppressed menses" and committed to asylums. Nowadays, while antipsychotic medications are a common treatment for both men and women, very little work has been done to ameliorate the hormonal fluctuations that seem to precipitate this form of the disease in female patients.

Other examples of how our hormones can dramatically impact our brains include the many women who develop depression for the first time during menopause—or women with previously controlled mental illnesses such as bipolar disorder or major depression, who experience a recurrence or worsening during menopause. Not to mention those women who feel suicidal when others have PMS. These are rare cases, but they do exist.

All this data shines a spotlight on something that has gone undetected for far too long. There appears to be an epidemic within an epidemic when it comes to women's brain health. Emerging research is pointing to the hormonal changes women experience in midlife as a possible trigger for many of the medical conditions known to affect women's brains more than men's. At the same time, menopause also increases susceptibility to heart disease, obesity, and diabetes—all of which happen to be risk factors for cognitive decline in turn. This is not to say that menopause is the cause of all evils. But while we have a fairly clear understanding of how to deal with diseases that affect other parts of our bodies, understanding the role that hormonal changes play in the female brain, and how to deal with that, is a neglected area that needs to be addressed just as urgently.

It is worth pointing out that men experience declines in testosterone with age, which result in the male equivalent of menopause, called andropause. Luckily for them, loss of fertility in men is a much more gradual process—Mick Jagger becoming a father for the eighth time in his seventies is a case in point. It is also relatively symptom-free. The two major symptoms men report are low sex drive and irritability. Also, while estrogen levels decline in men as well, their testosterone has the ability to convert into estrogen as needed, meaning that men never suffer the same severity of estrogen loss that women do.

At the end of the day, hormonal declines demonstrably affect women's brains more, and differently, than men's. Given the fact that women today spend roughly one-third of their lives in a post-menopausal stage, it is critical to consider how best to support the health of their brains in that part of their lives.

As many as 850 *million women* around the world have currently begun or are about to embark upon menopause. What if we supplied ourselves with the medical attention and care necessary ahead of time, well in advance of these hormonal changes that render us more vulnerable to cognitive and emotional symptoms? What if we were able to safeguard ourselves preventatively?

A CHANCE TO BEAT THE CLOCK

Historically, the connection between hormones and brain health has been overlooked, mostly because the world had yet to realize how hormonal changes impacted the brain. As we now know, many menopausal symptoms actually originate in the brain and are therefore *neurological* symptoms first and foremost. They must be taken very seriously, as they signal that something is happening inside the brain that, if left unchecked, may have unforeseen and unnecessarily tragic consequences in the years to come.

It is important to note that not all women going through menopause develop Alzheimer's, depression, or any other brain conditions—nor do all women show dramatic brain or cognitive changes. It has been estimated that about 20 percent of women don't develop any of the brain symptoms associated with menopause. However, the remaining 80 percent of women experience at least some of these unwanted "red flags," including a potentially higher risk of Alzheimer's. So as women approach midlife, there seems to be a critical window of opportunity not only to detect signs of higher risk to our brains, but also to then intercede with strategies to reduce or prevent that risk. Taking better care of our brains in the years leading up to and around menopause can effectively ameliorate the symptoms of menopause, while also dramatically reducing Alzheimer's risk for the years to come. As a society and as individuals, we urgently need to address this, because addressing the long-term health of any woman means understanding and addressing the effects of menopause on our brains.

What about post-menopausal and older women? Should they raise a white flag? Absolutely not. Age is but a number. It's all about what's in your mind and how you take care of your body and brain. That said, the sooner we all start taking care of both, the better. And it is never too late. In part 3 of this book, we will review several strategies aimed at optimizing cognitive health in women of all ages. It is never too late to start taking care of yourself. The goal is to match the right strategy to each woman's "hormonal age," as well as to a number of other important genetic, medical, and lifestyle factors. Whether you're sixty, seventy, or eighty (or older), engaging in preventative practices is an effective way to clear your head, strengthen your mind, and nourish your memories. If you or a loved one is experiencing memory loss or cognitive decline, it is my hope that following this book's recommendations will help alleviate the symptoms, improve emotional balance, and enhance resilience.

This seems like a good time to acknowledge that many women who are born with the XX genes are now choosing to undergo hormonal shifts in a transition from one gender to another. In 2020, society has come to recognize that gender is not the simple binary chromosomal distinction set forth at birth as once thought. There is, in fact, a fluidity and complexity to gender that was unspoken of for many years. The hormonal changes that take place for women who undergo hormonal treatment as they transition to the male gender are obviously quite distinct from those experienced by women who were born female and remain female. Unfortunately, hormonal transitions specific to the transgender journey haven't been well studied thus far, at least not in terms of their effects on the brain, which represents an important opportunity for future research. For those undergoing such transitions, it is my hope that for now, this book might convince you to initiate important conversations with your doctor about the effects of hormones, not only on your body but on your brain as well.

For all women, transgender or of the gender born, my recommendation for how to use this book is exactly the same. Let it serve as your loyal guide, laying the groundwork for frank discussions and meaningful decisions with your doctor. When we collaborate in this way, we can discover the very best courses of action available to all of us, personalized and essential to our future well-being.

CHAPTER 2

DISPELLING MYTHS AROUND
WOMEN'S BRAIN HEALTH

IN TWENTY YEARS OF RESEARCH, some of the most surprising, important, and neglected findings I've come across are about the real ways the female brain works. However, as long as a woman's brain lies far above and beyond her "bikini line," these vital differences often continue to go unaddressed. Case in point: Alzheimer's is a huge threat to women's health, and nobody talks about it. If there was a meteor that was going to hit several million people in thirty years, we'd presumably set aside resources and brainpower to stop it. Instead, most women are not even aware of the problem. The media doesn't report on it. Doctors aren't trained to address it.

So before we can talk about the reality of what's ahead for each woman, and for women as a whole, let's look at some enduring myths that have kept us, as a society, from recognizing, addressing, and preventing the unique risks to women's brain health.

This is a moment when the notion of bias has risen to the forefront of culture, and in many cases it is very real and necessary to confront. From a health-care perspective, there are a few biases that deserve large-scale and immediate attention, because like all preconceptions, their consequences can be widespread and disastrous. I am referring in particular to the general tendency to dismiss women's concerns due to gender ("you feel weird because you are a woman") or age ("you feel weird because you're getting older").

The double bias women suffer from is by no means the only misinformed perspective around aging. The field of Alzheimer's research, for one, suffers from a very similar problem. In fact, the disease is generally understood as the inevitable outcome of unlucky genes, aging, or both. You can just imagine how difficult it's been to gain a balanced perspective on how real Alzheimer's risk is for women—and just how important it is to do so.

As you'll notice, a large part of the discussion is focused on novel research in the field of Alzheimer's. That is primarily because Alzheimer's is the most extreme manifestation of a suffering brain, and ultimately, by understanding what leads to Alzheimer's, we will also understand what leads away from it. If we stay with the comparison of Alzheimer's to a stock market crash, the same way that economists who study stock market crashes also study what makes a healthy economy, so scientists who study Alzheimer's are actually learning what makes a healthy, resilient, long-lived brain.

While some of these discoveries are indeed specific to Alzheimer's, many of the most important ones have a far broader reach. They provide evidence for an uncomfortable but unavoidable truth: there are specific factors that make women especially vulnerable to a number of conditions that negatively impact overall brain health. Additionally, we now understand that even though both genders can experience cognitive changes, men and women tend to do so for different reasons. Sex differences in brain aging and dementia are only just being acknowledged, but the consequences of these findings are already changing the way we fight disease.

MYTH #1: GENES ARE DESTINY

There's always been a persistent sense that illnesses that affect the brain are due to genetics, and that if your mother or father had a specific disease, chances are you'll get it, too. But a slew of new research using next-generation medical imaging and genomic sequencing has completely upended our understanding of the role of aging and genetics in the development of many illnesses, Alzheimer's first and foremost. Today, it is clear that genes aren't destiny, and that aging isn't a linear path to inescapable disease.

The truth is, while some people do indeed develop diseases like Alzheimer's due to genetic mutations in their DNA, this typically happens to no more than 1 to 2 percent of the population. This is a much lower number than previously thought, and clearly contradicts the story that genes are destiny in this regard. We will discuss these genetic mutations and how to determine if you are carrying one in part 2. For now, let's just say that the vast majority of patients are not born with those mutations. For most people, risk has much less to do with "bad genes" and much more to do with the combination of our unique genetic makeup, our medical health, the environment in which we live, and all the choices we make on a daily basis.

This is not to say that our genes are not important. Our DNA is involved in every aspect of our lives, including making us women. However, from a medical perspective, it turns out that our genes are not as deterministic as we previously thought. Advances in DNA sequencing and the advent of genome-wide association studies (GWAS) have shed light on something called the "multigenic" nature of health and disease. This refers to the effects of interactive networks of multiple genes that influence our longevity and well-being, instead of a single "bad gene" triggering disease. Particular groups of genes work together to make you stronger and more resilient, while others tend to increase your risk of getting sick. These genes themselves don't make you sick. They indicate a higher risk—but a risk that can be modified.

Keep this fact close to heart; it is the game changer. Your genetics— your age, your gender, and your family—form the hand you've been dealt. But winning and losing have less to do with those cards than with the way you play the game: your environment, lifestyle, medical history, and, especially for women, hormonal health. Study after study shows that these factors act synergistically as powerful *epigenetic* forces that modify the way our DNA networks play out, by switching select genes on and off. While this doesn't change the structure of our DNA, it does change the expression of our genes throughout our lives, thereby influencing our chances of developing or not developing any given disease. As a result, we have come to appreciate that the underlying causes of most forms of cognitive decline, although sometimes genetic, are just as often linked to these other factors that are within our control.

From a scientist's perspective, it's important to remind everyone that we all once believed that conditions like depression, stroke, and even cancer were essentially unavoidable genetic outcomes. Instead, they have all turned out to result in great part from the interactions of genetic susceptibility and a large number of medical and environmental factors. Medical conditions known to affect brain health, such as heart disease, obesity, and diabetes, are also much more likely to arise from lifestyle factors than from genetic mutations. To give you a better sense of the scale of magnitude, it was estimated that 80 percent of all cases of cardiovascular disease and as many as 90 percent of all cases of type 2 diabetes in recent years were caused by nothing more than an unhealthy lifestyle. Consequently, they might have been prevented by paying more attention to things like dietary choices, weight control, and physical activity.

As it turns out, this is also the case for Alzheimer's. Recent population-based studies estimate that at a minimum, one-third of all Alzheimer's cases could be prevented by attending to key medical and lifestyle shifts. These shifts include a different approach to diet and exercise, conscientious intellectual and social engagement, stress reduction, better sleep, balancing hormones, avoiding smoking and toxin exposure, and management of cardiovascular health, as well as those factors leading to obesity and diabetes, to name a few. These practices work in powerful harmony to keep dementia at bay.

Research indicates that reducing each of these risk factors by just 10 percent could prevent nearly nine million cases of Alzheimer's by 2050. Depending on which literature you review, we may be able to prevent even more cases, while also minimizing the less severe cognitive problems that naturally occur with age. This is the discovery we've been working so hard to unearth. These are the numbers we've dreamed of. Independent of socioeconomic status or genetics, these very keys are accessible to anyone who chooses to take them in hand. The importance of these discoveries will become even clearer as we move on to the next myth surrounding women's health.

MYTH #2: IT'S JUST AGING—AND WOMEN LIVE LONGER

For many years, the collective mind-set has been that, since women tend to live longer than men, their longer life spans meant that they would simply "have more time" to exhibit Alzheimer's in higher numbers. In other words, it was a question not worth studying. As a scientist, and a general advocate for common sense, I approached this issue with a very simple question.

Do women actually live that much longer than men?

It turns out that this fabled longevity gender gap is in fact closing. Men are catching up. For example, life expectancy in the United States is currently eighty-two years for females and a little over seventy-seven for males, a difference of less than five years. In England, the difference is anticipated to be less than two years by 2030. In many other countries, the "big" difference in life spans isn't that big after all, and it's actually heading in the direction of no difference.

Interestingly, research shows that behavior and technology, rather than genetics, are the main reasons for the rapidly narrowing gender gap. At the beginning of the twentieth century, technological and medical progress did indeed lead to a gender disparity in mortality rates. As infectious disease prevention, improved medical technologies, better diets, and other positive health behaviors were adopted by people born during the early 1900s, death rates plummeted for both women and men. However, while women took full advantage of these improvements, men fell victim to the parallel rise of aptly called "man-made diseases." These include mostly alcoholism, smoking, gun violence, and road accidents, which tend to be more typically "male" health risks. Even the higher incidence of heart disease in men has been largely attributed to smoking, as well as to a poor diet. In other words, the consequences of male behaviors led to the belief that women had some biological advantage in the longevity department.

Rather, today's women are at risk of replicating the history of yesterday's men by taking on behaviors and stresses that were formerly considered a man's prerogative: smoking, drinking, and climbing corporate ladders. The impetus to "lean in" as female entrepreneurs working a hundred hours a week? Commonplace. Women raising small children while holding full-time jobs? Quite the norm. Women working not one but two jobs to support the family? Prevalent now for decades. A female president or prime minister? In some parts of the world, already the case. Perhaps related to these increasing demands, women over fifty now bear the same risk of heart disease as men. Mortality from lung cancer has almost tripled in women in the past two decades. The prevalence of obesity, anxiety, and depression has also increased significantly more for women than for men. Ditto for the risk of infections and a variety of hormonal conditions, from thyroid disease to infertility.

And while all this "progress" has been in process, men have learned to take better care of themselves, leading to the reduction in male mortality and the narrowing gender gap in life expectancy. When it comes to women's self-care, the opposite case is true. As our gender is the one that primarily straddles work worlds both inside and outside the home, our self-care has taken a back seat to both our care of others at home and our contributions in the workplace. In the broadest possible terms, men are being less injurious to their own health, and women have become more so.

For centuries, women have been seeking the same freedom of choice that men possess by virtue of gender alone. Although we have indeed pried open doors that once were shut to us, it seems we have been given entry under some onerous terms and conditions. Whereas men generally determined what was to be expected from them once home after a long day's work, as women entered the exterior workforce, we found ourselves maintaining our previous roles even as we assumed additional ones. Still today, we often do all this without adequate support or compensation, let alone acknowledgment.

What all this points to is that women's changing roles in society, and all the unhealthy behaviors, stresses, and struggles that have come from and with that, have been silently affecting not only our hearts, hormones, and waistlines—but our brains, too. It is in fact our brains that have been suffering to the point of precipitating our chances of developing a neurological disorder like Alzheimer's. One can just imagine what these same changes have done to our cognitive health at large, further highlighting the importance of our lifestyle and medical health above and beyond that of our age or genes.

Which brings us back to where we began: Can a couple of years' difference fully account for the fact that two out of every three Alzheimer's patients are women? Having taken a closer look, I think it seems unlikely. Although age certainly plays a role, statistical models that account for gender-dependent mortality rates broadly show the same 2:1 ratio at any age. In plain English, women with Alzheimer's outnumber men with Alzheimer's two to one regardless of their age, age at death, and differences in life span. The brain imaging studies discussed in chapter 1 lend further support to these findings by revealing that the problem isn't just that women live longer—it's that they seem to start getting the disease earlier. Specifically, around menopause. If you recall from the introduction, a woman as young as forty-five already has a one in five chance of developing Alzheimer's.

Furthermore, if the problem was just that women lived longer than men, then women would also be more likely to suffer from other age-related brain conditions such as stroke or Parkinson's disease. Only, quite markedly, they do not. The risk of stroke is equal for men and women, while Parkinson's tends to affect more men than women. Plus, if we look at the fifteen top causes of death in America today, men show higher death rates than women for fourteen out of the fifteen causes. Alzheimer's (ranking at number six) is the only disease that kills more women than men, across all age groups. In England and Australia, Alzheimer's and dementia have become the leading causes of death for women, knocking heart disease out of the top spot.

I want to underline that the point is not to ignore or discount male patients and their suffering—we have many male Alzheimer's patients and care about them just as deeply as our female patients. The point is that the Alzheimer's care that's available does not take into account gender differences in the development of the disease, and unfortunately overlooks female-specific risks. Only by providing specialized attention to both genders is medicine going to do what it's intended to do: ease human suffering and elevate human well-being.

So what are we to do about it?

MYTH #3: A CURE IS JUST AROUND THE CORNER

There is an unfortunate flaw in Western medicine's approach to health, in that it's based on the premise that there is nothing one can do to prevent a disease from settling in. Consequently, as a society, we typically wait until we're already burdened by an issue, then look to surgery or the latest and greatest pharmaceuticals to rid ourselves of whatever health problems we're experiencing. This approach works well as long as we are trying to fix a broken bone or fight a sudden bacterial infection. However, it isn't efficient for many other things, and it certainly doesn't work with our brains. Surgery is clearly impractical in this case, as we can't simply remove parts of our gray matter. Medications have also proved largely disappointing, with some of the best examples of pharmaceutical letdown hailing from the Alzheimer's field, which suffers the high of a 99.6 percent drug failure rate.

So far, a cure for cognitive impairment and dementia has eluded us. There are some FDA-approved drugs, such as acetylcholinesterase inhibitors (Aricept, Exelon, Razadyne) and memantine (galantamine), that help lessen symptoms for a few years. However, these drugs can't halt the disease's progression, nor are they in any way a cure. It is also worth mentioning that the most widely used Alzheimer's drug, Aricept, seems to work better for men than for women.

A new generation of disease-modifying drugs, engineered to act as vaccines, has been under development for quite some time. These drugs are designed to remove the Alzheimer's plaques (e.g., amyloid) from the brain, or prevent them from being deposited there in the first place. As of today, six Phase 3 studies, a level considered the gold standard of clinical trials, have been carried out. Each and every one of them has failed. The problem is, the clinical trials' lack of success wasn't because the drugs didn't do what they were supposed to do. The amyloid vaccines did actually work: after a few years of treatment, the brain plaques were gone. But in spite of this, patients did not improve. The treatment not only didn't decrease cognitive deficits, but in some cases, actually seemed make them worse.

Some scientists argue that removing the plaques is indeed the right strategy, but that the timing has been off. It is possible that initiating treatment during the early phase of Alzheimer's, when the disease is still contained, may yield better outcomes. As of now, several new clinical trials are testing vaccines for the prevention of Alzheimer's. If the results of these studies are positive, they will provide an incredible asset in our war against the disease. If they are not, we are back to square one.

THE REALITY: CARE AND PREVENTION EXIST! AND BOTH DIFFER BY GENDER

Thanks to the latest research, we can take advantage of the newly discovered window of opportunity to identify, address, and act upon our risk factors before symptoms have a chance to emerge.

Spurred by the new wave of data showing that Alzheimer's prevention is indeed feasible, it is becoming more common for medical providers to deliver direct clinical care to improve brain health, thereby reducing Alzheimer's risk, with a number of clinics focusing on both risk assessment and early intervention. Recent clinical trials have also provided persuasive evidence that targeted risk-reduction interventions can help us maintain cognitive function in old age. With the current failure of Alzheimer's drugs as a viable option, these findings offer us the much-needed alternative we've been striving for, empowering even the greatest skeptic not only with renewed hope, but also with the motivation to do what's necessary to safeguard ourselves and thrive throughout every stage of our lives.

This is particularly good news for women, as there is compelling evidence that women's brains can really benefit from specific medical and lifestyle practices, giving us the ability to reset the scales in our favor. These interventions are both safer and better tolerated than medications, yielding just as effective, and sometimes even better, results. The key is to tailor treatment toward each patient's unique risks and needs. In the next chapter we'll examine several risk factors that affect women's brains most—and how to address them.

CHAPTER 3

UNIQUE RISKS TO WOMEN'S BRAIN HEALTH

ONE OF THE MOST EXCITING developments in the area of health and wellness of the past decade has been the recognition that focusing on a person's uniqueness opens the door to far more effective strategies for disease prevention and treatment. This notion is at the basis of "precision medicine," a novel approach that looks at a full spectrum of health determinants that go above and beyond genetic predispositions to include things like how people live, where they work, which toxins they are exposed to, and how much stress they have in their lives, along with several aspects of their past and current clinical histories. With that awareness, one can attend to those specific risks and how they interact with one another ahead of time.

Cognitive health belongs to this same framework. Our ability to think clearly and keep a sharp mind results from complex interactions among a variety of factors, which, while including age and genetic makeup, is equally impacted by environment and lifestyle choices, as well as coexisting medical conditions such as obesity, diabetes, and heart disease. For women, in addition to taking the time to better manage our health in the first place, there is one often-overlooked key factor to keep an eye on—our hormones. Women's brains undergo shifts triggered by hormonal changes, which can render us vulnerable to aging and cognitive decline. Although this is not an absolute for all women, this amplified risk can be reduced by means of female-specific preventative medicine and lifestyle modifications.

We already have many of the necessary tools in place to assess both genetic and non-genetic risk factors for brain aging and dementia. Coupling this information with the latent power of our lifestyle choices, we now have in hand the keys to counteracting and reducing these risks. By taking into account our biological uniqueness and being proactive with specific choices tailored to support our signature needs, we are at the frontier of overcoming what has thus far been deemed insurmountable. And we're achieving this not through surgery and pharmaceuticals, but through prevention.

Our biological individuality includes, of course, being female. Research has shown us how women experience heart disease differently from men, resulting in radically different symptoms and outcomes. We need to look at brain health in a similar way. Women's bodies, brains, and lives differ from men's in a variety of ways that affect not only our overall cognitive health and mood, but also the factors that set off memory loss and dementia.

The field of Alzheimer's has once again provided the clearest evidence that women's brains need a different kind of care than men's brains, highlighting unique biological underpinnings to the gender disparity. It is now clear that men and women likely have different paths to dementia. We and others have identified over thirty genetic, medical, lifestyle, cultural, and societal factors that impact the risk of cognitive decline differently, depending on gender. Because of unique aspects of the female brain, some of these factors increase risk more dramatically in women than in men, while others escalate risk only in women. Importantly, hormonal changes in the years leading up to and after menopause have been shown to act as key underlying mechanisms that can activate these risks as well as existing predispositions. For many women, menopause is the turning point at which medical risks can become actual medical issues. It is also the time when our brains are particularly vulnerable to lifestyle and environmental stressors. While not all these risks may apply to you today, it is really important that all women understand what to watch out for, not only for their own future well-being, but also to help other women protect themselves along the way.

In this chapter, we will look into the genetic, medical, hormonal, and lifestyle risks that impact women most. Major culprits are described below and discussed in depth over the course of the book, together with effective recommendations to minimize and, even better, eliminate their negative effects on our brains. Because the truth is, memory loss doesn't begin according to a date on the calendar—it's determined in large part by all the choices we make and all the experiences we have along the way.

GENETIC RISKS

As previously discussed, for most people, the action of our DNA is not nearly as deterministic as once thought. However, there are factors ingrained in our DNA that, while not always being causative of disease, can still increase the risk of cognitive decline and dementia. These factors include whether you have a family history of dementia; some genetic risk variants; and, in some ways, your ethnicity.

Family History

Once we've checked the boxes for (a) aging in general and (b) being born female, having a family history of Alzheimer's is the next most important trigger for it as well as other forms of dementia. This is particularly the case for families affected by the genetic mutations that cause disease. In part 2, we'll find out how to determine if you or a loved one is possibly carrying one of these mutations. However, recent research breakthroughs indicate that optimizing one's medical care and lifestyle can do wonders for brain health, also for those possessing genetic mutations that cause disease.

Even if genetic mutations don't run in your family, if one or both of your parents have (or had) Alzheimer's, you are considered to be at risk. It is critical to underline here that having an affected parent doesn't mean that you will become affected too—but it does indicate that you have a predisposition, and therefore need to pay greater attention to your health. Something else to keep in mind is that having a mother who has suffered from Alzheimer's seems to confer greater risk than having an affected father, which is yet another often overlooked way in which women are at the very core of the problem in the absence of genetic mutations. While we don't yet know for sure how a family history increases risk, we do know that a healthy lifestyle can reduce the risk of developing dementia also for those with a higher genetic risk.

The APOE Gene

At present, the only established genetic risk factor known to impact cognitive health goes by the name of apolipoprotein E, or more simply APOE (pronounced ah-poh-ee). Thanks to the media, this gene has given doctors a lot of extra work, as it's been presented in such a way as to vastly oversimplify how it influences a person's likelihood of developing Alzheimer's. Let's get to the bottom of exactly what's what.

Everyone has an APOE gene, which is a normal part of our DNA. There are three different variants, or "alleles": epsilon 2, epsilon 3, and epsilon 4—which I'll abbreviate as APOE-2, APOE-3, and APOE-4. Each of these variants has different effects on health. The APOE-2 variant seems protective against dementia. The APOE-3 variant is broadly neutral. The APOE-4 variant has been linked to an increased risk of Alzheimer's. However, APOE-4 does not actually cause Alzheimer's—it simply increases risk. In spite of this, APOE-4 has been publicized as a dangerous genetic mutation, with some journalists even going so far as to label it "the bad Alzheimer's gene," although countless APOE-4 carriers live long, happy lives without so much as a trace of dementia in sight. At the same time, more than 60 percent of Alzheimer's patients don't carry the APOE-4 gene at all.

Nonetheless, there are two main reasons to take a person's APOE status into account. First, even though APOE-4 affects both men and women, women with APOE-4 seem more likely to develop cognitive impairment or Alzheimer's than men with the gene. Women with APOE-4 are also more likely than men to have a worse memory performance, greater brain shrinkage, and higher accumulation of Alzheimer's plaques already in midlife. But the most important reason to take this information seriously is that the effects of APOE-4 can be kept in check by using the program described in this book. In the next chapters, I will highlight all the tests and recommendations that work particularly well for those with APOE-4, and then we will delve into how to use genetic information to guide our customized choices of interventions.

Other Risk Genes

Over twenty additional "risk genes" or genetic variants have been linked to an increased risk of Alzheimer's. Their associations are not nearly as strong as APOE's, and need to be more firmly established. Nonetheless, something to pay attention to is that most of these genes have a similar effect in our bodies and brains: they influence our response to inflammation. As we'll discuss in "Medical Risks," below, chronic inflammation tends to affect women's brains more than men's, a fact that needs to be taken very seriously.

Ethnicity

If precious little work has been done to address gender disparities in brain health, even less has been done to acknowledge that women of color are at even more of a disadvantage. African American women are about twice as likely as white women to have strokes and to develop Alzheimer's or other forms of dementia. Likewise, women of Hispanic origin are one and a half times more likely to develop dementia, as well as heart disease and diabetes, than those who are white.

Tragically, knowledge about diagnosis, management, and treatment of these conditions is based almost exclusively on studies of white people, and mostly males at that. African Americans and Hispanics account for only 3 to 5 percent of Alzheimer's clinical trial participants, which further limits our ability to develop more specific interventions. However, there is an ongoing effort to produce high-quality data on large numbers of racial and ethnic minorities to better understand and treat any increased risks. The best evidence so far is reviewed in the next chapters.

MEDICAL RISKS

Several medical risk factors have been associated with a greater risk of cognitive decline and Alzheimer's for women than for men. These include chiefly specific risk factors for heart disease, obesity, and diabetes. Additionally, depression in midlife can impact memory as well as mood, and is believed to increase the risk of Alzheimer's more in women than in men. There is also emerging evidence that having suffered from traumatic brain injury or repeated concussions has more long-lasting negative effects on cognitive health in women. Thyroid disease is another big one, along with infections and chronic inflammation.

On the upside, all these conditions can be readily identified and often ameliorated, if not completely reversed, by means of appropriate medical care in combination with the lifestyle changes described in part 3. The sooner you address them the better, because often you can literally change your future.

Heart Disease

In many countries, cardiovascular disease (an umbrella term for many conditions that affect the heart, such as stroke, angina, and heart attacks) is the number one killer for both men and women. It is a major risk factor for cognitive decline and dementia as well, with as many as 25 percent of all dementia cases being attributed to stroke and transient ischemic attacks (TIA), or "mini strokes."

While men generally tend to suffer from heart disease more than women do, once a woman reaches the age of fifty, or about the age of natural menopause, her risk for heart disease matches that of a man's of similar age. On top of that, heart attacks are generally more severe in women than in men. In the first year after a heart attack, women are over 50 percent more likely to die than men are. Within the following five years, 47 percent of the women will die, develop heart failure, or suffer from a stroke, compared with 36 percent of the men.

Why is that? One theory is that before menopause, estrogen keeps the harmful LDL cholesterol low while improving the good HDL cholesterol, therefore protecting women's arteries from the buildup of plaque that contributes to heart attack and stroke. The menopausal drop in estrogen levels and the increase in LDL cholesterol are among the key players in a woman's increased risk of heart disease, although more research is needed to explore the mechanisms involved. Given that heart health is very much connected with brain health, and that what's good for the heart is good for the brain, taking care of our heart is crucial for safeguarding the brain as well. While heart disease and strokes are often treatable with medications and rehab, engaging in preventative practices and a heart-healthy lifestyle is arguably much more effective.

Metabolic Disorders

Type 2 diabetes is a risk factor for Alzheimer's, accounting for 6 to 8 percent of all dementia patients. It affects especially the elderly and post-menopausal women. Metabolic syndrome—a cluster of metabolic conditions including insulin resistance and abdominal obesity that increases risk of diabetes and heart disease—is also becoming an increasingly prevalent problem for post-menopausal women. Along with insulin resistance and pre-diabetes, all these conditions can affect both the body and the brain in a big way, mostly by causing inflammation and accelerating free-radical production. This is a big deal, as diabetes and obesity have both reached epidemic proportions in many countries. Today, almost half of the American population has either undiagnosed or diagnosed pre-diabetes or diabetes.

Our hormones are once again involved. Generally speaking, female hormones have a favorable effect on blood sugar levels, which in turn promote insulin sensitivity. Insulin is a hormone that helps remove sugar from the circulation by shuttling it off to our muscles and other hungry cells so that we can move our bodies and fuel our brains. Insulin resistance occurs when insulin stops being able to do its job as effectively. As women get older, this is in part caused by estrogen losing its grip on keeping our insulin levels down. As a result, sugar stays in our blood longer than it should, eventually getting sucked up by belly fat. Which is why the combination of menopause and insulin resistance can result in something no women are particularly fond of: weight gain. Pair that with a slower metabolism, and many women become prone to developing type 2 diabetes after menopause—a problem we'll tackle head-on in part 3.

Other Heart-Related Risks

Besides heart disease, diabetes, and obesity, other vascular risk factors to watch out for include high blood pressure, high cholesterol, and high triglyceride levels. What all these conditions have in common is that they affect your brain as surely as they affect your heart. They all can increase a woman's risk of stroke and also cause a number of problems in the brain. On the upside, they too can be improved, and often completely reversed, by means of the appropriate medical care and lifestyle changes.

Traumatic Brain Injury

Traumatic brain injury, or TBI, is a condition caused by a concussion (a blow or jolt to the head). This can affect blood and oxygen supply to the brain, while producing inflammation. TBI, especially if followed by a loss of consciousness, has been associated with an increased risk of memory loss and dementia later in life. But the immediate consequences of even a "mild" TBI can also be disabling, causing headaches, migraines, emotional swings, and disturbed sleep, as well as slowed thoughts and word recall, impaired decision-making, and a reduction in the ability to plan and function effectively. While these symptoms may resolve in a matter of months, in some cases they can last for years.

For decades, TBI research suffered from the same gender bias noted in other fields. The majority of research on brain injury focused on male-dominated sports such as ice hockey, boxing, combat sports, and football. Similarly, nearly all the brains donated to brain banks devoted to researching TBI were male, with the result that doctors treated concussions in men and women the same way. A ding on the head was a ding on the head regardless of whether or not you had one X chromosome or two.

But new research is disproving that notion. It turns out that women are more vulnerable, and respond differently, to TBI than men. Not only do women tend to receive more concussions than men in similar sports, but they also experience more symptoms and then take longer to recover. Hormones, along with the physiology of women's more delicate cranial bones and neck muscles, are possible reasons why women experience concussions differently. For example, female athletes tend to be at greater risk for concussion depending on which phase of their monthly cycle they are in. Recovery times also vary depending on hormonal levels.

While most research on TBI focused on athletes, it is important to acknowledge that another group of women has been suffering from concussions, though largely in silence: the survivors of domestic violence. Data on this topic is sparse, in part because domestic violence is still largely stigmatized and underreported. Nonetheless, domestic violence is estimated to affect at least 10 million people each year in the United States alone, with head and neck injuries being some of the most common issues, which we now know cause greater harm to women. While not discounting male survivors, direct experience of being subjected to domestic violence is greater among women. The gender difference is most striking for sexual violence, with women being five times as likely as men to experience sexual assault in their lifetime. Women also suffer more repeated and systematic violence, more severe assault and injuries, and more frequent hospitalizations than men. Clearly, this needs to change. This is not the book to offer strategies or solutions for domestic violence but to provide a different kind of advice. I want to emphasize that the support for victims needs to go beyond psychological and legal counseling (both very much necessary) to also include medical strategies to address any possible neurological consequences to the brain—chiefly, inflammation.

Inflammation

Inflammation can occur in a variety of forms. Whether a harmful bacteria or virus enters your body, you scrape your knee, or you have a tooth abscess, each of these events signals the body's defenses to kick into high gear. Our body possesses sentinel cells that alert the immune system to the presence of invaders. Chemicals are then released to ramp up the body to fight, surrounding "trespassers" and slowing their pace. Yet another team of bodyguards, called macrophages, releases cytokines, highly specialized germ fighters. A similar first-line defense exists inside the brain, where neural versions of macrophages called microglia are on constant patrol. They trigger inflammation to defend brain tissue against things that shouldn't be there, including viruses, bacteria, cancer cells, and Alzheimer's plaques. Once their mission is complete, the immune system calls them off, and all calms down and returns to normal.

Except when it doesn't. Sometimes, for various reasons, this inflammatory response can't manage to shut itself off, and chronic inflammation ensues. Unlike the acute inflammation that follows a sudden infection or injury, the chronic kind produces a steady low-grade overfiring that when left unattended long term can contribute to the development of many diseases.

There is now consistent evidence that low-grade chronic inflammation of the brain is related to the development of cognitive decline and even Alzheimer's. While inflammation doesn't cause these conditions, various studies have indicated that it may hasten the process, possibly by acting as a trigger. As luck would have it, this process seems to be worse in women. Research suggests that, in part because of hormonal differences, microglial cells are built differently in each gender, potentially leading to a less efficient immune response in women. Not surprisingly, a staggering 75 percent of all Americans diagnosed with autoimmune diseases such as lupus and rheumatoid arthritis are women.

At the same time, low-grade inflammation is a behind-the-scenes player for many of the medical risk factors for dementia we've encountered so far, including heart disease, obesity, diabetes, and concussions—which are all pretty bad news for women's brains. In addition, inflammation can severely exhaust hormonal levels in your body and brain.

What to do? Treating chronic inflammation is not as easy as it may seem. Anti-inflammatory drugs are widely available, but data on how efficient they are is quite mixed, especially when it comes to brain health. In general, clinical trials of nonsteroidal anti-inflammatory drugs (NSAIDs, like ibuprofen and naproxen) have shown no benefit at all, and sometimes even worsened symptoms in patients with dementia. Some new data suggests possible protective effects if NSAID therapy is started before the onset of symptoms, but the jury is still out.

For most people, keeping inflammation in check comes down to commonsense basics: avoid things that increase inflammation, and practice those things that are known to decrease it instead. As we will discuss in detail in step 3 in chapter 10, these include eating well (with a focus on anti-inflammatory foods), moving your body regularly, getting more rest, losing weight if necessary, and quitting smoking. In addition, seek out treatment for any inflammation-inducing culprits such as toxin exposure, high cholesterol, harmful bacteria, and even gum disease. Closely following these recommendations will help stop chronic inflammation before it runs rampant while alleviating it if it's already present. Speaking of bacteria . . .

Infections

We have long been aware that yet another cause of inflammation, systemic infection, can cause cognitive problems that resemble dementia. In the diagnostic workup of dementia, we routinely check our patients for bacterial and viral infections such as UTIs, herpes, and sexually transmitted diseases such as syphilis and HIV. Other conditions to watch out for are Epstein-Barr virus (EBV), Lyme disease, and babesia. Any positive findings we discover are addressed immediately, which typically ameliorates any cognitive symptoms present.

Infections such as these have traditionally been thought of as something to rule out in the process of diagnosis. After all, thanks to the brain's built-in defense system, called the blood-brain barrier, these pathogens can't usually make it inside the brain anyway. However, the latest research shows that we may have underestimated the problem, going so far as to have overlooked a key factor. As we age, the blood-brain barrier loses some of its oomph. As more viruses and bacteria manage to get through and reach the brain, it appears they might be able to accelerate the progression of Alzheimer's, perhaps even triggering its appearance.

This latest discovery is relevant to both men and women, but with one caveat: women are more susceptible to infections in the first place. For example, females generally suffer more severe flu symptoms than men do, even though they actually tend to harbor fewer viruses (while also complaining less!). Women are also at higher risk of developing a UTI than are men. One reason for this is that infections can throw off our hormonal balance, sending our cycles out of whack. This imbalance further weakens our immune response, making us more vulnerable to new germs—and more inflammation. I can't help feeling that the relationship between inflammation and Alzheimer's is going to be something that, more and more, takes center stage as we further unravel the associations between toxin exposures and the disruption they provoke in both the body and the brain. More on this soon.

Depression

Depression is a serious medical issue—one that impacts women very directly. In most cultures, it is quite common to blame a woman's poor mood on her hormones. Even when women are having a bad day or responding to extreme or aggressive external stressors, they are often chided or made fun of, with people blaming their mental state on PMS or some other form of hormonal swing. This is a conversation that's due for an update.

Contrary to popular belief, clinical depression is not a "normal part of being a woman" nor is it a "female weakness." Depressive illnesses are serious medical illnesses that affect more than 19 million American adults age eighteen and over each year—12 million of whom are women. Depression can occur in any woman, at any time, and for various reasons, such as developmental, reproductive, hormonal, and social factors, including stress from work, family responsibilities, financial issues, and of course the multitude of roles and expectations of women.

The result: Women are more than twice as likely to develop depression as men, a difference that emerges at puberty and worsens during menopause. While menopause does not cause depression, many women, even those who have never suffered from depression in their lives, experience depressive symptoms and emotional fragility during the transition. This is concerning because depression at midlife also happens to be a risk factor for Alzheimer's. While this is true for both genders, the risk seems higher in women. For example, in an examination of over 6,000 women, many of whom were of menopausal age, depressive symptoms were associated with a twofold increased risk of mild cognitive impairment and dementia later in life.

Importantly, depression is a largely treatable medical illness. From therapy to medication to healthy lifestyle changes, there are many different options available. Just as no two people are affected by depression in exactly the same way, neither is there a "one size fits all" treatment to cure it. What works for one person might not work for another. By becoming as informed as possible, you can find the treatments that can help you overcome depression and feel happy and hopeful again. More on this in part 3.

HORMONAL RISKS

Thyroid Disease

The thyroid is a small gland with a big job: it releases hormones called triiodothyronine (T3) and thyroxine (T4) that control the body's metabolism. Sometimes the thyroid produces too much of these hormones (hyperthyroidism), causing symptoms like weight loss, rapid heartbeat, and hand tremors; sometimes it makes too little (hypothyroidism), causing the opposite symptoms such as weight gain, feeling cold, and low heart rate, among others.

As it turns out, women are more likely than men to have thyroid problems. As many as one in eight women will experience them in her lifetime. Thyroid issues can also interfere with menstrual cycles, causing problems during pregnancy and menopause. At the same time, thyroid disease can cause cognitive problems that mimic symptoms of mild dementia, which is why, as we'll see in part 2, thyroid function is routinely screened for in the clinical assessment of dementia.

Pregnancy and Menopause

As mentioned throughout this book, our hormones influence our brain's health and well-being on a daily basis. These effects are generally subtle and tricky to pinpoint, except perhaps during ovulation or right before menstruation. If you're anything like me, you have some personal strategy when your time of the month happens (in my case, it's an emergency stash of chocolate). This book, however, is to help women develop strategies for the longer arc of an entire lifetime (and that still includes chocolate).

This is crucial given increasing evidence that lifetime estrogen exposure could be an important indicator of long-term cognitive health in women. In other words, the longer a woman has estrogens circulating throughout her body, and the longer the span of her reproductive years, the younger and healthier she and her brain seem to remain.

Most women have reproductive life spans of about forty years. Some have longer spans, which generally means they develop their cycle early, before age thirteen, and go through menopause later than usual, in their mid- to late fifties. At the other end of the spectrum are women who have relatively short reproductive spans, in some cases as short as fifteen years. Shorter spans can be due to starting menstruation later than usual while going through menopause earlier (whether naturally or due to surgery). Well, it turns out that the longer a woman is fertile, the lower her risk of age-related diseases—whereas a shorter reproductive span correlates with a potentially higher risk of cognitive decline and even dementia.

In the next chapters, we'll take time to go over the many factors that can strengthen your hormonal health, thereby delaying menopause. We will also review negative factors to beware of—in particular those known to hasten the process of early menopause.

Finally, the two most salient moments in a woman's reproductive life, pregnancy and menopause, are accompanied by massive hormonal changes that can have just as massive effects on the brain. Given how crucial both pregnancy and menopause are to women's health, and how much stigma there still is around their effects on a woman's mind, chapter 4 is entirely dedicated to these states (because you sure are "in a state"!).

RISKS RELATED TO ENVIRONMENT AND LIFESTYLE

Our body has a remarkable ability to recover from insults, as long as we aren't constantly weakening its defenses by introducing new offenders from the outside. Here's where our environment and lifestyle come into play. A polluted environment and an unhealthy lifestyle are nonstop sources of issues the body has to deal with, and both have a concrete impact on cognitive health. Notably, their impacts are different in women and in men. Here's a preview.

First off, a healthy diet is crucial in protecting our brains no matter our gender—but it turns out that women need a more specific diet, and in some cases, particular supplements as well. Further, lack of physical activity has been strongly associated with an increased risk of cognitive deterioration in both genders—but women tend to be less physically active than men, which can lead to their suffering more of the consequences of a sedentary lifestyle.

Lower education and lack of occupational attainment are other lifestyle factors known to increase Alzheimer's risk in both women and men. However, historically, women have had fewer opportunities for higher education and occupation, which may very well have contributed to the higher Alzheimer's prevalence in women we are seeing today. Of course, things are changing in most parts of the world, which will hopefully contribute to protecting new generations of women against this major disadvantage. At the same time, intellectual stimulation is just as crucial to keep our brains active, and a powerful preventative against cognitive deterioration. All these factors can be tweaked and corrected, particularly since you can control them yourself. In part 3 we'll see just how to do that.

We will also talk about stress, sleep, social interactions, smoking, exposure to toxins, and reactions to medications, as well as about the many cultural and societal factors that end up impacting women most. An obvious example of this is the "caregiver burden," a condition that affects more women than men, given that women are more likely to find themselves in the role of caring for family members, sick or otherwise.

How about men? Do they have any factors that increase only their risk while women are left unscathed? It is somewhat ironic that the main factor known to increase Alzheimer's risk in men more than in women is . . . the lack of a woman in their lives. Men who have never married or are widowed seem to have a greater risk of developing the disease as compared with married or "coupled" men, and also to un-married or widowed women. This is possibly due to the fact that, his-torically, women have been responsible for taking care of the family, not only by ensuring that everyone had a healthy meal and brushed their teeth, but also by specifically attending to their sick spouses whenever the occasion arose. Of course it is entirely possible (and logical) that being in a caring relationship is what really makes a differ-ence, rather than the gender of the person you're together with. None-theless, the data so far indicates that women are pros at taking care of others. It is my hope that this book will help all of us take better care of *ourselves.*

Okay, deep communal breath . . . You've made it through some tough stats here! I think we could all use a round of chocolate (or perhaps something stronger?) about now, but until then, here's some very good news. All the risk factors we've reviewed can be managed and, in many cases, completely reversed. In the next chapters, we will discuss a host of strategies proven to boost our memories, soothe our moods, keep our stress levels in check, and reactivate our metabolisms. These prac-tices, designed specifically for women, help us instead of hurt us, and so keep our female brains happy, well-nourished, and vitalized.

CHAPTER 4

THE BRAIN'S JOURNEY FROM PREGNANCY TO MENOPAUSE

WHEN I STARTED WORKING IN the field of Alzheimer's, I never would have thought that one day I'd be researching hormonal changes, let alone writing a book about them. Although it's long been known that hormones impact brain health, evidence of a firm connection between hormonal health and women's cognitive fitness is a relatively recent discovery. Our hormones have turned out to be even more of an ally, and their decline even more of a problem, than previously thought.

This is not to say that a woman's behavior is governed by her hormones. It is clear that our hormones do not dictate gender differences, and gender stereotyping is both limited and limiting in nature. Our biological heritage is but one force that interacts with many others, combining with emotional, cultural, and societal factors, not to mention our character and self-expression. With that in mind, acknowledging the powerful effects hormones can have on a woman's brain and body won't hold us back—it will instead empower us to make more informed decisions backed by science. Having better knowledge of how our brains really work is a vital step that can widen the breadth and sharpen the focus on women's health throughout all stages of life.

Let's look then at these mighty hormones and their effects inside our heads, from the ups and downs of pregnancy to the crash that follows menopause.

HORMONES FROM THE NECK UP

So far, we've mostly talked about estrogen, but three other key hormones also deeply impact the female brain and body as they fluctuate throughout the menstrual cycle. These are progesterone, the follicle-stimulating hormone (FSH), and the luteinizing hormone (LH).

As shown in figure 2, after the last day of a woman's period, her body starts preparing for the next ovulation. FSH stimulates the ovaries to produce a mature egg. This maturing process produces estrogen (mostly estradiol). During the menstrual cycle, estrogen is high when progesterone is low, and vice versa. Specifically, in the first half of the menstrual cycle, estrogen is nice and high, busy making us feel "sexy" while at the same time promoting the growth of the uterine lining so as to provide the egg with the support it needs to host a baby. Progesterone sits in the back, waiting for the happy news.

During ovulation, the mature egg is released into one of the fallopian tubes and travels to the uterus. If it comes in contact with sperm and is fertilized, a woman is effectively pregnant. But if the egg is not fertilized, another hormone, LH, peaks and then initiates the so-called luteal phase. Estrogen drops and naturally withdraws to give way to progesterone, which proceeds to dismantle estrogen's work, breaking down the uterine lining in the process. The thick lining and blood that were built up during the follicular phase will then be able to leave the body, and voilà, we're menstruating, and a new cycle begins.

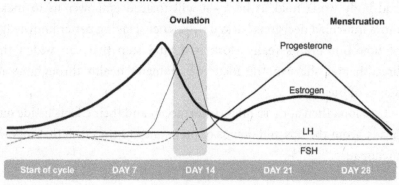

FIGURE 2. SEX HORMONES DURING THE MENSTRUAL CYCLE

Because of estrogen's energizing, mood-boosting effects in the brain, most women feel happier and generally more active during the first part of the cycle. During ovulation (in the middle of the cycle), as estrogen makes way for progesterone, many women feel tense or edgy at first, and much calmer afterward. That's because progesterone is a soothing and sleep-promoting hormone that has a multitude of effects throughout the body. Many of these effects can be attributed to its ability to counterbalance the action of estrogen, since these two hormones work in tandem, complementing and regulating each other. Imagine estrogen and progesterone sitting on either end of a seesaw, shifting rhythmically up and down over the course of your menstrual cycle. After age thirty-five, though, the amount of progesterone you make starts varying from month to month. When progesterone goes down, estrogen will rise on the seesaw. The problem is when these changes are so pronounced that progesterone ends up slamming into the ground. When progesterone levels are low or out of balance—for example, for women who suffer from PMS or, in general, during perimenopause—we tend to experience insomnia, anxiety, migraines, miserable periods, irritability, and even rage. And since it's also a natural diuretic, we get bloated, too.

While not a "female" hormone per se, testosterone is also involved. Men have approximately ten times more testosterone than women, though women produce some testosterone too. This hormone helps regulate sex drive while modulating bone and muscle mass and fat distribution. When testosterone levels are particularly low, women experience not only a loss of libido but also weight gain and low energy. The opposite can happen as well. For instance, women with polycystic ovary syndrome (PCOS), a common cause of infertility, produce a high level of testosterone that can cause menopause-like symptoms including irregular periods, difficulty sleeping, and insulin resistance.

The female brain is in continuous contact with all of our hormones and with our ovaries thanks to a highly specialized network called the hypothalamic-pituitary-gonadal axis, or HPG axis (figure 3). The network owes its name to two brain structures that are directly involved in the reproductive cycle: the hypothalamus, located deep inside the

FIGURE 3. THE FEMALE NEUROENDOCRINE SYSTEM

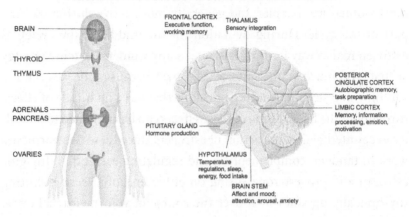

brain, and a tiny gland called the pituitary gland sitting just below the hypothalamus. The hypothalamus is in charge of stimulating estrogen and progesterone production in the ovaries, while the pituitary gland secretes both FSH and LH. This interplay of hormones circulating up and down the HPG axis is regulated by a feedback mechanism that reports to the brain in real time, day after day, throughout our lives as women.

The hypothalamus is on talking terms not just with the ovaries, but with many parts of the brain, too. These include especially the memory and emotional centers of the brain (the hippocampus and amygdala), as well as another region called the posterior cingulate cortex, responsible for storing memories of all the things you've done and the places you've been. The largest part of the brain, the frontal cortex involved in attention, language, and reasoning, is also tightly connected. And if you remember from chapter 1, these regions are all the more interconnected in women than in men.

Additionally, the HPG axis is in touch with two structures located in the most primitive part of the brain, or the brain stem. These are the raphe nucleus, our main source of mood-regulating serotonin; and the locus coeruleus, in charge of the fight-or-flight response. All these regions are part of the brain's estrogen network and quickly respond to variations in estrogen levels, which also helps clarify the extent to which our hormones are involved in most aspects of our cognitive and emotional life.

All is well within this intricate system as long as our hormones support and regulate one another in harmony. However, two major events have the power to disrupt this fine-tuned balance: pregnancy, with the subsequent arrival of a baby, and its nemesis, the onset of menopause and the end of our reproductive life. While these events are two entirely different stories, both can have a strong impact on our brains, and on our mental capacities in turn.

THE PREGNANT BRAIN: FLIP OR FLOP?

As many of us know only too well from personal experience, creating a human being from scratch is no small feat. Pregnancy heralds a period of remarkable change in a woman's body as we literally become the "starter home" to another person. While we have the profound pleasure of hearing a new heartbeat and sensing the first kicks and wriggles inside us, other things are occurring that don't inspire quite the same glee.

One of the hallmarks of pregnancy is an enormous surge in our sex hormones, with estrogen and progesterone ballooning to fifteen to forty times over their usual levels in an effort to prepare the body to carry a child. Our bellies are growing, ankles are swelling, backs are aching. At the same time, surges of oxytocin (aka the love hormone) cue the uterus for its upcoming contractions, while getting the breasts ready to produce milk. But the changes don't stop there. Women frequently report that bringing a new life into the world can also have a major impact on their brains. At some point during pregnancy, many women will ask themselves, "Is this little bundle of joy stealing my body? My life? And oh no, even my brain?" "Pregnancy brain" refers to the feeling of forgetfulness, inattention, and mental fogginess that sometimes accompanies pregnancy, just as "baby brain" refers to similar symptoms that occur once the baby is born. Can our hormones be hijacking our brains somehow?

The only other time that our bodies produce comparable levels of sex hormones is during puberty. Research has shown that this stage of life not only provokes hormonal changes in the body but also spurs dramatic structural and organizational changes in the brain. From prenatal development through adolescence, both boys' and girls' brains are busy growing neurons at light speed. A baby's brain contains more than 100 billion neurons, constituting about as many nerve cells as there are stars in the Milky Way. During a child's early years, synapses (the connections between neurons) further develop at the explosive rate of up to 2 million per second. As the child grows, many of these synapses are, however, discarded via a process of elimination called pruning. By early adolescence, about half of the original synapses are shed as a child's brain sculpts itself into its more mature form.

Thanks to new research, we now know that a similar "remodeling" takes place deep inside the pregnant brain. A seminal study performing brain scans on women before and after pregnancy found significant modifications in the areas of the brain associated with processing and responding to social signals. It's as if our brains were making space for new information to be gathered after a baby's birth. Interestingly, these striking changes, which were still present up to two years after their children's birth, were in the same brain regions that light up across our screens when new moms look at photos of their infants, and correspond directly to the degree of maternal attachment. These changes were so consistent that a computer algorithm based on this data could successfully distinguish pregnant women from a control group of women without children.

It is believed that this brain's makeover, so to speak, is associated with a maturation and specialization process that allows women to become more focused and attuned to their baby's needs. Basically, experiencing forgetfulness or brain fog during pregnancy doesn't mean you're losing your mind after all. You're actually in the process of building a whole new one! Your brain is busy refurbishing the new spaces and pathways that will allow you to become even more responsive to the myriad demands of motherhood. It's precisely the intensity of the remodeling going on that can lead us to notice shifts in memory and attention, which, all things considered, is no small wonder.

Is "Momnesia" Real?

Baby brain, or the cleverly coined "momnesia," is a much-noted phenomenon. Momnesia, however endearing a term, can be broadly described as "the state of mind where you are so overwhelmed with things to do, noise, and the needs of kids that you cannot remember one thing from one moment to the next." It refers to the rather disconcerting feeling of walking into a room to grab something, only to forget what it was you came for. Or leaving curling irons plugged in, or remembering at the last minute that a playdate or soccer practice is scheduled. Once I pushed an empty stroller all the way to the market because I had somehow forgotten that my daughter was at the park with the nanny. The examples are endless. This new "ritual" can become downright infuriating when performed a good many times a day. Lost keys, forgotten appointments, and misplaced bags are all common symptoms.

While not all studies agree, some evidence indicates that women can experience measurable changes in a variety of cognitive skills, memory first and foremost, both during and after pregnancy. For example, a cumulative analysis of fourteen different studies discovered that new moms generally experience reduced performance on memory tests that place a high demand on free recall and working memory. Free recall refers to the ability to remember items on a list, while working memory is your ability to keep many things in mind at the same time, similar to the RAM on a computer.

It is worth mentioning that memory difficulties were more pronounced depending on the number of children a woman had—a factor that didn't seem to have any impact on fathers . . . Whether these difficulties derive from the onslaught of multitasking that surrounds us as new moms or are due to shifts in our brain chemistry is a good question—one to which we can enthusiastically answer: both!

Nonetheless, even though most mothers may not feel as sharp as they used to, their brain's capacity is definitely unaltered. Your IQ hasn't changed a bit—but your priorities have. For example, the average mom tends to accumulate up to seven hundred hours of sleep debt (700!) in the first year with the baby, draining the brain of much of its latent power as it dedicates itself to caring for a child 24/7. Let's face it: when any one of us is getting but a fraction of our usual amount of sleep while at the same time juggling both the basic and the vital new to-dos of the day, even a top-notch noodle is doomed to suffer. A combination of sleep deprivation, shifting hormonal levels, and our newfound roles all combine in challenging us to keep it together.

Given the herculean tasks that confront motherhood at any stage, my best advice is to have respect for and awareness of this, and be gentle with yourself. Ask for help whenever possible to simplify any other areas of your life that can withstand it. Just as you think you've seen it all, life is about to get even more "interesting," however wonderfully so. As you tackle this very female version of Mission Impossible, it's a good time to reach for a game plan that's customized for you, one that just might make it *possible* after all.

A Heartfelt Arrival

Most of the changes that come with pregnancy, like the baby bump, exhaustion, and quirky food cravings, are healthy, temporary, and harmless. But two medical complications that may develop as a result of pregnancy can have long-lasting implications for the health of your heart—and therefore your brain—and need to be taken very seriously. These are

- high blood pressure during pregnancy (preeclampsia)
- gestational diabetes

Both conditions differ from "regular" high blood pressure and diabetes because each of these pregnancy-related conditions typically goes away once the baby is born. However, research suggests that they may signal a woman's predisposition to develop heart disease in the future, or more specifically, around menopause. For example, the Avon Longitudinal Study of Parents and Children looked at pregnancies in more than 3,400 women who were followed for nearly twenty years. Once they reached age fifty, those women who developed preeclampsia during their pregnancy had a 31 percent higher chance for heart disease than women who didn't. Those who developed gestational diabetes had a 26 percent higher risk of heart issues after menopause. Additionally, women with preeclampsia were more likely to deliver prematurely and give birth to underweight babies, while those with gestational diabetes were more likely to deliver overweight babies.

Luckily, preventative interventions can ensure that both mom and baby are healthy throughout pregnancy and for the years to come. These problems can often be avoided entirely by keeping an eye on healthy weight gain during pregnancy, exercising gently but regularly, and adopting a healthy diet before and during pregnancy. That said, women who are meticulous about all these factors can still develop preeclampsia or gestational diabetes. If you develop (or developed) either condition during pregnancy, it's a good idea to talk with your doctor about tracking your blood pressure, blood sugar, and insulin levels as you get older. Keeping cardiac risk factors such as weight and cholesterol levels under control is also important, as described in part 2.

Postpartum Depression: Sadness as the Stork Flies Home

While the birth of a baby can trigger a jumble of powerful emotions, ranging from excitement and joy to fear and anxiety, it can also spur something one might not expect: depression. Recent research indicates that as many as 70 to 80 percent of all new moms experience some depressive symptoms within the first two weeks of delivery. These so-called baby blues, which commonly include mood swings, crying spells, anxiety, and difficulty sleeping, are primarily attributed to the intense hormonal changes that come with childbirth.

However, about one in every ten new moms will experience something more serious, finding herself struggling with a deep sadness, steeper anxieties, and even the loss of a sense of self-worth for several weeks or more. This condition is called postpartum depression (PPD). If left untreated, it can severely affect a woman's ability to get through her daily routine. Another possible though unlikely condition is a mood disorder called postpartum psychosis. This extremely rare condition may include hallucinations, paranoia, and, rarer still, thoughts of harming oneself or others.

Both PPD and postpartum psychosis have long carried a social stigma. Instead of supporting and helping women heal from such trauma, society has historically turned against them, by categorizing them as "mad" and even going so far as to accuse them of being witches or victims of witchcraft. Quite remarkably, it wasn't until the late date of 1994 that the psychiatric community recognized PPD as an actual medical condition. It's no surprise, then, that women have felt apprehensive about discussing it publicly. In 2005, Brooke Shields lent her celebrity presence to PPD by sharing her experience battling the condition that women had silently suffered from throughout history. Now, over a decade later, PPD has become a household term and women are often given the assistance they need to progress through the depression and return to well-being. Pregnant women are routinely screened for it by their ob-gyns, and later by their pediatricians during infant checkups.

Suffering from PPD isn't in any way, shape, or form reflective of a character flaw or weakness. Quite the contrary. It is a physiological complication of giving birth, one that takes great strength of character to manage and overcome. If being a new mom has brought you feelings of anxiety or depression that seem more extreme than those that come from the challenges of the moment, what you're experiencing could be symptomatic of a recognized medical problem.

Whether you're experiencing the symptoms of PPD or reacting to the steep adaptation that motherhood requires, the best thing you can do for your baby, your family, and yourself is to check in with your doctor and tell it like it is. Rest assured, these conditions can now be effectively treated. The symptoms are more often than not the result of a medical problem with clear-cut solutions. Just last year the FDA approved Zulresso (brexanolone) as the first drug designed to specifically treat PPD. Hopefully, more therapeutic options will soon become available. The symptoms of PPD often respond best when treatment is started right away, so when in doubt, reach out for help sooner rather than later to be sure you get whatever assistance you need.

To all new moms, whether you experience shades of PPD, moodiness, or just sheer exhaustion, I hear you. The adjustment to motherhood can be very stressful as you learn to navigate your new role, balancing care for yourself and an infant, not to mention other children and family members, too. All of this inevitably adds up and takes its toll. I promise you, this traffic jam of demands doesn't last forever. But while you're knee-deep in them, the lifestyle changes and select supplements described in part 3 of this book can help you feel better and manage the symptoms as you go.

THE BIG M

Now let's move on to the other end of our reproductive years, where we encounter the "Big M," aka "the Change," or even "That Time." Whatever name it goes by, all women go through menopause—the time in a woman's life when her hormones wane as she loses her ability to bear children. Some women eagerly anticipate this moment, feeling liberated from pregnancy worries, premenstrual mood swings, and the monthly routine of tampons and cramps. For others, the thought of menopause comes with a prickly mix of emotions as they contemplate a distinct departure from their youth and attempt to broach the subject of their aging instead, struggling with what it all means in regard to their womanhood.

Whichever way you look at it, menopause signals the opening of a thus far historically unglorified chapter in a woman's journey, one that has the potential to take us on a wild roller-coaster ride beginning as early as our thirties and lasting easily a decade or more. From hot flashes and weepiness to insomnia and forgetfulness, menopause can be deeply disturbing for many. While some women sail through, barely noticing the shift, many others are plagued by hot flashes, aching joints, sore breasts, or a reduced sex drive—and an increased risk of developing a number of medical conditions that can negatively affect both the body and the brain.

In spite of the steep physical and emotional hurdles that often accompany menopause, speaking openly about it remains taboo. Unfortunately, as a result, some women feel as if they are alone in experiencing such changes, and many remain reluctant to openly discuss their symptoms. Often, when they do get up the courage to broach the subject, both family and doctors alike can be nonplussed or dismissive. Some women don't even realize that what they're experiencing has anything to do with menopause at all. Many are embarrassed to be suffering such symptoms in the first place and strive to hide them. In our youth-obsessed culture, there is something about the word *menopause* that signals negative associations with age, as if age is nothing more than a sign of deterioration and shame—rather than a marker of deeper wisdom, accomplishment, and perspective. As a result, menopause is an issue that is often avoided rather than confronted, thereby turning away curiosity, understanding, and support.

However, things are changing as more and more women open up about their experience in more overt, confident ways. Actress Kim Cattrall, better known as Samantha in *Sex and the City*, has given voice to many women's experience by describing menopause this way: "Literally one moment you're fine, and then another, you feel like you're in a vat of boiling water, and you feel like the rug has been pulled out from underneath you." *X-Files* actress Gillian Anderson said she felt her life was falling apart and that she could handle nothing for years before finally getting to the other side of menopause. Whoopi Goldberg was candid enough to discuss the loss of sex drive many women experience as hormones falter. Tales abound of sudden and embarrassing sweating in public places, lack of sleep, forgetfulness, and in some cases, even an acute sense of despondency.

In 2018, many of us were shocked at the news of the suicide of fifty-five-year-old Kate Spade, the celebrated designer. Only a few years before, fifty-year-old fellow fashion designer L'Wren Scott suffered a similar fate. One can't help but wonder if hormonal changes may have somehow played into their tragic demise.

Sadly, we will never know, but what we do know is that suicide rates for middle-aged women have gone up nearly 60 percent in recent years.

Clearly, something is afoot that can't be explained away as midlife crises or random misfortune. Although assessing these statistics requires a broad-scope look at the many complex and oftentimes hidden challenges women are currently confronted with in our society, this book begins to attend to this essential aspect of women's health, one that has thus far eluded our attention.

In the United States alone, approximately six thousand women are reaching menopause each day. Many are caught completely off guard. Thanks to how genuinely uninformed we are about menopause, many women remain baffled by what they experience, often feeling betrayed by their own bodies—not to mention by their doctors. The news that up to 80 percent of all women going through menopause have the potential to develop actual neurological symptoms (and an increased risk of dementia) raises the stakes even further.

However, it's not only those experiencing natural menopause who are at risk for the potential consequences of estrogen loss. Women are plunged into menopause daily because of surgery or cancer treatments as well. Here in the United States, about one in every eight women undergoes an oophorectomy (the surgical removal of the ovaries) prior to natural menopause. Similar rates are reported in Europe, while in China more than 250,000 hysterectomies (the surgical removal of the uterus, oftentimes along with the ovaries) are performed each year. Having had her ovaries removed may have saved Angelina Jolie's life, but this choice also meant her body would be subject to premature menopause.

Scientists have long known that, unfortunately, when a woman's ovaries (or even just one) are removed prior to menopause, she has a greater risk of memory decline and dementia—up to 70 percent higher in some cases. That's on top of a likewise increased risk of anxiety and depression—another issue that remains largely unaddressed in medical practice. Most women are not aware of this at all. To be fair, most doctors aren't either. But please take heart! As discussed in part 3, new research indicates that hormonal therapy after surgery appears to reverse those risks, at least for some women, suggesting that there may very well be a critical window for this therapy and subsequently for protecting one's brain from any adverse effects. Other solutions are also available, which we'll discuss in the next chapters.

Are Menopause Myths Holding You Back?

All this new research is forcing us to come to grips with the fact that almost everything we've heard about menopause so far, be it information handed from mother to daughter or from doctor to medical student, has been wrong, or at least misguided. Many patients have told me that one of their greatest challenges was finding information they could readily consume, and most important, trust. This chapter's goal is therefore to help women understand what's happening to their brains, as well as to their bodies, as we take control of our changing health-care needs.

One of the issues I've encountered in my own research is just how much misinformation about menopause is out there, making it hard to separate myth from fact. Before we start discussing solutions, it's urgent and helpful to bust a few common misconceptions about what menopause is and isn't.

MYTH #1: MENOPAUSE HAPPENS WHEN YOU'RE OLD.
Fact: The vast majority of women develop menopause in their forties and early fifties.

All women, somewhere in the neighborhood of forty-two to fifty-eight years old, go through menopause. In most industrialized countries, the average woman becomes menopausal at age fifty-one. Some women experience menopause earlier than usual, before age forty-two, which is sometimes referred to as "premature menopause." It can occur even earlier in women who have had their ovaries surgically removed, either alone or along with the uterus (hysterectomy), or whose ovaries stop working for other reasons such as cysts or reactions to cancer-fighting medications that strip the body of estrogen.

MYTH #2: YOUR PERIOD WILL JUST SUDDENLY STOP ONE DAY.
Fact: Your body takes years to go through menopause.

Many women believe that one day you suddenly stop having your period and that's that. Although there are some women who report barely noticing that their periods have disappeared, most only wish it were that simple. Menopause is defined as the final menstrual period, which is confirmed after a woman has missed her period for twelve consecutive months. But the hormonal changes leading up to menopause occur over a fairly long period of time, taking one to eight years for the ovaries to officially retire, ending your cycle once and for all.

When a woman's body is in the process of transitioning toward menopause, menstrual periods typically become less frequent and more irregular, and hormonal levels begin to fluctuate. This stage is referred to as perimenopause. Although a woman still experiences her periods during perimenopause, both the length of the menstrual cycle and the levels of circulating sex hormones become highly variable. On top of your period being all over the menstrual map, this can make for physical and emotional changes as well. Since periods can become less frequent during this time and one gets more used to missing them, in the end, it is often hard to know when they have actually stopped for good. This is of course much different for women who have their ovaries surgically removed, who, from one day to the next, go from having a regular cycle to finding themselves smack in the middle of menopause.

MYTH #3. AFTER MENOPAUSE, A WOMAN'S BODY STOPS MAKING HORMONES.

Fact: Menopausal women continue to produce hormones. But different ones.

Although hormone production significantly decreases after menopause, it doesn't ever stop entirely. For example, a little bit of estrogen is still being made. It is important to clarify that, although we tend to refer to estrogen as if it were a single hormone, in reality, there are three forms, or subtypes: estradiol, estriol, and estrone. Throughout this book, I use the term *estrogen* to refer to the combined effects of all three types, unless it's important to discuss each type specifically.

When doctors talk about "estrogen," they are usually referring to estradiol, which is the strongest of the three. Estradiol is produced by the ovaries during our reproductive years, and its levels are markedly reduced after menopause. Estriol is produced mostly during pregnancy. Estrone is the most prevalent estrogen in post-menopausal women. It is made by adipose fat rather than by the ovaries. So after menopause, we still have some estrogen going, mostly in the form of estrone. However, estrone is not nearly as potent as estradiol—hence the various symptoms and imbalances.

Myth #4. Menopause affects all women the same way.
Fact: Women experience menopause very differently.

All women go through menopause, but every woman's experience of menopause is different. Both the type and the extent of symptoms are extremely varied from woman to woman. Some women report no physical changes aside from irregular menstrual periods that stop when menopause is reached. Other women experience a multitude of symptoms from everyday hot flashes and night sweats to more extreme symptoms such as pain and even electric shock sensations.

An effective diagnostic approach to menopause has been complicated by yet another commonplace factor of Western medicine—the reliance on a one-size-fits-all approach, which is the continuation of the misunderstanding and marginalization of women's health that has existed since doctors first started treating women. Fortunately, there is an increasing understanding that each woman is unique and may experience menopause differently from other women—and therefore needs individualized treatments.

Myth #5. Menopause affects women only physically.
Fact: Menopausal women experience both physical and psychological shifts.

The reason women start losing estrogen in their forties and fifties (and in some cases even earlier) is that our neuroendocrine system is in transition. As the term indicates, this means that the brain (nervous system = neuro) and reproductive organs (endocrine system = hormones) are both involved and, therefore, equally affected. As mentioned before, many of the signature symptoms of menopause begin in the brain.

However, if talking about menopause is still taboo, its effect on mental well-being is totally not dinner conversation material. The result is that many women are terrified of going crazy but don't know whom to speak to about their concerns. I am here to tell you: You are not crazy. Your brain is changing, and so are your physical and emotional health. If you are experiencing these changes, know that they are a perfectly normal reaction to what's going on inside your brain and body. Unpleasant, for sure; daunting, even. But there is nothing wrong with you. Thankfully, there are ways to traverse this period of your life healthily and confidently thanks to a new understanding of and respect for this transition, one that this book is here to help you support and manage.

MYTH #6. WE HAVE NO CONTROL OVER MENOPAUSE.
Fact: While there are some facts of life we can't change, others are well within our control.

There are a number of factors that affect a woman's experience of menopause. Some of them are outside our control, whereas we can actually intervene with others. One factor you cannot change is that menopause is in part genetically linked, so you're quite likely to experience your menopause around the age your mother experienced hers. This isn't always true, as some women do deviate from this path. If your mother reached menopause at forty, but her sisters and your grandmother all experienced it around the age of fifty, it's hard to tell whether you'll follow her path or theirs. But more often than not, if most of the women in your family, your mother included, reached menopause early, late, or somewhere in between, you can eye your calendar with some degree of confidence.

The experience of menopause is also somewhat similar between mother and daughter. If your mom didn't have symptoms of menopause, chances are you won't either. If, instead, she did experience various symptoms, it is possible that you may, too—unless you actively take precautions to avoid the behaviors known to trigger these symptoms.

There are quite a few non-genetic factors that can accelerate and accentuate both the timing and degree of menopausal symptoms, while others may slow and steady the process instead. Our goal, of course, is to minimize the former scenario while maximizing the latter! For example, no lifestyle factor does more damage to your ovaries than smoking. If you smoke and your mother didn't, you'll probably reach menopause earlier than she did. On the other hand, if she smoked and you don't, you may experience menopause later than she did. Other lifestyle factors that influence the experience of menopause include your diet, exercise, sleep quality, stress levels, and even various medications. We will talk about all of these in part 3.

The Brain Symptoms of Menopause

Now that we have clarified what menopause is and isn't, let's take a closer look at the specific effects of menopausal changes on our brains. For those who still insist on using menopause as a cute punch line to a sexist joke (likely told by someone who has never experienced a night sweat), it's important to clarify that the menopausal ebb in estrogen doesn't just leave us fighting hot flashes, but also has us courting more serious issues such as a weakened memory and an increased risk of cognitive decline. The most common "brain symptoms" of menopause are reviewed below. Many, if not all, of these symptoms can be managed and often wholly reversed by following the program outlined in the chapters to come. Post-menopausal women will also greatly benefit from the lifestyle and medical decisions provided, all of them proven to protect and invigorate the mind at any age.

Brain Fog and Memory Lapses

It's quite common for women over forty to complain of "brain fog," exhaustion, forgetfulness, or difficulty concentrating. The memory lapses many women notice are real, and they can begin at a relatively young age, only to worsen as our hormone levels drop. Studies have shown that up to 60 percent of women report reduced focus and mental clarity as they go through perimenopause. Menopause-related cognitive changes happen to women in their forties and fifties, if not earlier—women in the prime of life who suddenly have the rug pulled out from under them. For some women, cognitive performance recuperates years into menopause. For many others, it does not, and may actually further deteriorate or even turn into a dementia diagnosis in later years.

Hot Flashes and Night Sweats

As any woman can attest to, there's nothing really "hot" about hot flashes. Hot flashes, along with their nocturnal counterpart, the night sweat, are a phenomenon called vasodilation—an indicator that your brain is undergoing a global warming crisis. The sweats are indeed a sign of the brain not doing its job correctly, in this case by failing to properly regulate body temperature. During a hot flash, some women experience an unannounced and sudden onslaught of heat so intense that it causes their face and neck to feel flushed and overheated; sometimes this is just as obvious on the outside as it feels inside. Other women go hot and then chilly instead. The hot flash can sometimes cause an irregular heartbeat or palpitations, and even headaches, shivers, and dizziness, which, all things considered, is really no picnic.

A typical hot flash can last anywhere from thirty seconds to ten minutes, although some can last more than an hour. The severity of the hot flash also differs among women. On average, a lucky 3 percent of women skate through menopause without ever breaking a sweat. Another 17 percent have mild, broadly tolerable hot flashes. But the vast majority of women suffer from hot flashes that can be severe and bring a considerable amount of stress to their lives.

Until recently, experts believed these sudden and intense waves of heat were a so-called temporary problem, affecting a woman for no longer than three to five years after her final menstrual period (which by anyone's standards strains at the definition of "temporary"). Instead, for many women, hot flashes continue many years post-menopause. This is particularly the case for current or former smokers and women who tend to be overweight, but also for those who are stressed, depressed, or anxious—which gives us even more of a reason to attend to all these problems. Seriously, if men had hot flashes, we'd have found a solution a long time ago!

Moreover, while most people persist in thinking of hot flashes as solely a quality-of-life issue, recent studies have called that theory into question too. It turns out that women who experience hot flashes earlier in life tend to have poorer endothelial function, a sign that their arteries are losing their ability to flex and relax, which can increase the risk for future heart disease. Since current diagnostic tests are not always accurate enough to predict heart disease for younger women, hot flashes may actually serve a positive purpose after all, acting as a red flag in helping to identify younger women who could benefit from early checkups. In the name of toasting a glass half full, we'll consider this a rather uncomfortable version of a silver lining.

Disturbed Sleep

On top of losing its grip over our internal temperature, our brain also falters at regulating our sleep-wake cycles, which points to hormonal declines as the trigger for many women's sleep issues. Insomnia is a prevalent symptom of menopause, frequently associated with night sweats, depression, and cognitive disturbances. Of course, if a woman is not sleeping well, her mood and eventually her mental equilibrium will no doubt be affected, too. Further, sleep is essential in the formation of memories and in cleaning out amyloid deposits that can lead to Alzheimer's, which makes resting our busy minds crucial for the long run.

Low Mood and Depression

Hormonal declines affect mood as well, oftentimes leading to depressive symptoms. Happy highs that are prone to turning into teary-eyed lows, or cheerful times followed by a string of crabby days, can challenge even the most even-keeled among us. This is a tricky area, however, since depressive symptoms caused by menopause can be difficult to distinguish from symptoms of depression due to other causes.

Aside from pregnancy-related depression, these include major depression, which probably has a stronger genetic component, and "situational" depression, which occurs after a particularly traumatic event, like a death in the family or losing your job. It's important to figure out which form of depression one is suffering from, because treatment can be very different depending on the cause. Far too often a woman will go to her doctor to discuss menopause and leave with a prescription for antidepressants. While antidepressants are needed in some cases, other strategies can and should be put in place to specifically deal with hormonal depression and its root causes.

INCREASED STRESS

Menopause can definitely cause stress, and stress can make all the brain symptoms of menopause a lot worse in turn. Stress itself originates in the brain, and our resilience to stress is largely in our hormones' hands. Let's back up and take a closer look at that. All sex hormones are produced through a series of sequential steps that start with cholesterol, that special kind of fat your doctor routinely measures in your blood. The body uses cholesterol to make a hormone called pregnenolone, which is also known as the mother of all sex hormones. Pregnenolone is in fact converted into progesterone, and progesterone can then be used to make estrogen or testosterone. This process tends to sing along without skipping a beat . . . as long as you are not stressed out. When you're under stress, another hormone steals the show. Enter cortisol, the number one stress hormone.

Here's the story. Your adrenal glands use pregnenolone, too, but to make cortisol. When you're under acute but temporary stress (e.g., you have an exam coming up soon, or there's a medical emergency that resolves quickly), your body will reroute some of its pregnenolone to increase cortisol production. Once the stressor is gone, cortisol production slows down and your body resumes its usual estrogen and progesterone production. But when you're under chronic stress, your cortisol levels skyrocket and remain high for prolonged periods of time. Your body has no choice but to keep making cortisol by stealing pregnenolone away from your sex hormones.

Several things happen to you then: your pregnenolone goes down (making you feel irritable), your progesterone plummets (keeping you awake at night), your estrogen subsides (giving you hot flashes), and your thyroid intervenes to slow down your metabolism (so now you are exhausted too). If you thought you were having problems before, now you're really in the soup. In the short term, too much stress leaves you drained, unhappy, and perpetually overwhelmed. In the long term, it can also lead to more serious problems like depression, heart disease, and an increased risk of dementia. Nobody wants that. It's important to always take steps to avoid or reduce stress. Your body and brain will thank you for it later!

Low Sex Drive

As the hormones that have been regulating the reproductive cycle, libido, and mood are ebbing, these lower levels can have a negative effect on women's sex life as well. Loss of desire is common in the years before and after menopause, peaking anywhere between the ages of thirty-five and sixty-four. Although these changes do not happen to all women, declining female hormones often lead to vaginal dryness, painful intercourse, difficulty becoming aroused, and an overall loss of sexual desire. If that weren't enough, hot flashes can make a woman feel unsure of herself and less desirable, carrying a huge impact on every aspect of her life, relationships included.

From a biological perspective, the actual loss of sexual desire is once again taking place inside our heads. The euphoric and pleasurable experience of sex stems primarily from the limbic system, that part of the brain that is also responsible for memory, affection, and mood. Therapies designed to support brain health and hormonal production, whether by means of counseling, medications, or lifestyle interventions, are therefore just as helpful to boost libido and stamina.

In the end, for many women, menopause is no joking matter. Over the last several years I have spoken to women in various states of emotional distress due to their menopausal symptoms, hearing the way that they have been treated by their doctors, colleagues, and even their own partners. I hear similar stories every day of every week, and I know that for every woman I work with, there are thousands of others out there having similar experiences. Surely it is time we started demanding solutions! And by solutions I mean evidence-backed recommendations, not some internet blog telling us to buy more supplements.

In parts 2 and 3 of this book, I will share a number of testing procedures that are indispensable to digging out the root causes of menopausal symptoms as well as other medical conditions known to affect our brains—and many recommendations to alleviate, and whenever possible, reverse the symptoms. Before we proceed, I want to draw your attention to a particular question I asked myself when I first started researching menopause.

Why Do We Have to Go Through This at All?

For anyone with ovaries, menopause is a fact of life, one we tend to take for granted. But menopause is a long-standing biological riddle, one that scientists haven't managed to fully explain. In fact, there are only two species on the entire planet that outlive their fertility: women . . . and whales!

When we look at this within an evolutionary framework, we could ask why we continue to live beyond the time we're fertile, while females of other species die once they lose the ability to reproduce. It would seem that if females continued to reproduce for the duration of their lifetimes, that would only maximize the passing on of their genes. So why are we built to do otherwise?

New research on whales—killer whales, no less—provides a clue: perhaps menopause is nature's way of avoiding a mother-daughter reproductive conflict. Killer whale societies are matriarchal, and sons and daughters live out their lifetimes with their mothers rather than their fathers. In addition, mothers stay close by to help raise their grandchildren. In this scenario, it is indeed advantageous for the mothers to lose their fertility, thereby eliminating any reproductive competition with their daughters and daughters-in-law.

This societal pattern in killer whales is similar to that of ancient humans. While living in hunter-gatherer societies, the men went hunting while the women stayed behind to raise the children. It is possible that avoiding reproductive competition might also underpin human menopause. Since women today are living far longer than their female ancestors, the time has come to roll up our sleeves and figure out how we can protect and invigorate our minds, even as our estrogens ebb.

Menopause: A Wake-Up Call

Until fairly recently, menopause was written off as the unnatural outcome of women's increased life expectancy, the unfortunate upshot of their living well beyond what nature intended. Subsequently, medicine met it with little more than a shrug. In recent years though, research has made tremendous progress in demonstrating that menopause is not only a pivotal aspect of women's health, deserving of proper attention, but also a wellspring of information destined to inform the future of women's health care.

When menopausal symptoms are attended to with adequate research and customized care, the host of potential issues that often accompany this hormonal shift can often be avoided. When it comes to a woman's cognitive health, menopause remains the only factor known to increase Alzheimer's risk in women and women alone, putting us at a distinct disadvantage based solely on gender. Between the way this hormonal juggernaut can produce symptoms that constrain women's quality of life for decades, and the fact that it puts us at risk for one of the most devastating diseases known to humankind, it warrants our fullest attention, and pronto.

Instead of keeping the blinders on when faced with the challenges of menopause, perhaps it's the wake-up call we've been waiting for, prompting us to take action. The choices we women make during this transition can have profound effects on our future health. In order to make the right choices, you want to identify your risk factors and predispositions so that you can personalize your plan with what will work best for you. I will assist you with this starting in the next chapter.

PART 2

TAKE ACTION: GET TESTED

CHAPTER 5

THE AGE OF PRECISION MEDICINE

WHETHER WE ARE STRESSED OR depressed, foggy from sleep deprivation, or bouncing back and forth between feeling exhausted and wired, our brains not functioning at their best can certainly be unsettling. Ultimately, when we struggle with these issues, we can find ourselves second-guessing our decisions or worrying unduly about the future. Though not everyone will experience all of these challenges at once, many women will hit "speed bumps" over the course of their lifetimes, confronted by a combination of these symptoms to a degree that is disruptive enough to give them pause. This can be due to the fact that, over time, our bodies and brains are going through various shifts and changes. It's up to us to make sure such transitions are attended to properly, and to gain access to the right strategies to address each symptom.

I cannot stress this enough: No two women are alike. What works for you may not work for your friend, your colleague, or even your own daughter—and vice versa. It is high time to abandon the one-size-fits-all approach that has dominated the field of women's health for centuries, in favor of a more dynamic model that focuses on women as individuals instead.

This concept is at the heart of precision medicine, an emerging approach for disease treatment and prevention that takes our personal, individualized variability into account. Precision medicine embraces a paradigm that allows us to break free from the algorithmic treatments bound by hit-or-miss, average-person practices. It offers a customized approach based on our own personal set of data: our genetics, our medical status, the specific environment in which we live, and the lifestyle choices we make. All these factors become equally informative, especially when it comes to prevention.

The idea is simple: we can maximize patients' chances of better health outcomes if we tailor treatments to what we know about their particular set of health and lifestyle "signatures," which not only determine their various strengths and vulnerabilities but can also cue their responses to a variety of interventions. All these factors have predictive values that help identify those risks specific to each person. This means they also allow for the development of a more effective personalized prevention plan, which can assist us in sidestepping what may have otherwise become future pitfalls.

So let's find out which risks and concerns *you* need to address to optimize cognitive health and protect your brain for a lifetime of use. First, we will focus on genetic risks. Then we will look at a variety of clinical conditions that can be addressed and are often completely reversible. Finally, in part 3, we will review a host of strategies proven to offset and minimize any impact of the identified risks.

GENETIC TESTING VERSUS CLEVER MARKETING

In the era of DNA testing, many people want to know their genetic future, as well as that of their children and entire families. While this is perfectly legitimate, there are different ways to go about it. One way is deeply rooted in science and carried out by certified clinical labs (CLIA labs); another way involves direct-to-consumer (DTC) genetic-testing companies and can range from reasonable to downright predatory.

Due to the price collapse of genetic testing and the FDA's gradual ease of the regulatory environment, DTC genetic-testing companies such as 23andMe, Family Tree DNA, MyHeritage, and ancestry.com are booming. According to industry estimates, the number of people who have had their genes analyzed with DTC tests currently exceeds 12 million.

The problem isn't the DTC tests that tell you about your lineage or whether you're likely to have blue eyes (which, incidentally, you already know). Those are based on measurable data. The problem is that many of the other tests run the risk of being only slightly more accurate than horoscopes, while others still are irresponsible at best. One that springs immediately to mind is the test that promises to improve your child's soccer ability with a personalized DNA-based program. Or another test that claims to predict your kid's ability to learn languages. Or yet another that will guess (because it's literally guessing) a person's chance of a high or low IQ.

As a scientist, I feel that the information provided by genetic testing could be of value—but that's assuming said information is accurate and reliable. Instead, even the largest and more reputable companies have been objects of criticism. For example, in 2008, the FDA cracked down on 23andMe, ordering the company to cease providing analyses of people's risk factors until the tests' accuracy could be validated. Basically, nobody actually knows just how reliable the reports are.

No matter what DTC companies try to sell you, aside from ancestry details and limited information about specific health risks, you really mustn't base your decisions on those findings. I say this because most DTC companies share limited information with users but let them download more of their raw data for informational purposes, in spite of the fact that the accuracy of the raw data is "not guaranteed." This is code for "the data may be wrong." Many users miss this vital point and go on to enlist the help of third-party services such as Promethease .com or codegen.eu to obtain user-friendly readouts of additional pieces of information, including genetic markers for diseases like cancer, Alzheimer's, and Parkinson's.

There are two major problems with this approach: first, the actual data is potentially incorrect. Second, the promised interpretation of the data is also potentially incorrect. That's because several of these third-party companies operate by leveraging content from free public archives for genetic variations, in spite of evidence that much of the available information may be inaccurate.

Just recently, an eye-opening study revealed that 23andMe misdiagnosed genetic markers of cancer risk, such as the BRCA gene (aka the "Angelina Jolie gene"), in a whopping 40 percent of cases—which makes the test only slightly more accurate than tossing a coin. Obviously, this sort of misinformation is disturbing on a number of levels. In the Alzheimer's field, genetic testing through DTC channels is not recommended, but many people use it to find out their APOE genotype. More on this below, in "Genetic Testing for Alzheimer's." For the time being, the bottom line is this: only genetic testing carried out by CLIA-certified labs meets quality standards and is worth your trust and money.

IF DEMENTIA RUNS IN YOUR FAMILY, ARE YOU AT RISK?

DNA testing has been used for decades for certain types of familial cancers and for brain diseases like Alzheimer's, multiple sclerosis, Parkinson's disease, Huntington's disease, and epilepsy. The result of a genetic test can confirm or rule out a suspected genetic condition, or help determine a person's chance of developing or passing on one.

Specifically for cognitive health, many people who are experiencing forgetfulness, memory loss, or difficulties with attention and language are concerned about their risk of Alzheimer's. Does having a parent affected by Alzheimer's imply that their children are eventually destined to suffer the same fate? If your mother or father has Alzheimer's, will you get it, too? How common is it to have the bad Alzheimer's genes?

These are very valid concerns. Alzheimer's is a complex disease, and its ins and outs can be confusing, which can be especially dismaying to patients and families trying to wend their way through the experience of developing the disease or caring for someone who has it.

As referenced at the beginning of this book, we now know that very few people develop Alzheimer's because of a rare genetic mutation in their DNA. These mutations are called "autosomal dominant," which means that a single copy of the mutation, inherited from one parent, is enough to cause the disease. So far, scientists have identified such Alzheimer's mutations in three genes: the amyloid precursor protein (APP) gene and the presenilin 1 (PSEN1) and presenilin 2 (PSEN2) genes. All three cause an overproduction of amyloid plaques, which in turn causes a particularly aggressive early-onset form of the disease that develops when people are in their thirties, forties, or fifties. This early-onset familial form is the only genetically determined form of Alzheimer's that is passed on from one generation to the next. A child whose biological mother or father carries a genetic mutation for early-onset Alzheimer's has a fifty-fifty chance of inheriting that mutation. If the mutation is in fact inherited, the child has a very strong probability of developing early-onset Alzheimer's, too.

Again, these mutations are less common than many people fear. In the majority of people, any genetic risk of developing Alzheimer's is linked not to rare genetic mutations but to susceptibility genes, in particular the APOE gene mentioned in chapter 3. It is very important to understand the difference between testing for a genetic mutation and testing for genetic risk factors, which we will do shortly. If Alzheimer's runs in your family and you are concerned about possibly being at risk, below you will find practical guidelines that will help you determine whether genetic testing is a viable option for you.

A Word About Pros and Cons

Before proceeding, take whatever time is necessary to fully understand the repercussions of having this test. If today you are a perfectly healthy forty-year-old who has seen a parent claimed by this disease, would you want to know if you face the same destiny? How will this knowledge change your life? Will knowing this help you or harm you?

Answers to these questions vary greatly. Many people, health-care providers included, argue that the test's value hinges entirely on having access to a cure. Since therapeutic options are scarce, the risks of any psychological harm in knowing you are at risk may very well outweigh any benefit gained. On the other hand, some people decide on the test hoping that effective treatment may be developed for them in time, while others are interested in clinical trial opportunities. Some people look at it as an opportunity to plan ahead, since long-term care and disability insurance, retirement, advance directives, and even a will can be major motivators to learning more about one's health risks. For others, simply knowing what the future has in store is reason enough to find out. Particularly as those with a family history of Alzheimer's approach the age at which their relatives began to suffer, it is understandable for them to feel anxious about their own potential risk. Some may believe they already have the disease, which can lead them to doubt their mental capacities prematurely, questioning every instance of forgetfulness or brain fog.

Whatever the motivation, it's true that knowing one's genetic status does have implications for the entire family. The decision is intensely personal and is ideally made after a period of research and self-reflection. It's also important to realize that while genetic testing can help you address some of these concerns, you don't actually need that information to put your finances in order, nor to help contribute to research. It is just as important to know that you don't always need DNA testing to rule out a genetic mutation with reasonable certainty. How? Keep reading.

The "Family History of Dementia" Questionnaire

Over the years I've noticed that defining Alzheimer's as "early" or "late" onset can be confusing to patients. Countless people have told me that their mother, father, or grandparent had "early-onset Alzheimer's," only for me to later find out that more times than not, their relatives did not exhibit symptoms of the disease until well after the age of sixty. From a diagnostic perspective, patients who develop Alzheimer's after age sixty are not early-onset, but rather late-onset patients. This is an important distinction because patients with a later onset of the disease are unlikely to carry the genetic mutations that cause it. As a result, Alzheimer's developed after age sixty is usually not caused by genetic mutations, and is therefore less likely to be transmitted from the parents to their children.

This is not universally the case, though, so a great first step in determining whether you or a loved one may be carrying a genetic mutation is to have an Alzheimer's doctor do a thorough family history evaluation. (If you are looking for an Alzheimer's doctor, see appendix A for guidance.) This evaluation is typically based on a family history questionnaire like the one included below, which is broken down into first- and second-degree family members. Use it as a guide to gather all the necessary information. The key facts you need to find are at what age symptoms began to occur and which types of symptoms were present (e.g., memory loss, confusion, depression, tremors, hallucinations). While collecting this information might be difficult and emotionally painful, it really is a crucial step. I find that families often have an uncanny ability to remember details about unexpected or peculiar behaviors when it comes to their relatives. Did any of your relatives routinely lose their keys or misplace objects like reading glasses? Did they tend to forget names or fail to recognize familiar faces or places? Did they repeat the same sentences over and over again, get confused about the time or day, or perhaps even forget what familiar objects were for?

Other things to find out include current age, age at the time of first symptoms, age at diagnosis, age at death, and the cause of death of relatives both affected and unaffected. Additionally, your doctor needs to know if any of your relatives suffered from conditions that can mimic the symptoms of dementia (e.g., ALS, epilepsy, brain cancer) or that may suggest different genetic links (e.g., Down syndrome). Write in the name and clinical information for all your family members, or as many as you can. Add as many columns as you need and go back in time as far as possible. For example, if one of your great-grandparents had dementia, by all means include this information in the forms.

If dementia runs in your family, this comprehensive information will help your doctor determine if the disease is more likely genetically driven or influenced by medical issues like cardiovascular disease or diabetes.

FIRST-DEGREE FAMILY HISTORY FORM

| | PARENTS | | CHILDREN | | | | SIBLINGS | | | |
	Myself	Mother	Father	Son 1	Son 2	Daughter 1	Daughter 2	Brother 1	Brother 2	Sister 1	Sister 2
Alzheimer's disease											
Parkinson's disease											
Huntington's disease											
Frontotemporal dementia											
Lewy body disease											
Pick's disease											
Vascular dementia											
Stroke											
Amyotrophic lateral sclerosis (ALS)											
Down syndrome											
Epilepsy											
Cancer (specify type/location)											
Heart disease (bypass, angina, etc.)											
High cholesterol											
Hypertension											
Diabetes (specify type 1 or 2)											

SECOND-DEGREE FAMILY HISTORY FORM

	GRANDPARENTS				RELATIVES			
	Maternal grandmother	Maternal grandfather	Paternal grandfather	Paternal grandmother	Maternal uncle	Maternal aunt	Paternal uncle	Paternal aunt
Alzheimer's disease								
Parkinson's disease								
Huntington's disease								
Frontotemporal dementia								
Lewy body disease								
Pick's disease								
Vascular dementia								
Stroke								
Amyotrophic lateral sclerosis (ALS)								
Down syndrome								
Epilepsy								
Cancer (specify type/location)								
Heart disease (bypass, angina, etc.)								
High cholesterol								
Hypertension								
Diabetes (specify type 1 or 2)								

Once you're ready, the guide below will help you to interpret the information:

- Genetic diseases are typically "multigenerational," which means that any genetic mutation would have affected at least one of your great-grandparents, grandparents, parents, and/or their siblings. If two or more of your closest relatives have or had Alzheimer's, and particularly if they developed symptoms at a young age (generally speaking, *before age sixty*, but especially if it was in their forties or fifties), a gene mutation, while not a certainty, is a possibility. In this case, ask your doctor whether genetic testing is advised.

- If only one of your parents and no other relatives have ever had dementia, and especially if the affected parent developed symptoms well *after age sixty*, you are unlikely to be carrying a gene mutation. In any case, it is always wise to discuss your family history with your doctor.

If your doctor determines that genetic testing is advisable, here is what you need to know. Genetic testing can be used in two ways: to confirm the presence of an Alzheimer's mutation in patients who are already showing symptoms, and as a means by which to assess risk in people without any symptoms at all.

GENETIC TESTING FOR ALZHEIMER'S
Diagnostic DNA Testing of People Who Have Symptoms

When a young or middle-aged person has symptoms of Alzheimer's and there is a family history of Alzheimer's before age sixty, doctors may suggest diagnostic DNA testing. Typically, this is done only if there is a previously known case of early-onset Alzheimer's in the family.

Diagnostic DNA testing is done most commonly on the PSEN1 gene, since mutations in this gene are the most frequent. Testing can be done through a commercial company called Athena Diagnostics (www .athenadiagnostics.com), or through some CLIA-certified labs affiliated with academic medical centers (wwwn.cdc.gov/clia). Sometimes DNA testing is done on the APP or PSEN2 genes, too. No commercial test is available for them, but testing can be done at some academic centers or as part of a clinical trial. If you enroll in a research study or clinical trial, the costs of genetic testing are typically covered by the sponsor.

As for the procedure, it is relatively simple. You will go for a blood draw, which is then sent out for testing, just like any standard blood test. If the test comes back positive, the doctor will then be able to identify the mutation that causes Alzheimer's in the family, which may prompt additional family members to test as well. If the test comes back negative, you don't have the mutation.

I cannot stress enough that genetic counseling, both before and after the test, is of paramount importance. Receiving genetic information without appropriate counseling can have an adverse and often unexpected psychological impact on some people, especially those with a predisposition to anxiety or depression. Thanks to the field having worked out a careful and conservative approach to genetic testing from the outset, such extreme outcomes have remained very rare. Nonetheless, even though the rate of catastrophic consequences is not high, they do occur. It is important to know yourself and to make sure you get all the help available to you before and after testing. It is particularly important to avoid rash decisions, so do consult with your spouse, your partner, or a trusted friend before going forward with the decision as to whether or not to test. If you decide to take the test, you can find a genetic counselor in two ways:

- Contact your nearest Alzheimer's support community, as described in appendix A.
- Search the online directory of the National Society of Genetic Counselors: www.nsgc.org.

Predictive DNA Testing for At-Risk Relatives

When a family member is found to be carrying a specific mutation, at-risk siblings, adult children, or other relatives can also find out whether they have inherited the mutation. About 10 percent of eligible relatives choose to get tested.

However, predictive testing is complicated because it deals with predicting the future of a currently healthy, symptom-free person, rather than testing someone who is presently ill. Guidelines are therefore even more strict. Specifically, if you are worried about your own risk due to a family member who has or had Alzheimer's, but this specific relative has not been tested for genetic mutations, predictive testing is *not* available to you. This is due to the relative in question needing to be tested first. If it turns out that they indeed have a genetic mutation, then you will be able to get tested, too. However, there are many instances where the relative with Alzheimer's has died, so they can no longer be checked for genetic mutations. Another possibility is that the affected relatives are living but refuse to have the test. In either of these cases, your doctor won't be able to request the test for you.

If you are eligible, take the test and learn whether you are indeed at genetic risk for Alzheimer's. If you are, what are the next steps? First off, counseling is a must. Secondly, support and advocacy groups exist to help you connect with other patients and families, as well as with the research, resources, and services in place to assist you (see appendix A for more information). Many organizations have experts who serve as medical advisers or provide lists of doctors and clinics that can help. Equally important is the option to enroll in clinical trials that focus on genetic heritability. Currently, two large clinical trials, the Dominantly Inherited Alzheimer Network (DIAN) and the Alzheimer's Prevention Initiative's (API) Autosomal Dominant Alzheimer's Disease (ADAD) trial, are testing the effectiveness of amyloid-clearing drugs in volunteers carrying genetic mutations for Alzheimer's (see appendix A). These studies are open to enrollment, and more trials will hopefully become available soon.

APOE Testing

If you remember from chapter 3, the APOE gene is the only established genetic risk factor for late-onset Alzheimer's. Let me reiterate that APOE is *not* a bad genetic mutation, but it does influence Alzheimer's risk. Currently, APOE testing is used in research settings to identify study participants who may have an increased risk of developing Alzheimer's. This knowledge helps us look for early brain changes and compare the effectiveness of treatments for people with different APOE profiles. However, this test is not effective in determining any one person's risk, and is therefore not recommended for clinical use. Here's why.

There are three APOE varieties, or alleles: E2, E3, and E4. Everyone has two alleles, so there are six possible combinations: E2/E2, E2/E3, E2/E4, E3/E3, E3/E4, or E4/E4. People with the E2/E2 combo have the lowest risk of Alzheimer's, while those with E4/E4 have the highest risk. E4/E4 carriers are also more likely to develop symptoms at an earlier age, though still typically after age sixty. A study of 17,000 dementia-free people estimated that if you are sixty to seventy-five years old and have two copies of the APOE-4 gene (i.e., E4/E4), then you have a 30 to 55 percent risk of developing mild cognitive impairment or Alzheimer's by age eighty-five. If you have only one copy of the APOE-4 gene, you have a 20 to 25 percent risk of developing either condition by age eighty-five. If you don't have the gene, however, your risk is still 10 to 15 percent.

You can see why information about APOE status doesn't help much in terms of predicting future dementia. Also, in the case of genetically determined Alzheimer's, the impact of genetic mutations outweighs that of APOE-4, so testing doesn't add much information for those patients either.

Nonetheless, from a precision medicine perspective, knowing your APOE status can be helpful—but only if your doctor knows what to do with this information. There are many, often contradictory approaches to counteracting the effects of APOE. There is increasing evidence that APOE-4 carriers respond to some treatments differently, and sometimes better than non-carriers, as you'll see in part 3. Participating in clinical trials focused on APOE also deserves a thought. For example, the ongoing API Generation study also aims to test two experimental drugs for the prevention or delay of dementia specifically in people with two copies of the APOE-4 gene (see appendix A for more information).

So for those of you who do want to find out, there are three ways to learn your APOE status:

- **Ask your doctor to run the APOE test.** The plus is that you will be tested by a certified lab, which limits the chance of any errors in testing. Results are received directly from your physician, who will either address your concerns or refer you to a specialist to do so.

- **Enroll in a research study or clinical trial that focuses on APOE status.** The advantages are that you will be tested by a certified lab, and the costs of genetic testing will be covered by the sponsor. Clinical trials also provide novel medications that may counteract the effects of APOE-4.

- **Order a DTC test such as those offered by 23andMe.** By ordering the test yourself, you keep this information private, but will not receive guidance from a specialist. Another downside is that there's a higher chance of testing errors. If you already used DTC channels to find out your APOE profile, I would recommend getting a second opinion via a CLIA lab (www.cdc.gov/clia).

If you are interested in finding out your APOE status, keep in mind that genetic counseling is important in this case as well. For some people, learning that they are APOE-4 carriers becomes a strong motivator to take better care of themselves, with no or minor short-term psychological risks. For others, it can be a very frightening and disconcerting experience instead. You are the only one who knows how you will react to the news, although even you may not know for sure how the information will ultimately impact you. This is why I encourage you to take your time to do the appropriate soul-searching prior to deciding to be tested, and to enlist the help of a trusted counselor or doctor for any questions that come up.

CHAPTER 6

MEDICAL HISTORY AND LABORATORY TESTS

AT THE RISK OF BELABORING THE POINT, I want to emphasize that taking care of yourself is of the utmost importance, no matter what your DNA is or isn't. In this regard, there are ways that scientists can help, and there are ways that doctors can help—but if you're like most any woman I've ever met, you know that we also need to learn to help ourselves. Where cognitive health is concerned, many of our worst worries can be avoided by showing ourselves proper TLC.

Managing our medical status is crucial to this aim. In fact, some medical conditions can increase the risk of Alzheimer's or worsen its symptoms. These are chiefly heart disease, diabetes, obesity, and depression, which all can in and of themselves affect cognitive performance, dampening our mental acuity and clouding our memories.

Further, more than forty medical conditions have been identified that can cause or mimic the symptoms of dementia, thereby misleading people into thinking they are slipping into some form of mind-robbing disease. Fortunately, most of these conditions are treatable and often completely reversible. Two common examples are vitamin B12 deficiency and an underactive thyroid (hypothyroidism). Our minds can be dramatically affected by these and other influences, such as infection, inflammation, and metal poisoning, to name but a few—which all are within our control to address. Getting the right diagnosis is crucial because, in many cases, symptoms subside when the underlying problem is treated. So it is imperative to recognize these manageable conditions and deal with them pronto.

Regular medical checkups combined with the recommendations included in part 3 of this book, such as a healthy diet, moderating alcohol consumption, avoiding cigarettes, keeping stress and inflammation at bay, and consistently exercising, among others, can not only improve but also reverse most if not all of these conditions. Some of these shifts you can actually attend to yourself, while others will require a doctor's help. But if you really let that fact sink in, many of you may be taking a huge sigh of relief about now.

These next chapters focus on developing a comprehensive risk management plan that starts with compiling a clinical and medical history. This includes your current and past medical problems and concerns, including any medications, your family's medical history, your current lifestyle choices, and your exposure to environmental hazards. This information will provide the framework for your specialized treatment plan by highlighting any specific areas of concern. We will start by outlining what a typical clinical evaluation for brain health involves, including select tests that you can easily get done with your doctor's assistance. In the next chapter, we will use these test results to further refine your personalized risk assessment.

For all tests, reference values are included in table 1.

TABLE 1. KEY MEDICAL AND LAB TESTS FOR ALZHEIMER'S PREVENTION AND MANAGEMENT

INDEX	TEST	REFERENCE VALUES		
		Optimal	Borderline	High risk
Central body fat	Body mass index (BMI)	18.5–25	25–30	>30
	Waist-to-height ratio	0.42–0.48	0.49–0.5	Over 0.5

Hypertension (high blood pressure)	Blood pressure (mmHg)	<120/80	120/80–140/90	140/90
Metabolic markers	Fasting blood glucose (mg/dL)	70–99	100–125	<70 or >125
	Fasting blood insulin (mcU/ml)	<5	5–15	>15
	Hemoglobin A1c (HgA1c, %)	4–5.7%	5.7–6.4%	>6.4%
Lipid markers	Total cholesterol (mg/dL)	<200	200–240	>240
	HDL cholesterol (mg/dL)	>60	50–60	<50
	LDL cholesterol (mg/dL)	<100	100–160	>160
	Triglycerides (mg/dL)	<150	150–200	>200
	Lipoprotein A (Lp[a], mg/dL)	<30	30–50	>50
Thyroid function	TSH (μIU/mL)	<0.27	0.27–4.2	>4.2
Homocysteine	Homocysteine (mcmol/L)	<10	10–14	>14
Nutrients	Vitamin B12 (ng/L)	190–900	150–190	<150
	Folate (ng/L)	5.8–32.8	3–5.8	<3
	Omega-3 DHA (mcg/mL)	>100	60–100	<60
	Omega-3 index	>8%	4–8%	<4%
Inflammation	Hs-CRP (mg/mL)	<1	1–3	>3

Hormones		Follicular phase	Ovulation	Post-menopause
	Estradiol (pg/mL)	12.4–233	41–398	<138
	Progesterone (ng/mL)	0.06–0.89	0.12–12	<0.05–0.13
	FSH (mcIU/mL)	2.4–12.6	14–95.6	7.7–58.5
	LH (mcIU/mL)	3.5–12.5	4.7–21.5	25.8–134.8
		6–8 a.m.	4 p.m.	Bedtime
	Cortisol (mc/dL)	10–20	3–10	<5

LET'S GET PHYSICAL

This first step involves assessing your weight, height, waist circumference, and blood pressure. These parameters will help clarify if you are at risk for cardiovascular disease, obesity, or diabetes.

Check Your BMI

Being overweight or obese can increase your risk for heart disease and diabetes, which in turn increase your risk of Alzheimer's. Incidentally, increasing weight is also one of the surest ways to get hot flashes. In a meta-analysis of over 4,000 women, obese women reported experiencing almost 80 percent more hot flashes than their slimmer peers. Just being overweight is enough for the incidence of menopausal symptoms to increase by 13 percent.

Your body mass index (BMI) can give you an idea of what a healthy weight range means for you, and can help you set a weight-loss goal if you need to lose weight. Keep in mind that men and women have a different target BMI, which further differs by age. Generally, an age- and gender-adjusted BMI between 25 and 30 is classified as overweight, and a BMI over 30 is considered obese. This online BMI calculator from the Centers for Disease Control and Prevention is ac-

curate and easy to use: www.cdc.gov/healthyweight/assessing/bmi
/adult_bmi/english_bmi_calculator/bmi_calculator.html.

Find Your Waist-to-Height Ratio

The waist-to-hip ratio is the most commonly used indicator of central body fat, aka belly fat, a marker of heart disease risk at all ages, but particularly important around menopause. To calculate it, measure yourself around the smallest part of your waist, being careful to not hold in your stomach! Then take a measurement at the widest part of your hips. Divide your waist measurement by your hip measurement. For example, a person with a thirty-inch waist and thirty-eight-inch hips has a waist-hip ratio of 30/38 = 0.78. In general, for women, the ratio should be no greater than 0.8; the number for men is 1.0. If you are above that, it means that you are at risk. However, since women's hips are classically wider than their waists, this test can lead to underestimating adipose fat and therefore risk of heart disease in women.

A more accurate measurement is your waist-to-height ratio, which is calculated by dividing your waist size by your height. If your waist measurement is less than half your height, you're not likely to be at risk. Specifically, for women, a waist-to-height ratio between 0.42 and 0.48 is considered healthy. These rules bend somewhat after menopause, as some weight gain around the waist is normal. But as a rule of thumb, a five-foot-four (sixty-four-inch) woman should aim to keep her waist less than thirty-two inches, while a five-foot-nine (sixty-nine-inch) woman should ideally keep her waist measurement under 34.5 inches.

Measure Your Blood Pressure

High blood pressure (hypertension) is a well-known risk factor for heart disease and stroke. It can quietly damage your body for years before symptoms develop. If left uncontrolled, you may wind up with a disability, a poor quality of life, or even a fatal heart attack. What is perhaps less known is that hypertension is also a common cause of vaginal dryness and reduced sexual desire in women. From a neurological perspective, effective management of hypertension, especially in midlife, is important to also reduce the risk of future cognitive declines. If your blood pressure is chronically high, lowering it can lower the impact of mild cognitive impairment, which is the next best thing in the study of dementia prevention. Additionally, some studies suggest that APOE-4 carriers might particularly benefit from blood pressure management.

There is less evidence for an association between low blood pressure (hypotension) and an increased risk of heart disease or dementia. Nonetheless, low blood pressure can cause dizziness, weakness, fainting, and a risk of injury from falls, which needs to be addressed, too.

Treatment and lifestyle changes can help control your blood pressure to reduce your risk of life-threatening complications. So have your doctor measure your blood pressure at regular intervals, ideally every six months to a year, especially if you are post-menopausal. Blood pressure readings are made up of two numbers, for example, 140/90. The first number is your systolic blood pressure, or the highest pressure reached when your heart is busy pushing the blood throughout your body. The second number is your diastolic blood pressure, which is the level of pressure maintained as your heart relaxes between beats. Here are some things to look out for:

- If your blood pressure is 140/90 or higher over a number of weeks, you may have hypertension. Time to work with your doctor to lower it.

- If your blood pressure is between 120/80 and 140/90, it is slightly higher than it should be. Lowering it a bit is your goal.

- If your blood pressure is chronically lower than 90/60, you may have hypotension. Talk to your doctor about the appropriate treatment.

LABORATORY TESTS

In the clinical workup of dementia, but also for dementia prevention, blood and urine samples are routinely collected to rule out infections and to check how organs, such as the liver or kidneys, are functioning. Always ask your doctor to make sure you don't suffer from infections, especially UTIs, which are frequent in women. Silent UTIs in particular are tricky to spot because they don't trigger obvious symptoms like burning or itching, but can seriously cloud your head.

In more specialized centers like ours, several additional lab tests are performed to measure lipid and metabolic markers known to impact cognitive function (see table 1). These tests can help determine if you have insulin resistance or diabetes, high cholesterol or high triglycerides, or nutrient deficiencies, which all can both mimic the symptoms of dementia and increase its risk. Lab tests can also help assess your hormonal levels. As much as you can, always know your numbers!

Get a Fasting Glucose and Insulin Test

These tests help you find out if you have diabetes or could be at risk for it:

- Fasting blood glucose should be under 90 mg/dL, or even better, in the 75–80 range. If your level is 100–125, you are considered in the pre-diabetes range and may be insulin resistant. If it's over 125, you may have diabetes.

- Optimal fasting insulin is lower than 5 microunits/ml. Anything higher indicates insulin resistance.

- Have your doctor measure hemoglobin A1c in addition to fasting glucose. The A1c test reflects your average blood sugar level for the past two to three months, rather than on the day you do the test. This is helpful because sometimes an A1c test can detect diabetes where a glucose test hasn't. The healthy range for hemoglobin A1c is 4–5.7 percent.

Women with the APOE-4 gene need to pay extra attention to these metabolic markers. There is evidence that, especially as they go through menopause, APOE-4 carriers with insulin resistance tend to experience more severe memory decline as compared with those with a regular metabolism.

Get Your Fats Checked

If you have an abnormal amount of fat in your blood (dyslipidemia), you may be at risk for both cardiovascular disease and insulin resistance. This is especially the case if you have high total cholesterol (over 240 mg/dL), particularly low HDL cholesterol (below 50 mg/dL for women or 40 mg/dL for men), high LDL cholesterol (over 160 mg/dL), and/or high triglycerides (over 200 mg/dL).

Additionally, some studies have indicated that a type of cholesterol called Lipoprotein(a), or Lp(a), may do a better job at predicting cardiovascular risk for women. This is particularly true for those who have a past history of heart disease, or for women with a family history of early-onset heart disease or sudden death in the family. The research is still ongoing, but it looks like women who would be considered at low risk for heart disease based on standard examinations may instead harbor higher risk related to elevated levels of Lp(a). For example, if your total cholesterol levels are normal but your Lp(a) is high, your risk is also high.

APOE-4 carriers should pay extra attention to their lipid levels too. Besides being a risk factor for Alzheimer's, the APOE-4 variant increases risk of heart disease, likely due to its negative effects on raising LDL cholesterol. Higher circulating LDL can lead to an increased formation of plaques in the vascular system and reduced circulation, effectively delivering a one-two punch to cholesterol and blood flow at the same time.

Generally, patients with out-of-range values are advised to lower their lipid level, especially LDL cholesterol. This can be sometimes achieved by means of drugs such as statins, but also by following the drug-free lifestyle recommendations described in part 3.

Check Your Thyroid

Thyroid disease, especially having a sluggish thyroid (hypothyroidism) can cause symptoms similar to those of menopause, as well as high cholesterol, weight gain, and fatigue. It is also a cause of reversible cognitive disturbances.

The thyroid-stimulating hormone (TSH) has long been part of the screening laboratory test for dementia. Optimal TSH levels range between 0.27 and 4.2 mcIU/mL. Levels below 0.27 and above 4.2 may be indicative of thyroid dysfunction. Other tests measuring available thyroid hormones circulating in the bloodstream (Free T4, Free T3) are also helpful indicators of thyroid function. Your doctor may also want to test for TPO and TGB antibodies to rule out autoimmune conditions that attack the thyroid, such as Hashimoto's disease and Graves' disease. In case of a positive test, speak to your doctor about available treatments, and also make sure that you follow the hormone-balancing recommendations outlined in the next chapters.

Homocysteine, a Marker of Vascular Risk

A high level of homocysteine is not only a risk factor for heart disease, stroke, and hardening of the arteries, but for dementia as well. Homocysteine levels above 14 micromol/liter are considered high. However, new research shows that the risk of developing dementia is nearly doubled in people with homocysteine levels at or above 13. This indicates that our brains are more sensitive to this substance than previously imagined. Optimal homocysteine levels are below 10. If your level is higher, make sure you work with your doctor to lower it.

The good news is that since homocysteine levels are in part regulated by specific B vitamins, high homocysteine is reversible by eating a healthy diet rich in these vitamins, or by taking specific supplements, as described in chapter 11.

Don't Skip Your Nutrients, Especially the B Vitamins and Omega-3s

Deficiencies of some B vitamins, especially B6, B12, and folate (B9), can lead to problems with brain function, the nervous system, and other aspects of your health. Besides altering homocysteine levels, low B-vitamin levels can provoke cognitive decline and even mimic the symptoms of dementia. For example, low levels of B12 can cause pernicious anemia, a condition that can lead to fatigue, fuzzy thinking, confusion, moodiness, and slowness. Researchers believe that up to 15 percent of people in the United States have some vitamin B12 deficiency. It's therefore important to check your blood levels if there are any signs that they may be low. Sometimes, a test that measures MMA (methylmalonic acid) is used as a follow-up to help diagnose an early or mild deficiency in case of a B12 test result that is at the lower end of the normal range.

Omega-3 fatty acids work to protect your brain cells from the wear and tear that naturally occurs with aging, while also providing support for the cardiovascular system. Adequate omega-3 levels have been associated with reduced brain shrinkage, preserved memory, and a reduced risk of dementia in late life. Not all doctors check omega-3 levels, but we believe this measurement to be helpful for Alzheimer's prevention.

The so-called omega-3 index is another important measurement. A higher omega-3 index indicates that you consume a balanced amount of omega-3s and omega-6s. This is favorably associated with a reduced risk of many chronic diseases, especially cardiovascular disease. Because Americans as a rule consume far too few omega-3s from fish or fish oil, it's no surprise that an estimated 95 percent (with the exception of folks from Alaska) have a low omega-3 index, putting them in the high-risk category. In general, in countries with high fish consumption, such as Asia and Northern Europe, this is less of a problem.

Most people who eat a balanced diet should have adequate B vitamins and omega-3s. But there are exceptions. After age fifty, our metabolism naturally slows down and absorption of vitamin B12 may decrease as a result. Further, gastritis, Crohn's disease, celiac disease, and immune disorders such as lupus may cause your B12 levels to go down. Several types of medication might also affect your B12, especially drugs to help treat acid reflux, peptic ulcers, and indigestion, like antacids (e.g., Tums) and proton-pump inhibitors (e.g., Prilosec,

Prevacid), as well as Metformin, a drug for diabetes. Vegan and strict vegetarian diets can also lead to deficiencies in both B12 and omega-3s. Additionally, women are particularly at risk of folate deficiency during pregnancy, as a growing baby absorbs lots of folate from its mother. Birth control pills are also known to deplete your B vitamins, and so is heavy drinking.

In all of these cases, talk to your doctor about having your vitamin B and omega-3 status checked. In chapter 11, we will discuss whether nutritional supplementation may be helpful to you, and under what circumstances.

C-Reactive Protein: A Marker of Inflammation

There are several parameters we can measure in blood to detect the presence of inflammation. One of the most reliable tests is known as the CRP test. CRP, or C-reactive protein, is one of the chemicals produced by the immune system to fight harmful substances in the body, and it's also one of the chemicals that leads to inflammation. The CRP test measures the amount of this protein in the blood. Although it doesn't tell where the inflammation is or what's causing it, this test is a good way to determine if something is off. In particular, high-sensitivity CRP (hs-CRP) can detect insidious low-grade inflammation, and is often used to assess risk of heart disease as well.

High Cortisol: Too Much Stress

You probably don't need a blood test to find out if you're under stress. However, stress can be insidious, especially if you've been suffering from it for a long period of time, in which case an objective measure might help motivate you to take the problem seriously. The Stress Screener in chapter 7 is a good starting point to determine if you need to seek your doctor's guidance. If so, it might be helpful to also have your cortisol (e.g., the main stress hormone) checked.

Cortisol can be measured via your blood, urine, and saliva. The blood test is far more accurate, and is typically done twice in the same day, once in the morning and again later in the afternoon. That's because cortisol levels change a lot in the course of a day. High cortisol levels can also indicate the presence of infections or Cushing's syndrome, a medical condition characterized by weight gain, bruising, thinning of the skin, and even cessation of menstrual periods. That said, if you feel under stress, as so many of us are, you may as well skip the blood test and just take action. Chapter 13 provides several stress-busting recommendations to get you started.

Your Sex Hormones: To Check or Not to Check

When a woman suspects she's in perimenopause, it's an excellent time to have a complete medical examination by a qualified health professional, either an ob-gyn or an endocrinologist (see appendix A for how to find one). The diagnosis of perimenopause can usually be made by reviewing a woman's medical history, her menstrual history, and any signs or symptoms.

Blood tests typically aren't needed to diagnose menopause. But under certain circumstances, your doctor may recommend tests to check your levels of estradiol, FSH, and LH. Your estradiol levels decrease, while FSH and LH levels increase as menopause occurs.

The best way to measure your blood hormone levels is to have your doctor do it. Over-the-counter home tests to check FSH levels in the urine and saliva are available but unfortunately they're not particularly reliable.

However, not even the most accurate blood tests can tell you for sure whether you're in menopause. For example, since FSH levels rise and fall during the course of your menstrual cycle, they can be low one day and then quite high the next. More important, you can be in perimenopause even if your FSH levels are low. The same goes for estradiol levels, which can fluctuate widely during each month. Also, if you are taking birth control pills or have an IUD, or if you're taking breast cancer medications, the test results may not give you an accurate picture. If you are concerned about your menopausal status, I recommend that you fill out the Menopause Screener in chapter 7 and seek your doctor's guidance.

COGNITIVE TESTING

Mental cognitive status tests are a key step to evaluating memory, thinking, and problem-solving abilities in an objective way. Some tests are brief, while others can be more complex and time-intensive. More comprehensive cognitive tests are often given by a neuropsychologist, and only specialized centers and licensed clinicians have access to these rigorous tests. Online cognitive testing and brain teasers are widely available, but are currently not recommended for diagnostic purposes. We'll look into this in more detail later.

For now, I want to draw your attention to an important fact. Men and women differ in the way in which they experience cognitive changes. In fact, the early signs of cognitive decline, and even of Alzheimer's, are easier to spot in men. This is due to the fact that, throughout our adult life, women outperform men in a variety of cognitive tasks. This is especially true of verbal memory—the ability to recall words and stories, and to access language verbatim. Studies that compared memory performance between men and women at different stages of life showed that the only period when women start displaying measurable decline in memory performance on cognitive testing is after menopause. But in spite of this, many post-menopausal women continue to have an edge over their male counterparts in midlife as well as in old age, and sometimes even into the early stages of Alzheimer's.

While this is certainly good news, there is one downside to this advantage. The thing is, verbal and associative aspects of memory are one of the major cognitive measures used to diagnose a memory disorder, and one of the primary reasons people seek medical help. While to some extent we are all resigned to the idea that we may lose our keys or misplace our belongings, we are much less tolerant of how failing to come up with words or remember conversations can impact our social and work lives. However, since women tend to be better at this function than men and reference values are not always gender specific, this may hinder a doctor's ability to recognize and diagnose Alzheimer's. Women may also wait longer to go see a doctor, with the result that by the time they are finally diagnosed, the disease has had a chance to grow more severe, while male patients are diagnosed sooner. We are left to wonder how many women remain undiagnosed until the deficits are so severe that treatments no longer have a chance to work.

Hopefully, soon enough we'll have tests that work *for women*. In the meantime, pretty much everyone agrees that looking at a patient's brain is much more informative and accurate than cognitive testing alone.

BRAIN IMAGING

Our brains possess something akin to a fingerprint. While the architecture of the brain—with its various partitions into lobes, functional areas, and specific structures—may be roughly the same in all of us, there are significant variations when it comes to the size, shape, activity, and molecular composition of our brains. This tremendous variability is never more evident than when viewing brain scans.

I have been doing brain imaging for over fifteen years, inspecting and quantifying thousands of scans—and not a single day goes by when I do not stand in awe of the uniqueness the scans reveal, each patient's brain different and distinct from the next. The brain's individuality not only is based on our unique genetic makeup but is also shaped, molded, and "written upon" by our backgrounds, education, and experiences. Add to that the many foods you've been exposed to, your cultural environments, all the places you've explored, and all the joys and sorrows of your life, and it only makes sense that no two brains could ever be alike. In my opinion, brain scans are absolutely essential to understanding a person's brain and any individual risk factors that may affect cognitive function. And let's not forget that a brain scan can detect Alzheimer's many years before symptoms emerge.

Several types of brain scans are widely used in clinical practice and research. A typical clinical examination starts with computerized tomography (CT) or magnetic resonance imaging (MRI), both of which take pictures of the inside of your brain to reveal its structure and anatomy. These scans are particularly helpful to rule out a variety of conditions that can cause cognitive changes very similar to those observed in dementia patients. Four of these conditions in particular pose greater risks to women: brain tumors, aneurysms, white matter disease, and atrophy.

According to the American Brain Tumor Association, about 80,000 adults and children are diagnosed with a primary brain tumor each year. The chance of developing a brain tumor is very small, with a lifetime risk of 1 percent or less. However, there is variability in the risk of developing a brain tumor for males and females. In particular, meningioma, the most common primary brain tumor, is more common in women than in men, in part because of its interactions with our sex hormones. Most meningiomas are slow-growing and benign, but even those can sometimes cause cognitive issues that can be mistaken for Alzheimer's. Fortunately, meningiomas can usually be managed and sometimes removed without risk of severe damage to the brain, especially if caught soon enough—which would be impossible to do without a brain scan.

Aneurysms are another condition to watch out for. Think of an aneurysm as beginning with a weak spot in the wall of a blood vessel inside the brain. With continued flow of blood to the vessel, the spot gets worn out and starts bulging, almost like a small bubble. While many aneurysms don't cause symptoms, in some cases, they can grow big, leak, or explode. Bleeding in the brain, known as hemorrhagic stroke, is very serious and requires urgent medical care. Among all causes of stroke, ruptured brain aneurysms occur twice as often in women as in men, especially between fifty and fifty-nine years of age, often in correlation with the fall in estrogen levels that comes during menopause. In terms of prevention, brains scans make it possible to detect these risks, and the positive medical and lifestyle changes described in part 3 can significantly reduce the odds of a brain aneurysm leaking or popping and, more generally, of stroke.

Now on to white matter disease. This condition results from the wearing away of brain tissue in the largest and deepest part of the brain: the white matter. This tissue contains millions of nerve fibers that connect different parts of the brain and spinal cord and that signal nerve cells to talk to one another. A fatty material called myelin protects the fibers and gives white matter its milky color. Your white matter helps you think fast and walk straight, and keeps you from falling. When it becomes diseased, the myelin breaks down, impairing nerve communication. White matter disease has been associated with increased odds of negative outcomes, especially for women, once again in particular those undergoing menopause. However, there are ways to prevent and even reverse this condition, chiefly the heart-healthy practices we'll review in the next chapters.

Finally, let's talk about brain atrophy. MRI scans are key to determining if your brain is aging well. Over time, certain parts of the brain may shrink ("atrophy"), especially those important for learning, memory, and planning, as well as other complex mental activities. That's what we're on the lookout for when inspecting an MRI scan of an aging person. Is the brain as large and full as it should be relative to its peers? Are there any signs of atrophy? Some scans can show signs of cortical thinning or ventricular enlargement, which occur when the brain is losing tissues. Brain shrinkage could be an early sign of Alzheimer's, or an indication that your brain is aging faster than desirable, the latter being a common finding in some women in menopause. As we now know, age-related neuronal loss can be due to a number of medical and lifestyle factors we can not only modify but even completely eliminate.

Personally, I am a big fan of another brain imaging technique, called positron emission tomography, or PET. PET offers the unique ability to look at the brain's energy activity, as we saw in chapter 1, as well as to examine a variety of other parameters like a brain's neurotransmitter portfolio, uptake of essential fatty acids, inflammation, and a multitude of important chemicals needed for brain health. But most important, PET is currently the only technique that allows us to determine if a patient is suffering from Alzheimer's by detecting the presence of another major brain problem: amyloid plaques.

The ability to spot Alzheimer's hallmark signs in the brain is crucial for clinical purposes, especially for patients with an uncertain diagnosis. "Uncertain diagnosis" means that a patient is showing symptoms that could be caused by Alzheimer's as well as by another form of dementia, and the doctor is not sure which one is which. For example, patients with a diagnosis of Alzheimer's who show speech difficulties (aphasia) or disinhibition—typical symptoms of another condition called frontotemporal dementia (FTD)—could have either Alzheimer's or FTD, as these conditions possess some common features. Does the patient really have Alzheimer's, or is it FTD instead? Since Alzheimer's plaques are not found in the other form of dementia, a positive PET scan revealing them would confirm an Alzheimer's diagnosis. On the other hand, a negative PET scan showing no Alzheimer's plaques would effectively rule out Alzheimer's as the cause of the dementia symptoms present.

Believe it or not, almost 20 percent of patients with a diagnosis of Alzheimer's turn out *not* to have Alzheimer's, as determined via their PET scans. Use of PET scans can lead to a change in diagnosis in as many as 69 percent of cases—and a change in patient treatment plans in about 25 percent of cases. Clearly, this information can prove extremely valuable.

PET is also the only technique able to detect early Alzheimer's brain changes in people at risk for the disease. PET scans are particularly good at detecting the presence of Alzheimer's plaques decades before patients manifest any actual symptoms of the disease. These so-called predictive scans are currently not FDA-approved, which means that you can't simply ask your doctor to prescribe one. The only way to get these scans is by participating in research studies like ours, or in clinical trials. Participating in brain-imaging research is a great opportunity to receive a top-notch brain health evaluation, establish a solid baseline to use for comparison with later assessments, and obtain invaluable information that you wouldn't otherwise have access to. For example, finding out that you have (or don't have) a brain tumor, aneurysm, or other life-threatening brain condition is frankly quite priceless. If you are showing signs of cognitive impairment, or are at genetic risk for Alzheimer's (as described in chapter 6), clinical trials are also particularly attractive because in this case you can kill two birds with one stone: you have access to both the information provided by the PET scan and a treatment that might turn out to be successful. Plus, you will also be offered counseling, which is, of course, crucial. If participating in a clinical trial is of interest to you, a list of ongoing studies is included in appendix A. Just keep in mind that, for now, most clinical trials are restricted to people age sixty or older.

I am a firm believer in the value of brain imaging for disease prevention. Even though these techniques are currently available at only a few specialized clinics and research centers, it is my hope that we may soon make them much more accessible. With regard to women's health, I look forward to the day when we will routinely peek inside a woman's head and use her brain as our guide to providing the best recommendations specific to optimizing her health. Much in the same way a current female's middle-age health-care routine includes mammograms, a more evolved women's health-care system will demand careful attention with respect to brain aging, a full focus on the function of hormones in protecting it, and precision strategies to prevent Alzheimer's from becoming a woman's unnecessary destiny.

In the meantime, addressing the risk factors we can detect, and reacting with our current research's know-how, are unquestionably the best strategies we have today. It is my mission to ensure that every one of us receives the support her brain deserves to function to its maximum, age gracefully, and make the all-too-frequent occurrences of dementia a thing of the past.

CHAPTER 7

FILL OUT THE QUESTIONNAIRES

THE BEST WAY TO DETERMINE what your brain needs for optimal health would be to conduct several thorough exams, not the least of which would be the brain scans mentioned in the previous chapter. However, you may not have access to a brain scan to take a look at what's actually going on inside your head. The series of questionnaires I've included below will help you find out which aspects of your medical status and lifestyle choices need addressing first and foremost.

The questionnaires will prompt you to take a careful look into your general health, along with the various choices you make on a daily basis, to get a clearer picture as to which ways you are supporting your brain health and which ways you may inadvertently be sabotaging it. Taking care of our brains is difficult because the clues don't arrive in the form of jeans that fit or firmer abs. Use the questionnaires to establish your "baseline" and overall health profile as related to the major risks to women's brains: Alzheimer's, menopause, inflammation, and medical risk factors such as heart disease, diabetes, and depression. And let's not forget stress!

Taking these tests is a convenient way to learn how close or how far away your daily life is from one that's optimized for long-term brain health. This information can help you identify whether you need to see a doctor, and how to go about getting the help that's right for you. When it comes to women's health, one size *does not* fit all. Having as much information as possible with regard to your own health status can be extremely helpful in guiding you to take powerful steps toward gaining balance and achieving your goals.

Read each question carefully and answer as accurately as possible. Some of the questions include the physical and lab measures we discussed in the previous chapter. If you haven't done these tests in a while, refer to the most recent results or skip the question for now and take the test again once you have the information. Always make sure that you receive copies of your medical records and blood test results from your doctor. Don't be afraid to ask—you are entitled to receive this information.

After finishing the tests, read the interpretation of your scores below each test. Just keep in mind that a questionnaire is not a diagnostic tool. Always consult a health-care professional for further assistance.

TEST YOUR RISK OF DEVELOPING ALZHEIMER'S

QUESTIONS	YES	NO	DON'T KNOW
Are you a woman?			
Are you older than 60?			
Do you have a family history of Alzheimer's?			
Do you have a mother, father, sister, or brother diagnosed with Alzheimer's or other dementia?			
Are you an apolipoprotein E (APOE) epsilon 4 carrier?			
Have you ever had a head trauma or traumatic brain injury (TBI)?			
Do you practice (or have you consistently practiced) sports or other activities that cause frequent injuries (e.g., football, boxing, working in construction)?			

Do you suffer or have you suffered from depression for long periods of time (over 6 months)?			
Have you ever been diagnosed with herpes, syphilis, or any other infectious disease?			
Do you currently smoke or have you quit smoking less than 5 years ago?			
Do you currently take recreational drugs or illegal substances (e.g., cocaine, amphetamine, LSD), or do you have a history of taking such drugs?			
Have you taken benzodiazepines (e.g., Valium [diazepam], Ativan [lorazepam], Restoril [temazepam], Xanax [alprazolam]) for over 6 months?			
Have you taken antidepressants (e.g., sertraline [Zoloft], fluoxetine [Prozac, Sarafem], citalopram [Celexa], escitalopram [Lexapro]) for over 6 months?			
Do you have a personal history of alcoholism?			
Have you been told by a doctor that you have cardiovascular disease (e.g., heart disease)?			
Have you been diagnosed with high blood pressure?			
Have you been told by a doctor that you have diabetes?			
Have you been told by a doctor that you have pre-diabetes or insulin resistance?			
Is your BMI greater than 25?			
Do you have low B vitamin and/or low omega-3 levels, as measured by a blood test?			
Are you in menopause, either naturally or due to an ovariectomy or hysterectomy (i.e., surgical removal of the ovaries or uterus)?			
Is your diet high in fatty foods, sugar, and/or processed food (e.g., hamburgers, bacon, ham, sausage, cheese, butter, ice cream, cookies)?			

Do you eat less than 2 servings of fruits and vegetables in a typical day? (Note: 1 serving is the size of a small apple or 1 cup of vegetables.)			
Do you lead a sedentary life (i.e., do you spend less than 2 hours per week doing physical activities like walking, running, exercising at the gym, or even dancing)?			
Are you concerned that your memory is not as good as it used to be (e.g., your memory is worse than it was 10 years ago)?			
Do you have difficulties recognizing people or remembering names, appointments, or where you placed objects?			
Do you need multiple reminders to do things you used to do on your own, like chores, shopping, or taking medication?			
Do you feel that your memory is noticeably declining?			
Do you feel sad, down in the dumps, or prone to crying more often than in the past, and without any apparent reason?			
Do you repeatedly forget important appointments, family occasions, or holidays?			
Do you become fatigued when reading compared with in the past?			
Do you have trouble doing routine calculations, managing finances, or balancing a checkbook?			
Have you lost interest in your usual activities such as hobbies, reading, or social occasions?			
Do you become easily and unexpectedly irritable, agitated, or suspicious? Or have you started imagining (i.e., hearing, seeing, or believing in) things that are not real?			

If you answered yes to 22 or more questions, your risk of developing Alzheimer's is high. It is recommended that you contact your doctor for further evaluation. A neurological or geriatric consult can determine the best course of preventative action. Be sure to discuss how to lower your risk, and make sure you follow the recommendations in part 3 of this book, which will help you manage your risk.

If you answered yes to 11 to 21 questions, your risk of developing Alzheimer's is moderate. You might want to contact your doctor for further evaluation. To start, make sure you follow the recommendations in part 3 of this book, which will help you lower your risk.

If you answered yes to 10 or fewer questions, your risk of Alzheimer's is low and further assessment is not needed at this time. However, if you are concerned, do not hesitate to discuss this with your doctor.

TEST YOUR RISK OF DEVELOPING HEART DISEASE

QUESTIONS	YES	NO	DON'T KNOW
Are you older than 55?			
Are you African American, Mexican American, or Native American?			
Have you ever had any of the following conditions: heart attack, stroke, transient ischemic attack (TIA), peripheral artery disease (i.e., reduced blood flow to your arms and/or legs), or abdominal aortic aneurysm (i.e., enlargement of the lower area of the aorta, the major artery of the body)?			
Have you ever had any of the following procedures: coronary bypass surgery, angioplasty, or stent placement (i.e., a procedure to open narrowed or clogged arteries by placing a small tube [stent] in the artery to keep it open)?			
Have your parents, siblings, or children had any of the above conditions or procedures at an early age (younger than 55)?			
Have you been diagnosed with high blood pressure?			

Do you currently take high blood pressure medication?			
Have you been told by a doctor that you have diabetes?			
Is your BMI greater than 25?			
Is your waist-to-height ratio higher than 0.5?			
Do you have high total cholesterol (>200 mg/dL)?			
Do you have high LDL cholesterol (>130 mg/dL)?			
Do you have low HDL cholesterol (<50 mg/dL)?			
Do you have high CRP levels, as measured by a doctor?			
Do you currently smoke or have you quit smoking less than 5 years ago?			
Have you smoked over 100 cigarettes in your life?			
Do you often feel angry, aggressive, or in a bad mood for no good reason?			
Is your diet high in saturated fat, sugar, and/or processed food (e.g., hamburgers, bacon, ham, sausage, cheese, butter, ice cream, cookies)?			
Do you eat less than 2 servings of fruits and vegetables in a typical day? (Note: 1 serving is the size of a small apple or 1 cup of vegetables.)			
Do you lead a sedentary life (i.e., do you spend less than 2 hours per week doing physical activities like walking, running, exercising at the gym, or even dancing)?			
Have you ever been diagnosed with high blood pressure during pregnancy (preeclampsia)?			
Are you in menopause, either naturally or due to an ovariectomy or hysterectomy (i.e., surgical removal of the ovaries or uterus)?			

If you answered yes to 12 or more questions, your risk for heart disease is high. It is recommended that you contact your doctor for further evaluation. A cardiological consult can determine, through a series of tests, whether you are suffering from or headed for heart disease. Be sure to discuss how best to take action and follow the recommendations in part 3 of this book, which will help you lower your risk.

If you answered yes to 6 to 12 questions, your risk of having heart disease is moderate. Make sure you follow the recommendations in part 3 of this book to start lowering your risk. Consider contacting your doctor for further evaluation.

If you answered yes to fewer than 6 questions, your risk of having heart disease is low and further assessment is not needed at this time. If you are concerned, and especially if you have a family history of heart disease, do not hesitate to discuss this with your doctor.

TEST YOUR RISK OF DEVELOPING DIABETES

QUESTIONS	YES	NO	DON'T KNOW
Are you older than 60?			
Are you African American, Mexican American, Native American, Native Hawaiian, Pacific Islander, or Asian American?			
Do you have a mother, father, sister, or brother diagnosed with diabetes?			
Do you have a family history of low blood sugar, diabetes, high blood pressure, or high cholesterol?			
Have you been diagnosed with high blood pressure?			
Have you ever been diagnosed with insulin resistance?			
Is your BMI greater than 25?			
Is your waist-to-height ratio higher than 0.5?			
Do you have high total cholesterol (>200 mg/dL)?			

Do you have high LDL cholesterol (>130 mg/dL)?			
Do you have low HDL cholesterol (<50 mg/dL in women)?			
Is your diet high in fat and sugar? (See chapter 10 if you're not sure.)			
Do you experience sudden and/or frequent cravings for sugar and other high-carbohydrate foods?			
Do you experience fatigue suddenly or on a daily basis?			
When you eat sweets, do you again crave them 2–3 hours later?			
Do you experience feelings of shakiness, nervousness, or headaches that are relieved by eating sweets?			
Are you bothered while sleeping by increased perspiration or excessive thirst?			
Do you lead a sedentary life (i.e., do you spend less than 2 hours per week doing physical activities like walking, running, exercising at the gym, or even dancing)?			
Have you ever been diagnosed with gestational diabetes during pregnancy?			
Are you in menopause, either naturally or due to an ovariectomy or hysterectomy (i.e., surgical removal of the ovaries or uterus)?			

If you answered yes to 14 or more questions, your risk of developing type 2 diabetes is high. It is recommended that you contact your doctor for further evaluation. Through a series of tests, your doctor can determine whether you are suffering from diabetes or pre-diabetes. Be sure to discuss how best to take action, and follow the recommendations included in part 3 to restore your energy levels and reboot your metabolism.

If you answered yes to 7 to 13 questions, your risk of having type 2 diabetes is moderate. It is recommended that you contact your doctor for further testing. Through a series of tests, your doctor can determine whether you at risk for insulin resistance or pre-diabetes. Be sure to discuss how best to take action and follow the recommendations included in part 3 to lower your risk.

If you answered yes to fewer than 7 questions, your risk of having type 2 diabetes is low and further assessment is not needed at this time. However, if you are concerned, and especially if you have a family history of diabetes, do not hesitate to discuss this with your doctor.

TEST YOUR RISK OF DEVELOPING DEPRESSION

When answering the questions below, choose the answers that you feel best indicate how you have been feeling over *the past month*.

QUESTIONS	YES	NO	DON'T KNOW
Are you unhappy with the way your life is overall?			
Do you feel that you don't have enough social and emotional support?			
Do you find yourself down or sad without a specific reason?			
Do you experience mood swings?			
Do you feel tired or have a lack of energy for no specific reason?			
Do you have little interest or pleasure in doing the things you usually enjoy?			
Do you feel down, depressed, or hopeless?			
Do you have trouble falling or staying asleep, or have you been sleeping too much?			
Do you have a poor appetite or have you been eating more than usual?			

Do you feel bad about yourself or feel like you are a failure?			
Do you have trouble concentrating on things, like reading the newspaper or watching TV?			
Do you ever feel that you would be better off dead or that you should hurt yourself in some way?			
Were you diagnosed with or have you suffered from postpartum depression?			
Do you experience or have you ever experienced PMS-related depression?			
Are you in menopause, either naturally or due to an ovariectomy or hysterectomy (i.e., surgical removal of the ovaries or uterus)?			

If you answered yes to 8 or more questions, your risk of suffering from depression is high. It is recommended that you contact your doctor for further evaluation. For women in particular, if you answered yes to the last three questions, it is likely that hormonal changes may be involved in the feelings of depression you have been experiencing. Make sure you follow the recommendations in part 3 of this book, which will help you ameliorate these symptoms.

If you answered yes to 4 to 7 questions, your risk of suffering from depression is moderate. If you are concerned, and especially if you are perimenopausal or menopausal, or if you have suffered from depression in the past, discuss this with your doctor. The recommendations in part 3 of this book will help you manage any symptoms and hopefully get rid of them.

If you answered yes to fewer than 4 questions, your risk of suffering from depression is low and further assessment is not needed at this time. If you are concerned, and especially if you have suffered from depression in the past or have a family history of it, do not hesitate to discuss this with your doctor.

MENOPAUSE SCREENER

QUESTIONS	YES	NO	DON'T KNOW
Are you over 35?			
Have your periods become irregular (i.e., skipped periods)?			
Have your periods become heavier (i.e., heavier flow, flooding)?			
Have your periods become lighter (i.e., light flow, spotting)?			
Has your cycle become shorter (i.e., less than 28 days apart or less than it used to be)?			
Have you experienced phantom periods (i.e., skipped one or more periods)?			
Was your last menstrual period over 12 months ago?			
Do you suffer from disruptive hot flashes (intense and sudden waves of heat accompanied by excessive sweating)?			
Do you suffer from night sweats (intense and sudden waves of heat accompanied by excessive sweating at night)?			
Do your breasts feel much more sensitive or tender than usual?			
Do you suffer from vaginal dryness or painful intercourse?			
Has your desire for or enjoyment of sex decreased?			
Has your complexion gone through noticeable changes (e.g., drier than usual, acne, eczema, etc.)?			
Have you experienced changes in hair growth (e.g., unwanted facial hair or hair on other parts of your body)?			
Is the hair on your head clearly thinning?			

Question			
Are you experiencing digestive problems (bloating, gas, diarrhea, constipation, nausea, or heartburn)?			
Are you experiencing incontinence (sudden and unexpected release of urine and/or feces)?			
Have you been gaining weight for no clear reason?			
Do you feel bloated and uncomfortable, especially toward the second half of your cycle?			
Do you have PMS symptoms around the time of your period, or without having a period (cramps, bloating, headaches, irritability)?			
Do you suffer from stiffness or achy joints?			
Have you been diagnosed with osteopenia or osteoporosis?			
Do you feel more tired than usual or have difficulty sleeping?			
Do you have difficulty concentrating or remembering things?			
Do you often feel forgetful, fuzzy-minded, or confused?			
Do you suffer from headaches around the time of your period?			
Are you experiencing uncharacteristic mood changes (e.g., sadness, irritability, etc.)?			
Are you experiencing depressed moods or feelings of hopelessness?			
Are you experiencing easy tearfulness, crying for no good reason, or easily getting emotional?			
Do you feel overwhelmed or out of sorts?			
Are you feeling anxious, more so than what you would consider normal?			
Are you having panic attacks?			
Have you suffered from a hormonal imbalance in the past (thyroid condition, PCOS, insulin resistance, diabetes)?			

Are you taking some form of prescription birth control?			
Do you suffer from infertility or subfertility (can't carry a pregnancy to term)?			
Have you received any medical treatment, such as a hysterectomy or chemotherapy, that caused or precipitated menopause?			
Do you currently take hormone replacement therapy or are trying to get off it?			

If you answered yes to 18 or more questions, you appear to exhibit many symptoms of hormonal imbalance. Chances are you are in perimenopause or menopause. It is recommended that you contact your doctor for further evaluation. Also make sure you follow the recommendations in part 3 of this book, which will help you normalize these symptoms by ameliorating hormonal levels.

If you answered yes to 9 to 17 questions, you appear to exhibit some symptoms of hormonal imbalance. This is a great time to contact your doctor for further evaluation, while following the hormone-balancing recommendations in part 3 of this book.

If you answered yes to fewer than 9 questions, you appear to exhibit very few symptoms of hormonal imbalance and further assessment is not needed at this time. Keep in mind that this is the best time to prepare for what's ahead by closely following the preventative recommendations outlined in the next chapters.

STRESS SCREENER

When answering the questions below, choose the answers that you feel best indicate how you have been feeling over *the past two to three months.*

	OFTEN	SOME-TIMES	RARELY
Do you experience any of the following symptoms: headaches, chest pain, muscle tension, nausea, or changes in sex drive?			
Do you worry excessively and feel overwhelmed with responsibilities?			
Do you struggle to focus on tasks or stay motivated?			
Do you experience irritability, sadness, or anger?			
Do you have little appetite or find that you are overeating?			
Do you struggle to regulate how much caffeine, alcohol, or tobacco you use?			
Do you withdraw from others or feel overwhelmed in groups of people?			
Do you suffer from frequent colds and flus?			
Do you suffer from indigestion, acid reflux, or ulcers?			
Do you have sugar cravings, especially after dinner?			
Have you developed a muffin top? Have you been gaining weight around your waist?			
Do you have heart palpitations?			
Do you have a hard time falling asleep and/or staying asleep?			
Have you been experiencing anxiety attacks?			
Do you feel fatigue or burnout (e.g., you use coffee to keep you going)?			
Have you been feeling very negative in the way you see life and people?			

Have you experienced a loss of stamina, especially in the afternoon and evening?			
Are you worried about decreased problem-solving skills?			
Have you been struggling to get over simple colds, flus, or infections?			
Do you find yourself "eating emotionally" (e.g., eating unhealthy foods or eating when you're not hungry, as a response to stress or difficult feelings)?			
Do you feel dizzy after getting up from a seated or supine position?			
Do you find yourself crying for no good reason or getting easily emotional?			
In the morning, do you feel like you can't get out of bed or you only "wake up" after 2 cups of coffee?			
Do you experience decreased stress tolerance?			
Do you suffer from low or unstable blood sugar levels?			
Are you suffering from anxiety or depression?			
Do you have tension headaches?			
Do you have high blood cortisol levels, as measured by a doctor?			

If you answered yes to 18 or more questions, you are at high risk of experiencing health consequences due to stress, or you may be experiencing them already. It is likely that you also suffer from high cortisol levels. It is recommended that you contact your doctor for further evaluation and testing. It's vital to manage stress in your lifestyle to safeguard your health by closely following the stress reduction strategies outlined in the next chapters.

If you answered yes to 8 to 17 questions, you are likely experiencing a degree of stress-related health effects. While you may not be having serious health consequences yet, it's important to lead a healthy lifestyle that includes stress-reduction techniques. Manage your stress with a healthy diet and good-quality sleep, and learn to manage your emotional well-being by closely following the recommendations outlined in the next chapters.

If you answered yes to fewer than 8 questions, your stress level is low, and it seems unlikely that you have high cortisol levels. However, if there is stress in your life, or if you sometimes feel wiped out and overwhelmed, make sure to keep it at bay with the healthy diet, exercise, sleep, and stress-reduction techniques outlined in the next chapters.

TAKE A LOOK AT THE BIG PICTURE

Now that you have completed the questionnaires, mark your results as high, medium, or low risk in the table below.

RISK	ALZHEI-MER'S	HEART DISEASE	DIABE-TES	DEPRES-SION	MENO-PAUSE	STRESS
High						
Medium						
Low						

Here are some examples of why this is helpful. One of our patients, Ms. KS, age fifty-three and just diagnosed with menopause, got the following results:

RISK	ALZHEI-MER'S	HEART DISEASE	DIABE-TES	DEPRES-SION	MENO-PAUSE	STRESS
High	X		X		X	
Medium		X				
Low				X		X

In Ms. KS's case, it is crucial to address symptoms of menopause and diabetes that may be contributing to the increased Alzheimer's risk. Given the connection between menopause and insulin resistance, stabilizing her insulin and glucose levels is a key step in her management plan.

Another patient, Ms. MV, age forty-five and perimenopausal, obtained the following results:

RISK	ALZHEI-MER'S	HEART DISEASE	DIABE-TES	DEPRES-SION	MENO-PAUSE	STRESS
High	X			X	X	X
Medium		X	X			
Low						

In Ms. MV's case, we need to address the high stress level that may be worsening the brain symptoms of menopause and affecting her mood by impacting hormonal health. Stress, depression, and menopause are all known contributors to Alzheimer's risk.

Now that you have identified your own risks, move on to the next chapters to find customizable recommendations that make specific sense for your particular risks. These recommendations are aimed at providing lifestyle guidelines that can be done at home and on a day-to-day basis. We will also review prescription medications that may be helpful and are warranted for some women.

Nonetheless, my advice is always to start with lifestyle changes and follow those recommendations for *at least three months* before turning to medications. Select those that address your specific risks to unlock maximum benefits for your individual needs and see how you feel. Today, every woman is finally in a position to take her health into her own hands and optimize her lifestyle choices to fortify her brain and maximize the longest, healthiest, most memory-rich life possible.

PART 3

TAKE CHARGE: OPTIMIZE YOUR BRAIN HEALTH, MINIMIZE YOUR RISKS

CHAPTER 8

HORMONES, ANTIDEPRESSANTS, AND OTHER MEDS: DO *YOU* NEED THEM?

BY THE TIME YOU HIT YOUR FORTIES, estrogen replacement therapy has probably crossed your radar. If you are in your late forties and approaching menopause, you might be thinking that it's time to explore more deeply just what estrogen therapy, or the newly coined menopause hormonal treatment (MHT), is all about. What if you've already reached menopause—could MHT be right for you even once menopause has begun? How about if you're in your sixties instead? Did you opt into taking hormones or did you decide on another route? Whatever the case, how do you know if you made the right choice?

Whether to use prescription medicines for menopause is one of the most complex health-care decisions facing women in midlife today. Traditionally, there was much less question: as soon as menopause hit, it was time to go on hormones. Even as recently as fifteen years ago, women at menopause were automatically offered a prescription for MHT, which is indeed the most obvious course of action for treating menopause symptoms. MHT replaces the estrogen, or both the estrogen and progesterone, that the ovaries cease to produce in menopause.

While replacing these hormones makes sense in principle, the ever-shifting landscape regarding the benefits versus the risks of MHT has made the choice a challenging one for providers and patients alike. In fact, many women are downright frightened of MHT due to reports that the treatment can increase one's risk of cancer. Let's take a look at how this news came about and whether it's accurate.

HORMONAL THERAPY FOR MENOPAUSE: HOW IT ALL BEGAN

Menopause has historically been treated with everything from opium to acupuncture, from prayer to surgery. It wasn't until the 1930s that estrogen was discovered, revealing the link between estrogen loss and menopause. The push to find a solution picked up speed then, ultimately leading to the FDA's approval of estrogen treatment for menopause symptoms in the 1940s. The thought was that by replenishing the estrogens a woman's body was no longer producing on its own, replacement hormones would protect us against heart disease and bone loss (osteoporosis) while soothing disruptive hot flashes.

In 1942, Wyeth Pharmaceuticals introduced Premarin, an estrogen pill that quickly became a national bestseller. Premarin sales soared until the 1970s, when it was linked to an increased risk of endometrial cancer. However, combining estrogen with a progestin (a synthetic form of progesterone) seemed to make the treatment safe and effective once again, leading to the release of a second pill, called Prempro. Prempro, containing both estrogen and progesterone, was a logical evolution of the therapy since the two hormones work together as partners in a woman's body. Estrogen, among other things, promotes the growth of cells in the breasts and uterus, while progesterone's job is to keep this cell growth in check. By the 1990s, the American Heart Association, the American College of Physicians, and the American College of Obstetricians and Gynecologists were all convinced that the new MHT formulation was perfectly fine for post-menopausal women.

This conviction was in part informed by observational studies showing the protective effects of MHT on heart health as well as overall mortality. For example, the Nurses' Health Study, one of the largest prospective investigations into the risk factors for major chronic diseases in women, reported an 11 percent reduction in the risk of coronary artery disease in women who used MHT as compared with those who had never taken the hormones. This garnered a lot of attention since, in the United States, coronary artery disease is not only the most common type of heart disease but also the leading cause of death in both men and women.

MHT went on to become widely used before the government had a chance to test it in formal clinical trials. Finally, in 1993, the National Heart, Lung, and Blood Institute launched the Women's Health Initiative, a fifteen-year multiphase trial of over 160,000 post-menopausal women designed to formally test MHT efficacy, with a particular focus on the prevention of heart disease. By then, it had become standard practice to add a progestin to estrogen therapy for any woman with an intact uterus in order to guard against uterine cancer, which had been associated with the estrogen-only version of the drug. For women who had had a hysterectomy, standard practice recommended the use of estrogen alone. This was due to the fact that no longer having a uterus lowered the risk of cancer growth. The Women's Health Initiative included two large-scale randomized clinical trials designed to reflect this distinction.

The first clinical trial, called the estrogen-alone study, involved women who had had a hysterectomy and were given Premarin, the estrogen-only therapy. The second trial, the estrogen-plus-progestin study, was designed for women who still had their uterus and were therefore prescribed the combination estrogen and progestin therapy, Prempro. Between both studies, thousands of participants were randomly assigned to receive either of the two hormone medications or a placebo. The trials were to proceed for many years.

Then a bombshell hit the medical establishment. In 2003, both trials were abruptly shut down when early data showed that MHT was doing exactly the opposite of what was intended. Not only was the treatment failing to reduce the risk of heart disease, but both regimes were showing an increased risk of stroke and blood clots. If this wasn't enough, the estrogen-plus-progestin therapy also increased the risk of breast cancer.

The news was shocking, completely overturning what doctors had believed for more than a half century. Almost overnight, nearly 80 percent of the American women who had been using these therapies stopped cold turkey, while at the same time kicking off several lawsuits. Sales plummeted. MHT was now considered deadly. To make matters worse, news broke that MHT was also linked to an increased risk of dementia, further terrifying women about the long-term effects of the treatment. All of this quickly snowballed and further drug development for menopause came to a dramatic halt.

Instead of the crisis spurring on new research to successfully deal with the challenges discovered, a void of any such activity grew in its place. To this day, the Women's Health Initiative, the now-infamous study that took place over twenty years ago, still stands as the world's most comprehensive source of information regarding the risks and benefits of MHT. With no better sources to turn to, women around the world remain understandably fearful of MHT and are left feeling conflicted and apprehensive about how to successfully navigate what should be yet another vital chapter of their lives.

THE "WINDOW OF OPPORTUNITY"

Within a few years of the collapse of the Women's Health Initiative, investigators came to the conclusion that the initial interpretations of the study's results were, at least in part, incorrect. Upon closer inspection, criticisms were raised regarding both the validity of the studies' approach and the relevance of the findings.

The most outstanding shortcoming was that the trials were conducted predominantly on women in their sixties and seventies, therefore many years into menopause. It later turned out that many of these women already suffered from the very conditions that MHT might have preempted had they begun the therapy earlier, especially with regard to heart disease. Since women's arteries typically begin to harden after menopause, being administered MHT so late in the game likely made the therapy less capable of reversing or ameliorating symptoms that had already begun developing. MHT also seemed to increase the risk for blood clots, a condition to which older women are more susceptible. This, in turn, contributed to an increased occurrence of heart attacks.

The questions of dosage and frequency also raised some eyebrows. For instance, as was typical of the times, only high doses of hormones were tested. Questions as to whether different dosages, different forms of the hormones, or different methods of administration would have been safer or more effective were left unexplored. A further hitch was that it was considered safe to put women on estrogen and leave them on estrogen, for life. This has since been reassessed. The current thinking is that MHT should be primarily used as a short-term solution, and even then, only for some women.

Equally unfortunate was the fact that for decades, physicians treated menopause using a one-treatment-fits-all approach. Many professional medical societies now agree that the blanket use of estrogen is, indeed, a mistake. The medical community now acknowledges that just as the experience of menopause varies so extremely among women, so should any treatment plan be adapted to address these variations. Unfortunately, though, the results of the Women's Health Initiative were broadly applied to all women and all MHT regimens.

Insights such as these have spurred more thought—thought that merited further investigation, especially as so many more questions have come into the picture. One example of this that seems obvious in hindsight is whether hormone use presents different risks and benefits for women younger than those studied in the trials. Is there an optimal age at which to initiate MHT or an ideal duration for the therapy? Are there formulations and methods of application that would prove safer and more effective?

In recent years, data from the Women's Health Initiative has been reanalyzed, and several of the original conclusions have been updated and revised. One such development refers to the concept of a "window of opportunity" for when to first administer the treatment. This idea has received greater attention of late, as we've come to recognize that the risks and benefits of administering these hormones seem to vary according to two essential parameters in particular: a woman's age and how long she's been in menopause.

The importance of these factors became particularly clear thanks to follow-up analyses of data collected after the trials were interrupted, which showed exceptional and contrary results to those initially cited. This reassessment revealed that women who initiated MHT when they were younger than sixty years of age, or otherwise within ten years of the onset of menopause, had a lower mortality rate than those who did not take MHT. A subsequent pooled analysis of thirty clinical trials also showed that women who began MHT before age sixty had a 39 percent lower risk of death than those who didn't.

Further, a new clinical trial of over 600 women, called the Early Versus Late Intervention Trial with Estradiol (ELITE), provided fairly conclusive evidence that MHT has the potential to slow down the progression of atherosclerotic plaques when therapy is initiated soon after menopause. This has been linked to a 32 percent reduction in the number of heart attacks and cardiac deaths. Additionally, early use of MHT has now been linked to a decrease in the risk of deaths from hip and bone fractures due to osteoporosis.

For another twist: Some experts now believe that in the absence of contraindications like cancer, estrogen-alone therapy can potentially be a lifesaver for prematurely menopausal women, especially those who have had a hysterectomy. For those of you who haven't had the need for a hysterectomy, you might be surprised to learn that hysterectomies are the second most common surgery among women in the United States, and the most common cause of early menopause. Surgical menopause differs from natural menopause in many ways. Women who have this surgery tend to be younger, many in their early forties rather than in their fifties, and the subsequent surgery-provoked drop in their estrogen levels is sudden rather than gradual. This leaves patients more vulnerable to the negative effects of hormonal depletion, which may result in an increased risk of heart disease, osteoporosis, and cognitive decline—and perhaps even premature death. While more research is needed to establish a firm association, data shows that over the ten-year period following the end of the Women's Health Initiative, a minimum of 18,601 and a maximum of 91,610 postmenopausal women who had had a hysterectomy died prematurely from heart disease, possibly because they did not take estrogens.

Overall, ongoing research points to the possibility that, when applied judiciously and for an appropriate period of time (as determined by a patient's personal medical history), MHT may have some wide-ranging benefits. However, since this evidence comes from observational studies and reexamination of clinical trials designed to look at other questions, more research is needed to conclusively answer these questions.

In the meantime, many doctors remain broadly unprepared to address women's concerns regarding MHT. The number one question for every woman approaching menopause in this day and age is whether or not to take estrogen and perhaps risk cancer. If they reject estrogen, how are they supposed to manage the daily interference of hot flashes without any support? Where are they to go for relief of menopause-related depression, anxiety, and lack of sleep? How about the risk of dementia? Which doctors are equipped to assist us properly? As women, we are all looking for solutions to help us deal with menopause efficiently and effectively. In spite of how great the need, the advice and solutions we seek have been largely unavailable to us.

This chapter is dedicated to providing answers to many of the most pressing questions. First, we will examine the actual bottom-line risks and benefits that exist around MHT. We will then discuss whether hormonal therapy could be right for you, or if other solutions might be better suited to freeing you from the symptoms of menopause.

MHT NOW: RIGHT TIME, RIGHT PLACE

Is MHT Really a Cancer Risk?

It is no wonder that the possibility of developing cancer is at the very core of why most women decide against MHT. Clearly, it is a question that needs to be taken very seriously.

As mentioned at the beginning of this chapter, the link between hormonal therapy and cancer was provided by the Women's Health Initiative. In the estrogen-plus-progestin trial, taking MHT resulted in a higher incidence of breast cancer than taking a placebo. However, the estrogen-alone study showed exactly the opposite effect: treatment was associated with a 23 percent reduced incidence of breast cancer in women who had undergone a hysterectomy. Even many years after the Women's Health Initiative was interrupted, the risk of breast cancer for participants remained remarkably low. Clearly, there is a conflict in these results that deserves to be addressed.

It's important to note that both trials were shut down not due to cancer risk, but because MHT use led to an increased risk of heart disease. However nuanced and ultimately confusing the results of these studies were, the media highlighted the correlation with cancer, to the point of generating public panic around the cancer risk for all women. Now, many years later, we have a better understanding of the factors that influence cancer risk with MHT use.

First off, whether or not you've had a hysterectomy figures prominently in how you assess your choices. As mentioned before, estrogen-only therapy is generally considered safe for women who have had a hysterectomy, whereas estrogen-plus-progestin is a safer choice for those who haven't. However, cancer risk is high in women with a personal history of breast, uterine, or ovarian cancer. For these women, MHT is *not* recommended, as it can increase the risk of recurrence. Generally, breast cancer survivors, as well as women with a family history of cancer, should consider non-hormonal therapies, such as those we will discuss in the next chapters.

In women without a history of cancer, risk is mainly dependent on the duration of MHT use, as the risk increases the longer a woman is on the therapy. Although data is still limited, risk also seems to grow higher depending upon the type of progestin used: medroxyprogesterone acetate (MPA), the type of progestin that was used in the Women's Health Initiative trials, has been shown to raise one's risk considerably, whereas other progestins such as micronized progesterone carry lower risk.

For those who haven't had a hysterectomy, it is also important to distinguish between "relative risk" and "absolute risk" of cancer as related to MHT. When you go to the doctor and have a discussion about the risks of anything health related, more often than not, the estimates your doctor gives you are based on what is called *relative risk*. Relative risk is a general estimate of risk relative to someone else, typically to a group of patients not taking the drug. *Absolute risk* is instead an estimation of whatever degree of risk exists for any given individual.

Let's look at an example of each of these terms. There will be math, but stay with me.

Suppose you read in the news that there's a new drug that does wonders in reducing hot flashes but, as a side effect, increases the risk of cancer by 50 percent. Sounds pretty scary, right? But that's an estimate of relative risk. It indicates that the risk of cancer increased by 50 percent in a group of patients who took the drug as compared with another group of patients who did not take the drug. In actuality, whether or not this is really bad news depends on two factors: how many patients were in the study to begin with, and how many *untreated* patients developed cancer. For example, let's say that, among a group of one hundred patients who did not take the drug, two developed cancer anyway. And let's say that, when reading the fine print, you discover that among the other group of one hundred treated patients in the study, three developed cancer. In other words, this new drug actually increased cancer occurrence by just one case relative to what could have happened anyway—from two cases up to three. Suddenly that impressive-sounding 50 percent jump no longer packs as much of a punch.

However, if the drug had increased the number of cancer patients from twenty to thirty, that's a problem! Although a 50 percent change is the case in both examples, in absolute terms, it's the actual number of lives affected that matters more than a percentage quoted. Keep these numbers in mind as we look at the actual data on MHT and cancer risk.

The estrogen-plus-progestin arm of the Women's Health Initiative study (this is the combo linked to cancer) estimated that for every 10,000 women who took hormones for a year, the incidence of breast cancer was thirty-eight cases in the treated group as compared with thirty in the untreated group. That's a 26 percent increased relative risk in women who took MHT. But in absolute terms, this means that if 10,000 women took hormones for a year, treatment would result in only eight more cases of breast cancer as compared with if no one took the hormones. Even though just one additional case is too many, eight cases out of 10,000 are much less frightening odds than those implied by "a 26 percent increased risk of cancer." Whenever we are attempting to understand data and its interpretation, it is precisely these sorts of distinctions that are worth our time and effort.

Many years and many studies later, the general belief is that the increase in cancer risk induced by MHT might be small enough to allow women to reconsider it, providing these women do not have a preexisting high risk of cancer and are prescribed the right formulation for the right amount of time. Each patient should be evaluated as a candidate for MHT on an individual basis so that their overall balance of risks and benefits can be weighed and taken into account.

The last section of this chapter describes how to calculate your cancer risk and contains flowcharts to help you determine the best kind of therapy for you based on your own risk factors.

How About MHT and Alzheimer's Risk?

Now let's turn to another delicate issue: Does hormonal therapy increase the risk of dementia?

There is no other medication specifically prescribed for women that has received greater attention in the field of dementia research than MHT. In spite of this, most of the evidence still comes from the all-too-familiar Women's Health Initiative study that, rather unnervingly, continues to inform most of our decisions.

This is due to the fact that the study also consisted of an additional branch called the Women's Health Initiative Memory Study (WHIMS). To date, this remains the largest and longest randomized placebo-controlled trial of the effects of MHT on dementia risk. In order to test whether MHT was effective for dementia prevention, the WHIMS focused on post-menopausal women who were age sixty-five or older at the time of enrollment. The trials included an estrogen-only arm for women without a uterus and an estrogen-plus-progestin arm for women with a uterus. The estrogen-alone segment found no significant impact on dementia risk. However, for the estrogen-plus-progestin segment, there was a doubling of the risk of dementia with MHT use.

So, on top of increasing the risk of heart disease and cancer, estrogen-plus-progestin therapy was detrimental to cognition, possibly by accelerating existing brain issues in those older women.

However, given recent reports of beneficial effects of MHT on heart disease in younger women, it is possible that starting MHT earlier might be protective against dementia as well. Indeed, evaluations of the combined statistics of over eighteen studies have shown that, among younger fifty-to-fifty-nine-year-old women, those who took hormones had a *30 to 44 percent reduced risk of Alzheimer's* as compared with those who did not take hormones. So that's good news.

More evidence that MHT may have value for dementia prevention comes from studies of women who have had hysterectomies. As previously mentioned, surgical removal of the uterus, in particular when the ovaries are also removed, has been linked to an increased risk of future dementia. However, a study of 1,884 women showed that women with hysterectomies who started estrogen-alone therapy within five years of surgery and continued until the natural age of menopause had a lower risk of dementia as compared with those who did not take the drug. Additionally, randomized clinical trials of younger women with hysterectomies show that those who used estrogen-alone therapy saw general beneficial effects on memory performance and brain activity as compared with non-users and also with those who had discontinued treatment.

Not-so-glowing reviews come instead from two new randomized clinical trials that showed no cognitive improvements in women who started MHT within six years of menopause onset. If nothing else, cognition didn't get worse, and MHT did not increase the risk of dementia in either trial.

More clinical trials are needed to specifically look at MHT effects in younger women, especially those of perimenopausal age. The brain imaging findings described in chapter 1 encourage further investigation of the potential efficacy of estrogen-based therapies in supporting healthy brain aging if initiated prior to the onset of menopause.

TO RECAP

At the end of this chapter you'll find flowcharts that will help you determine if you or a loved one may benefit from MHT in regard to a variety of risks, including heart disease, cancer, and dementia. Feel free to skip to the charts if this is a burning question. Here I am going to summarize the data so far. Although the evidence regarding the risks associated with MHT use is obviously complex, some things seem clear:

Estrogen-only therapy is generally safe for women without a uterus:

- For women who undergo a hysterectomy prior to menopause, starting estrogen-only therapy within a five-year window from surgery and continuing treatment until what would have been the natural onset of menopause appears to potentially reduce the risk of heart disease and dementia. Caveat: these hormones should not be taken indefinitely. This is a discussion that must be addressed directly with your doctor.

- The value of MHT is less clear for women who have had a hysterectomy prior to menopause and are currently over five years post-surgery, or otherwise past their natural age of menopause. So for example, if one had surgery at age forty-two and is now fifty (about the average age of menopause), starting MHT is probably not helpful for dementia prevention. It may still be helpful for other issues, though, so be sure to discuss these with your doctor.

- Women who have had only their ovaries removed and not their uterus need both estrogen and progestin. That's because estrogen alone can increase the risk of cancer in the uterus. See below.

Estrogen-plus-progestin therapy has varying effects on women with a uterus. Whether these effects can be considered potentially positive is dependent upon age, as well as other specific factors, some of them indicated here:

- MHT may be helpful against cognitive decline in eligible women within five years of menopause.

However, more work is needed to establish a firm association. Caveat: estrogen-plus-progestin therapy can increase breast cancer risk, especially when taken for longer than three to five years. Breast cancer risk is higher in the first two to three years of use but seems to go back down to average risk levels about two years after you go off the treatment. As risk is influenced by a number of factors, this is a discussion that must be addressed directly with your doctor.

- MHT seems to increase the risk of dementia if initiated after age sixty or more than five years after the onset of menopause. So if you are younger than sixty but stopped getting periods more than five years ago, MHT is probably not helpful.

- MHT is not helpful (and may be detrimental instead) for women with a diagnosis of Alzheimer's.

- Although more evidence is needed, some studies suggest that estrogen-plus-progestin therapy could potentially have a more negative impact on women with the APOE-4 gene. As a result, APOE-4 carriers should be especially prudent when considering this option and should make a point of bringing these specific findings to their doctor for discussion.

PROTECTING THE BRAIN (AND THE HEART) FROM CANCER THERAPY

In 2018, I wrote an op-ed in the *New York Times* about the menopause-Alzheimer's connection. I did so with the intention of raising awareness about hormonal health as a strong, yet largely overlooked determinant of a woman's overall brain health. I expected that it might stir up a number of reactions, but what caught me by surprise was how many emails I received from breast cancer patients in particular.

Breast cancer is recognized as a major public health crisis in our world.

Here in the United States, one out of every eight women ends up dealing with breast cancer in her lifetime. Between 60 and 80 percent of all breast cancers are related to sex hormones, like estrogen. The cells in estrogen-receptor-positive (ERP) cancers have protein receptors that attach to estrogen, which helps them grow. As a result, treatment of these cancers is aimed at blocking or suppressing estrogen to prevent the cancer from recurring.

That is why I received so many responses from the breast cancer community. Having made the connection between a lack of estrogen and an increased risk of Alzheimer's, both current patients and survivors were concerned that their cancer medicines might be at unfortunate odds with their brain health. Currently, 3 million American women are breast cancer survivors. Due to the nature of their anti-cancer medications, they also happen to be estrogen depleted.

I am by no means a cancer expert but felt compelled to look into this issue. The drugs used to fight cancer extend life for millions of people and sometimes eradicate the disease completely. However, they can harm the ovaries and provoke amenorrhea, or lack of menstruation, whether as a temporary effect or a permanent one. Specifically, there are two major types of chemotherapies: estrogen blockers and aromatase inhibitors. As the name implies, the job of "estrogen blockers" is to block estrogen receptors. They work like a broken key in a lock. By sticking to the estrogen receptors (the lock), they prevent the normal key (estrogen) from fitting anymore, thereby stopping the tumor in its tracks. Aromatase inhibitors stop estrogen production throughout the entire body instead, including inside the brain. Women of pre-menopausal age are likely to get started on an estrogen blocker, which is usually tamoxifen (brand names: Nolvadex and Soltamox). Women who are already post-menopausal are usually given an aromatase inhibitor such as Arimidex, Aromasin, and Femara.

Although these drugs' effects on cognitive function are not yet entirely understood, both the loss and blockage of estrogens can result in a wide variety of brain symptoms. For example, estrogen-blocking tamoxifen triggers hot flashes in approximately 40 percent of the patients. Complaints regarding memory issues and brain fog, often referred to as "chemo brain," are also very common in breast cancer patients. It further complicates things that these symptoms can be hard to tell apart from other factors, like the effects of surgery or radiation.

That said, there is no clear evidence that chemotherapy increases the risk of dementia—although unfortunately the available data is far from conclusive. Some studies report minor to no negative effects on cognitive function, nor an increased Alzheimer's risk, while others raise some concerns. Given the scarcity of data, we just don't know for sure.

We do know, however, that some chemotherapies may increase the risk for heart disease, a connection that is also often overlooked. Quite a few of these drugs can be hard on the heart, like tamoxifen, Adriamycin, Herceptin, and some aromatase inhibitors. Though the risk seems fairly low, it is real, particularly for women over sixty-five.

To be clear: **nobody is telling cancer patients to decline treatment**. Far from it.

I am sharing this data because women want to know—and *need* to know. Not to endanger their lives by going off cancer meds, but to demand information about these incredibly important and largely understudied issues, *and* to demand better and safer treatments that take into account their bodies as a whole. It's quite important that patients be well-informed about their medical health overall—and just as important that their oncologists be aware of those other risks, too. Now more than ever, prevention is key. Given the weight of evidence regarding the role of estrogen in the brain, cancer survivors should gather all the facts available and discuss options with their doctors. We want patients to undergo the best treatment available. At the very least, this should include regular screenings for heart and brain function, too. I am here to help you with this. The guidelines included in part 2 are designed to detect possible risk factors for cognitive decline and heart disease. This knowledge can be crucial in preventing future issues, as well as in tailoring treatments to balance the risk of cancer recurrence with the risk of other problems. At the same time, the key recommendations included in part 3 can assist cancer patients and survivors in safeguarding their brains and hearts as they make progress through their healing journey.

THE NEW GENERATION OF HORMONES
Oral versus Topical

Hormones are administered in different forms. Some are given orally or locally at high doses, and are systemic in nature. Others are taken topically or "transdermally," meaning they're designed to be absorbed through your skin.

The disastrous Women's Health Initiative tested systemic hormones only. With systemic therapy, hormones enter the bloodstream and travel to all parts of the body. These come mostly in the form of a daily pill or patch and tend to be popular choices. Intrauterine devices (IUDs) that deliver larger doses of hormones to the entire body are another option. (Note: Copper IUDs do not contain hormones.) Hormonal injections into a muscle or just under the skin are also available. One pro of systemic therapy is that the hormones are able to reach your brain, too, helping to relieve a variety of menopausal symptoms. The cons are that the hormones reach your other organs as well, possibly increasing the risk of unwanted by-products, including cancer.

When it comes to topical hormonal therapies, the action of the hormones remains more localized. Topical formulations include creams and oils that are applied to the skin, vaginal creams, and low-dose vaginal rings or inserts (like Estring and Vagifem). Most vaginal rings deliver low doses of hormones and are considered topical therapy, but if you're unsure about the type of ring you have, check with your doctor. The rings or inserts are commonly used to treat what is called vaginal atrophy, a major cause of vaginal discomfort characterized by itching and dry, uncomfortable sex—and even urinary incontinence.

There are a lot of questions around whether topical hormonal products are as efficient, and as risky, as oral MHT. It's important to note that even though these products are very different from the systemic therapies tested in the Women's Health Initiative, they still carry the same physician's-warning labels that cite an increased risk of heart disease, stroke, and cancer. As a result, women remain equally cautious.

Currently, only 25 percent of women with vaginal atrophy end up accepting this treatment for it.

However, new studies suggest that topical estrogen may carry a lower risk of blood clots than systemic estrogen, making it preferable for women at risk for heart disease and diabetes. Additionally, an examination of nearly 46,000 women found that those who used low-dose vaginal estrogen had a 61 percent lower risk of heart disease than did those who used nothing. They also had a 60 percent reduction in hip fractures. So it looks like topical treatment is not only helpful for vaginal atrophy but may also have other health benefits. On the downside, it does not help with hot flashes and night sweats. Regarding the question of its effects on dementia risk, we are still without the data necessary to yield any answers.

Bio-identical Hormones

Historically, estrogen formulations were made of conjugated equine estrogens, or CEEs. Not to put too fine a point on it: these estrogens were extracted from the urine of pregnant horses, as the name Premarin ("pregnant mare urine") implies. CEEs are still the most used estrogen formulation for menopausal hormone therapy, either alone or in combination with a progestin. Other commonly used hormones include synthetic estrogens and progestins.

More recently, natural or "bio-identical" hormones are being widely discussed. The term refers to compounds that are made from plants, typically soybeans or wild yam root, but have the same chemical structure as hormones produced in the body. Pharmaceutical companies make some bio-identical hormones that are FDA-approved and sold in standard doses. These include a wide variety of patches, gels, and creams available by prescription.

You can also get customized bio-identical hormones made through a pharmacy. In a practice known as "custom compounding," bio-identical hormones can be made at any dose, based on your personal needs as requested via a doctor's prescription. The idea is that taking natural hormones in customized doses may be more effective and better tolerated than typical MHT drugs. Although this idea is perhaps a logical one, and one that leans toward the concept of the precision medicine model we've discussed, there is a snag for now.

At this time, custom-compounded formulas are not FDA-approved. This is not surprising, since FDA-approved drugs are made in standardized dosages that have been tested in clinical trials, so their effects and side effects are predictable and manageable. Given that custom-compounded hormones are by definition the opposite of standardized (the dosage varies from person to person), unlike the FDA-approved treatments, they have not been tested to prove that the active ingredients are absorbed properly or provide predictable hormone levels in one's blood and tissue. Therefore, although bio-identical hormones are often presented as risk-free, we cannot consider them safer than government-approved ones, as both their efficacy and risks are still untested. So for now, whether hormones are coming from horses, plants, or test tubes, it is better to assume that their risks are pretty much comparable, and to proceed with the same careful recommendations discussed throughout the chapter.

The Birth Control Pill: Friend or Foe?

As women, we may choose to take hormonal contraceptives for various reasons, whether it be for endometriosis, painful menstrual cramps, or to avoid getting pregnant. The available hormonal contraceptives— implant, injection, and the pill, patch, ring, IUD—all deliver a small dose of estrogen, progesterone, or both to our bodies. By doing so, they suppress our body's natural hormones and prevent pregnancy. Some methods stop the body from ovulating, while others also affect the cervical mucus, making it difficult for the sperm to find an egg, or rendering the lining of the womb less "hospitable" to a fertilized egg so that it cannot manage to implant itself there.

Many considerations around the risks and benefits of hormonal contraceptives can be accessed via other resources—for example, the National Institute of Child Health and Human Development: www .nichd.nih.gov/health/topics/contraception. As far as our discussion is concerned, let's cut to the chase: Will using contraceptives affect how we end up experiencing menopause? Can these contraceptives hurt our ovaries? And finally, could they negatively impact our cognitive performance?

While birth control can stop ovulation, it doesn't stop the loss of follicles. Consequently, birth control is neither causing nor precipitating menopause. What it can do, though, is mask signs of menopause, including the menstrual irregularities that might have given you the first clues that you're nearing menopause. In fact, if you're taking the pill during perimenopause, or even after menopause, you may still have periodic bleeding due to the hormones in the medication itself. This so-called withdrawal bleeding is not an actual period per se, though it can certainly look and feel like one. So when and if menopause were to co-occur, you would be missing the telltale sign of your actual period winding down or disappearing, since the contraceptive would be suppressing your period (or lack thereof) while potentially supplying you with withdrawal bleeding instead. This confusion can undoubtedly make it challenging to know when and if menopause has begun. So many women have told me that as soon as they went off birth control, they went straight and hard into menopause, symptoms and all—most definitely a disconcerting experience.

Given everything we've discovered about the relationship between hormones, menopause, and brain health, a larger question remains: Can the use of birth control affect the health of the brain? Oddly enough, even though more than 100 million women take the pill worldwide, there have been only a handful of studies dedicated to its effects on the brain.

Whether due to this fact or not, there is currently no clear evidence that birth control increases or decreases the risk of cognitive decline or dementia. However, there is evidence that it affects mood. Sometimes it does so in positive ways, as when successfully prescribed to alleviate PMS symptoms. Some perimenopausal women using hormonal contraceptives also report the welcome relief of fewer and less intense hot flashes, along with reduced mood swings. But in other instances, therapy has the opposite effect, increasing the risk of depression. A recent study of over 1 million women age fourteen to thirty-four showed that all common forms of hormonal contraception were associated with an increased likelihood of developing depression. While the increase in risk itself was reasonably small, higher risks were linked to the progesterone-only forms, especially with some IUDs. So if you suffer from or have a tendency toward depression, the IUD might not be the best option for you, unless it's the non-hormonal, copper-based option. I'd recommend you discuss this with your ob-gyn.

Although the general belief has been that the IUD acts locally and has no effect on the rest of the body, it turns out that this information is incorrect. If what is thought of as a "localized" therapy can affect your brain by triggering depression on the one hand or alleviating mood swings on the other, it would behoove us to take a closer look at what the effects of other systemic therapies, like the pill, may have on the brain. In fact, women on the pill are 25 percent more likely to be given antidepressants than non-users.

Having access to contraception has been an invaluable resource to women. The overarching positive impact of birth control led the Centers for Disease Control and Prevention to declare family planning one of the top ten most important public health achievements of the twentieth century. But while this progress has dramatically improved women's health and quality of life, it urgently deserves updated, ongoing attention to fully explore the safest methods by which to deliver these benefits. In the meantime, accessing these choices prudently and informing ourselves to the very best of our ability is advisable when considering any medication. Going forward, we need to develop a voice that's heard, one that demands careful examination of all current birth control options and encourages whatever studies are necessary to create new and improved formulations.

ANTIDEPRESSANTS AND OTHER MEDICATIONS

Women who are not good candidates for MHT (like cancer patients and those at risk for cancer) or those who prefer to stay clear of hormones often seek out non-hormonal therapies to relieve menopausal symptoms. There are some options on the market, starting with antidepressants. In June 2013, the FDA approved an antidepressant called Brisdelle as the first non-hormonal therapy for the hot flashes associated with menopause. Sadly, Brisdelle is not terribly efficient at reducing its target symptoms. In fact, the drug seems to lessen the number of hot flashes in women who have ten or more hot flashes per day by only one or two incidences. Although I guess it's better to have eight rather than ten hot flashes a day, I'm sure we were all hoping for better odds than that.

By the same token, there are other medications that were originally approved for treating depression and even seizures that have actually proved more effective for treating hot flashes. These include

- Selective serotonin reuptake inhibitor (SSRI) antidepressants such as paroxetine (Paxil), citalopram (Celexa), and escilatopram (Lexapro). It looks like fluoxetine (Prozac) may also help in some but not all cases.

- Serotonin-norepinephrine reuptake inhibitor (SNRI) antidepressants such as venlafaxine (Effexor) or desvenlafaxine (Pristiq) also show promise.

- The anti-convulsants gabapentin (Neurontin) and pregabalin (Lyrica) have shown some success.

- The alpha-adrenergic agonist clonidine (Catapres) may also have a positive effect.

Just a word of caution that antidepressants are the number one drug in the country—and women are the major users. Women are nearly twice as likely as men to be prescribed an antidepressant, a disparity that becomes even more pronounced after age forty. There are some concerns that doctors may be too quick to give women antidepressants instead of digging deeper into the root cause of their patients' concerns. For example, menopausal changes often trigger symptoms of depression, which are unlikely to resolve by simply taking antidepressants.

Below, let's take a look at who might benefit most from these medications.

MAKING AN INFORMED DECISION

Now that we have examined in detail the available options, let's talk about solutions. Do you need MHT? Should you take it? And if so, what kind? Are antidepressants a better option? How about not taking drugs instead?

Below you will find specific guidelines to determine whether or not MHT is an option for you. This information will also provide you with a jumping-off point to help you evaluate the pros and cons with your doctor. Many women going through menopause don't require hormonal support. Menopause is, after all, a natural process, and some women traverse it quite gracefully without any need for medical intervention. For other women, however, symptoms can be so severe and disruptive that the proper introduction of hormones, when applied judiciously, can be a godsend. On the other hand, there are many women for whom MHT is not at all advised, and, thankfully, other solutions are available for consideration.

Before we dive in, there's one more thing to consider. Unless you're a scientist, you may not know that estrogen isn't just estrogen. There is, in fact, an estrogen that exists solely inside the brain, different from the one that is produced in the ovaries or with body fat. Remember, brain estrogen possesses many more functions beyond reproduction, and therefore it functions quite independently from estrogen deployed elsewhere in the body. The estrogen made in the body protects mostly our heart and bones, whereas the estrogen manufactured in the brain protects particularly our memories, thoughts, and feelings. Brain estrogen has a call-and-response relationship with body estrogen, responding to its actions and inactions via the HPG axis that connects our brains to our ovaries. Aside from this sort of interbody back-and-forth, the brain makes a lot of its estrogen in-house and has its own hormonal ecosystem.

Part of what makes this complex is that we have ways to measure estrogen in the body (via a blood test), but we don't have good ways to measure estrogen in the brain. To this day, the latter remains a proper black box. But don't worry, we are working on resolving that right now! I hope that soon, perhaps even by the time you read this book, some of the groundwork will have been tested for getting meaningful information on estrogen activity within the brain.

Meanwhile, consider this: The "hard-to-reach" nature of the brain is another reason why MHT has variable effects on cognitive function, which makes it difficult to predict what kind of response you will have.

That said, a few things are clear. For example, who should *not* be put on MHT. If you currently have any of the conditions listed in table 2, or if you've ever suffered from these conditions in the past, MHT is not going to be your cup of tea. For a quick rundown, women with a history of cancer (such as breast, uterine, or endometrial cancer) should not take MHT, and neither should women with a history of coronary artery disease, stroke, or heart attack. The same goes for those suffering from blood clots, deep vein thrombosis, or severe liver disease. It goes without saying that MHT is not indicated for those of you who are pregnant or trying to get pregnant. As you can see, this rules out a lot of women.

TABLE 2. CONTRAINDICATIONS TO HORMONE THERAPY FOR MENOPAUSE

SYMPTOM	WHAT TO DO
Unexplained vaginal bleeding	Avoid MHT
Pregnancy (confirmed or suspected)	Avoid MHT
Liver disease	Avoid MHT
History of breast, uterine, or ovarian cancer or other estrogen-dependent tumor	Avoid MHT
History of heart attack, angina, coronary bypass surgery, angioplasty/stent, stroke, or transient ischemic attack (TIA)	Avoid MHT
Blood clots in the legs or lungs	Avoid MHT

Known blood clotting disease and/or testing positive for factor V Leiden	Avoid MHT
Untreated hypertension	Avoid MHT
One first-degree relative or more with breast cancer or at risk for breast cancer	Consider non-hormonal therapy
High triglycerides	Avoid oral estrogen; consider transdermal estrogen
Gallbladder disease	Avoid oral estrogen; consider transdermal estrogen

If you make it through the above contraindications, then your age (especially in relation to menopause) and your hysterectomy status as well as many other factors (including things like your medical and family history, whether you smoke, and your need for contraception) all impact this decision. Less obvious considerations, such as the cost and coverage of the therapies, all play a role in evaluating their risk-to-benefit ratios and should be carefully weighed by both you and your doctor as a team.

Let me underline that the primary indication for MHT remains relief of hot flashes, night sweats, and vaginal dryness. MHT is not recommended for prevention of heart disease, Alzheimer's, cognitive decline, or any other conditions. Perhaps this will change as we gather new information, but for now, MHT is not the best treatment for any of these concerns.

The figures below summarize the best available evidence and recommendations regarding MHT for menopause. These decision-making diagrams, however helpful, are not intended by any means to replace your doctor. They simply aim at providing the first step in assisting you to better address an otherwise complicated topic with your health-care provider. Between the two of you, you can then reach whatever personalized treatment decisions are safest and make the best sense all around. This includes deciding whether prescription medications are appropriate to start with and, if so, choosing the best course of treatment.

Before we start, make sure you have this information handy:

- Are you menopausal? If this question surprises you, let me surprise you even more. Many women find that they really don't know or can't seem to know for sure whether they've begun, are in the middle of, or have completed menopause. To be honest, it is not as cut-and-dried as one might think. To help you better discern the difference between an interruption of your menstrual cycle and the Big M, review the following conditions that can interrupt your cycle, often leading women to not be certain whether they're experiencing an interruption or actual menopause:

TABLE 3. POSSIBLE CAUSES OF ABSENT MENSTRUAL CYCLE

Unexpected pregnancy	Just when you thought you were old enough to have unprotected sex . . . surprise!
Intrauterine device (IUD) system; injectable birth control	Some IUDs and injectable birth control may cause the uterus to stop bleeding without causing menopause. In this case, your estrogen levels remain normal until you reach natural menopause.
Birth control pill	Hormonal contraceptives don't stop the loss of follicles, so even if you're not bleeding, birth control doesn't cause or precipitate menopause.
Endometrial ablation	This procedure eliminates the lining of the uterus, which often results in stopping or greatly reducing most uterine bleeding without causing menopause. Estrogen levels remain normal until you reach natural menopause.
Primary ovarian insufficiency (POI)	POI is a condition in which younger women have only occasional periods or no periods at all, even as early as teenagers. Early menopause is possible.

Hysterectomy	Women who have had their uterus removed (hysterectomy) but still have their ovaries stop having periods but don't really go through menopause until their natural age at menopause. However, surgery interferes with the blood flow to the ovaries, which may cause low hormones and subsequent lack of bleeding (amenorrhea).
Oophorectomy	Having both ovaries removed (oophorectomy, or OVX) will cause instant menopause even if the uterus is not removed. Having one ovary removed will likely not cause menopause until the natural age, but it may cause the symptoms of menopause at a younger age.
Chemotherapy and radiation	Both of these treatments can result in temporary or permanent menopause. Although this is not the same as natural menopause, it can lead to many of the same symptoms.

- Determine your age at menopause: you are in menopause if it's twelve months after your last menstrual cycle. If that's you, write your age at menopause here: _____.

- Calculate your cardiovascular risk score (e.g., your risk of heart disease or stroke in the next ten years) using the American College of Cardiology (ACC) / American Health Association (AHA) heart risk calculator: www.cvriskcalculator.com. Write your ASCVD risk score here: _____.

- Calculate your risk of breast cancer using the National Cancer Institute's Breast Cancer Risk Assessment Tool: www.cancer.gov/bcrisktool. Is your score high, medium, or low? Write it here: _____.

Now that we have the key data, we are ready to discuss which treatment might be best for you. Figure 4 will help you determine the best course of action. Answer the yes-or-no questions and follow the arrows. If it turns out that you are better off not doing MHT, the

FIGURE 4. TREATMENT-DECISION FLOWCHART

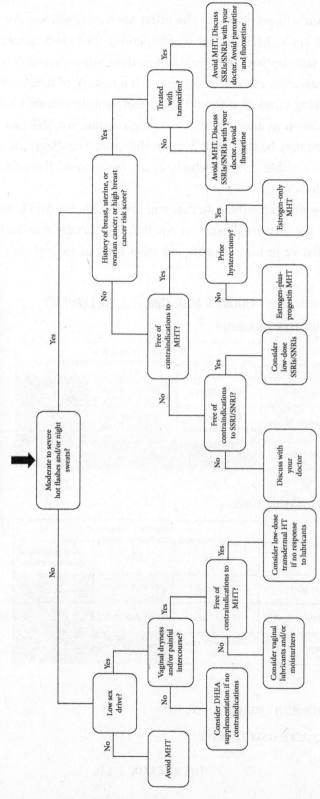

diagram will point you to the safest alternative choice. For example, as you know, MHT is not recommended for breast cancer patients. Some safer options may include low-dose antidepressants, clonidine, or gabapentin. However, women with a history of breast cancer who are taking tamoxifen should avoid SSRI antidepressants, which have been shown to interfere with the drug's action. An SNRI such as venlafaxine may be the safest drug in this case. The diagrams will guide you to a viable choice—which, again, you should then discuss with your doctor.

If the diagrams indicate that you are eligible for MHT, move on to figure 5 to further determine whether the therapy may be helpful to you relative to brain health and what kind of formulation might be

FIGURE 5. MHT: TAKE IT . . . OR LEAVE IT?

NO PRIOR HYSTERECTOMY

CVD risk score		Years since menopause			Dementia risk
		≤5	6–10	>10	
	Low (<5%)	EPT is indicated	EPT is indicated	Avoid EPT	Higher
	Medium (5–10%)	EPT is indicated (consider transdermal)	EPT is indicated (consider transdermal)	Avoid EPT	Moderate
	High (>10%)	Avoid EPT	Avoid EPT	Avoid EPT	Lower

PRIOR HYSTERECTOMY

CVD risk score		Years since surgery			Dementia risk
		1–5	5–10	>10 or past natural age at menopause	
	Low (<5%)	ET is indicated	ET is indicated	Avoid ET	Higher
	Medium (5–10%)	ET is indicated	ET is indicated	Avoid ET	Moderate
	High (>10%)	Discuss with your doctor	Discuss with your doctor	Avoid ET	Lower

EPT: ESTROGEN + PROGESTIN THERAPY

ET: ESTROGEN-ONLY THERAPY

best. Remember that the duration of use should be dictated by individual symptoms and related risks. The benefits are more clear for women who initiate therapy before or close to the onset of menopause. The risks, on the other hand, get steeper with continued use and/or advancing age.

Hey, hold on! Before you run to a pharmacy, prescription in hand, I encourage you to run an experiment instead. I encourage you to try managing your symptoms without medications first. I'm not asking you to continue on without help—I am going to share precious keys that should allow you to produce comparable, med-free effects in the upcoming chapters. Consider giving these alternatives a chance prior to introducing MHT into your body. I know, I know, you just made it through all those charts and graphs unscathed . . .

I must reiterate that prescription medicines come with many potentially dangerous side effects of their own, and the last thing any of us needs is to accidentally exchange one negative side effect for another. Another reason to look beyond estrogen replacement is the fact that estrogen is not always a friendly and helpful substance—especially when it's not your own. It doesn't cost much to start with the safer strategies that focus on ameliorating hormonal levels by means of diet, exercise, and other natural therapies. These methods are known to boost hormonal production in the brain as well as in the body, while improving memory, sharpening our minds, and supporting resilience, all the while reducing risk of dementia for all women, no matter what stage of the game they're at. Remember, too, that even if you have opted in on MHT, eventually you may need an alternative. As soon as one goes off MHT, hot flashes often resume, even years after menopause. So any which way you slice it, alternative options are your friend—the friend that's in it with you for the long haul.

Whether or not you're eligible and interested in MHT, these next chapters unveil scientifically validated, non-pharmacological therapies for menopausal symptoms. These solutions target those symptoms originating inside your brain, which are the symptoms that bother the majority of us most. Ideally, I would like you to commit to following these recommendations for *at least three months* before turning to MHT or antidepressants (unless there are other medical reasons to do otherwise). For many patients, changing lifestyle habits can be of tremendous help in managing unpleasant symptoms like hot flashes and night sweats, without any need for inviting the side effects of taking new medications. With this kind of win-win . . . it's a no-brainer!

CHAPTER 9

FOOD MATTERS FOR YOUR GRAY MATTER

IN OUR SOCIETY, WE TEND to focus more on using our diet to whittle our waistline than caring about how it's impacting our health. We often lose track of the fact that what we eat will determine if we have the vitality to enjoy our lives unimpeded or shoot us in the foot instead. While worrying about how to achieve a "good body" on the outside, we often lose sight of the fact that our diets are busy creating our state of health on the inside, our brain included. Food is intended to support all of our systems and, whether or not we're conscious of it, directly affects the health of our brain, day in, day out.

We all intuitively use food to soothe our moods and clear our heads. Feeling blue, we may reach for chocolate; when we're tired, we pour another cup of coffee. There are endless examples of how the food we eat impacts our frame of mind, thereby creating a domino effect that affects our thoughts, memories, and actions.

As it turns out, of all the organs in the body, the brain is the one most vulnerable to the ravages of a poor diet. From its signature architecture to the unusual means by which it performs, the brains cries out for the proper fuel like no other entity in our body—a topic I explored in great detail in my first book, *Brain Food*. More briefly, the brain is the most metabolically active organ we possess, and consequently the hungriest, demanding over 20 percent of your body's total energy haul. But what sets it apart even further is that the cells inside our brains are irreplaceable. Unlike those in the rest of the body, where cells continuously renew and replace themselves, the vast majority of our brain's cells remain with us from start to finish. This certainly sheds some light on why extra care and nourishment is paramount for the brain to successfully deliver a lifetime of performance on our behalf.

Meal after meal, the foods we ingest are broken down into nutrients, absorbed into the bloodstream, and drawn up into the universe of our nervous system. Once they arrive, their job is to replenish depleted storage, trigger the proper cellular reactions, and, finally, to become themselves part of the very fabric of our brain. This is something to consider the next time you reach for a candy bar instead of an apple. Whichever one you choose will become part and parcel of how your brain will function.

A slew of new research, including my own, shows an important correlation between a healthy diet and a healthy brain. When consumed in the right amounts and from the right sources, food has marked and measurable beneficial effects on brain health and function. The right diet does ensure that our brain remains stronger longer, and shows more resilience and activity, regardless of age. In addition, a healthy diet can be a powerful ally in boosting our energy levels, supporting heart health and hormonal harmony while warding off the wide range of common ailments that affect the majority of adult women, from slow metabolism to insomnia and anxiety. Further, what we eat is a powerful epigenetic lever for switching hundreds of thousands of genes on and off, which can help minimize the genetic risk of developing a mind-destroying disease like Alzheimer's.

Unfortunately, though, the field of nutrition suffers from the same shortsightedness as does scientific research in general. There is a chronic lack of acknowledgment regarding how gender affects our distinct needs and requirements when it comes to adequate nutrition— unless a woman is pregnant, that is. Not only do men and women differ in the way their bodies and brains function on a day-to-day basis, but these differences sometimes demand different dietary requirements as well. In this chapter, we will review the research on gender disparities in diet and nutrition for brain health. In chapter 10, you'll find specific guidelines as to which foods and nutrients to focus on, and what to avoid at all costs!

APPLES, PEARS, AND WHY ENERGY MATTERS

The fact that diets don't deliver the same results for a man as for a woman is probably obvious to any woman who's ever tried to lose weight. When a woman says, "I'm going on a diet," she's usually not messing around. You might catch her increasing her intake of everything and anything remotely green, from raw broccoli to wheatgrass juice. She might even go so far as to completely give up sugar, bread, and butter. Watch her shrink the portion sizes upon her plate while she devises new and healthy meals for her entire family. She then hops on the scale hopefully, only to find there's little to no change at all. Maybe a few ounces or pounds have come off, but not the much-anticipated and well-deserved weight loss she's slaved over. Meanwhile, her husband quit drinking soda for a week and it looks like he's dropped ten pounds. Oh, the injustice. Do men really have an advantage in the diet department, or is it just an optical illusion?

As it turns out, it might be a bit of both. Men and women have rather different metabolic requirements that influence not only their general health and well-being but also the way they respond to diets. Not to mention, our shape.

It is well known that genetic and hormonal factors are implicated in how body fat distribution differs between the genders. Generally, men tend to have more visceral fat, which is stored around the organs in the belly, while women tend to have more peripheral, subcutaneous fat, stored along the hips and backsides. This gives rise to the "apple" and "pear" shapes. Men's apple physique may make it easier to notice when they trim down since it's so localized. On the downside, the apple shape is more dangerous since too much belly fat is a risk for heart disease, stroke, diabetes, and even certain cancers.

Although women's pear physique is less risky from a health perspective, from puberty to menopause, women generally have a higher percentage of body fat than men. That's even when we take in fewer calories by eating less. A healthy range of body fat for women is 20 to 25 percent, as compared with the 10 to 15 percent recommended for men. In other words, the body fat percentage of a normal-weight woman is similar to that of a man who would be classified as overweight. Men tend to be leaner than women because they generally have more muscle. The more muscle you have, the more fat you burn. Furthermore, the predominantly male hormone, testosterone, increases protein synthesis and lean body mass, which in turn raise a man's metabolism. Like it or not, guys are burning more calories than us all day long, even while doing nothing at all. It is this accelerated metabolism that is also responsible for their bodies responding faster and more noticeably to diets.

A woman's estrogen, on the other hand, is not doing her any favors in the weight-loss department. Not only do women have a higher percentage of body fat than men, but on top of that, estrogen reduces a woman's ability to burn that fat. In fact, we are particularly talented at gathering *and* storing it!

When we were hunter-gatherers, and even later as an agrarian society, our bodies developed the ability to store energy as fat, knowing that the next famine could very well be our last. This ability was most likely intended to assist us in having a healthy pregnancy and for the nursing that comes afterward. With food dangerously scarce, that was indeed a great advantage to the prehistoric woman. This is much less of an asset for us as modern women. We now face a dense oversupply of energy-laden foods and endless opportunities to eat them, but we are still saddled with bodies that haven't yet made the evolutionary adjustments necessary to burn off such "abundance."

Women's bodies, as a result, are fat-accumulating, carb-running machines. This is in part thanks to estrogen's positive effects on insulin, the hormone that helps remove sugar from our circulation, granting us the ability to maintain steady blood sugar levels. Even when eating healthy high-carb diets, most women tend to burn these extra carbs right away (whereas men will store them in their muscles, in the form of glycogen).

Everything goes pretty well until a woman approaches her forties and hormone levels begin to flag. Then two things become more likely: her metabolism slows down at the same time that her insulin goes wonky. Interestingly, in this case, her brain is just as much to blame as her diet. The decrease in estrogen is also working its mischief inside the hypothalamus, reducing the brain's ability to burn carbs and regulate adipose tissue distribution. This all adds up to increasing weight and a thickening waistline. As a result, many women end up with a five-to-ten-pound weight gain as they transition into menopause. This is not a random event that happens by accident. This happens quite fatefully in the female body, as it's programmed to store even more fat as soon as estrogen begins to decrease. This time around, belly fat's the answer. Why's that? Because visceral adipose fat produces estrone, the backup form of estrogen for post-menopausal women.

Wait, is this a good thing, then?

Sometimes the road to hell is paved with good intentions. This increase in belly fat goes hand in hand with an increased risk of heart disease, diabetes, and obesity—all observed after menopause. I'm sure the irony of this is not lost on you. In the same moment our brains and bodies are demanding an increase in calories and nutrients, many women end up struggling to shed the additional weight instead.

The challenge for women is to keep a steady metabolism—no small feat. It is of utmost importance, then, that we find a means by which to provide ourselves with the most plentiful supply of energy while at the same time making sure things don't get out of control. This is where paying attention to our diet becomes more critical than ever.

It goes without saying that weight gain is an issue for the entire human race, not just women. However, a woman's body is literally built to change far more than a man's. Let's face it, it downright metamorphoses. After assuming its childhood form, it sprouts a dramatically new body at puberty, one that continues to develop and differentiate itself before turning into nothing short of a mobile home during pregnancy. It rapidly reconfigures itself into yet another physical form post-pregnancy in service to the baby, and then does so again, once it's not. At menopause, it's time to do so all over again, and as if all that were not enough, it happens once more, in old age.

However magnificent we are in this respect, it's not always fun being such a shapeshifter. Superpowers such as these require respect and attention that often go ungarnered. It's high time to be kind and caring to ourselves as we better address how to undergo each of these peculiar twists and turns in the healthiest way possible.

"IN A WORLD FULL OF TRENDS, I WANT TO REMAIN A CLASSIC"

Hats off to model, designer, and entrepreneur Iman for this famous quote, pointing out that the latest trends often fall short of those that stand the test of time. This is just as true in the field of nutrition. Society tends to swing from one extreme diet to another, sometimes for no apparent reason at all, other than a celebrity or the media advocating for yet another diet craze to sweep the nation. Whether it's veganism or gluten-free, fat-free or keto, the search for the "miracle diet" is never-ending. We need to be alert to the fact that many trendy diets are not based on actual science—unless, of course, we're talking about the science of marketing.

Worse still, hardly any of these diets, and perhaps none at all, adequately consider the female physiology. If there's one thing we've learned from clinical trials, it's that when it comes to women, diets that are based on going to extremes don't work in the end. Not only will they not produce the results they promise, but they may also tamper with the delicate integrity of our highly specialized bodies and brains.

We return once again to a now familiar study, the Women's Health Initiative that generated so much confusion around MHT all those years ago. Ironically, much of what we know about which diets don't work for women comes from the same study. Among its various branches, the trial also included a dietary modification arm (WHI-DM), which remains the largest clinical trial of dietary interventions in women.

The study started in 1993, during the peak of the low-fat, high-starch diet craze. You could not walk down a single supermarket aisle without seeing the terms "low-fat" or "fat-free" emblazoned across the vast majority of products. The powers that be declared fat was evil, and as a result, low-fat was "the only way to go," the latest cure for all that ailed us whether it was heart disease, cancer, or the obesity epidemic. As a product of the times, WHI-DM researchers applied this low-fat approach in their studies.

Over 48,000 post-menopausal women enrolled in the trial. Of these, about 40 percent were randomly assigned to a low-fat diet. The rest of the women continued their usual diets. For the low-fat group, the intervention was designed to lower a participant's total fat intake to only 20 percent of their total calories. Eight years later, the researchers looked at how many women in each group had developed heart attacks, strokes, and other forms of heart disease. In addition to totaling the occurrences of breast and colorectal cancer, they looked at things such as weight gain, cholesterol levels, and, of course, hot flashes. The results were once again disappointing. Women on the low-fat diet had no increased resistance against cancer or heart disease. Also, they persisted in having the usual frequency and degree of hot flashes, and not unremarkably, they had not lost any appreciable amount of weight.

However, the WHI-DM was controversial from the start. Among other concerns, the vast majority of women were in their sixties and seventies when the study began. At this point in their lives, it may have been too late for dietary changes to reduce the risk of heart disease and other chronic conditions. But mostly, the diet plan in and of itself was called into question. Back then, going low-fat usually meant going very high carb, ingesting a total of six servings of grains a day. Worst still, in the hope of reducing their fat intake, these poor women had most likely loaded up on the latest low-fat and fat-free foods, which we now know to be highly processed and loaded with hidden sugars and additives.

In my experience, it is also unwise to go on a strictly low-fat diet around menopause, the moment when a woman's body is deliberately calling for more fat to make more estrogen. It is now known that when women adopt very low-fat diets, their estrogen levels often dramatically drop.

In the end, this expensive trial did highlight an important truth: beware of following trends! The WHI-DM was another nail in the coffin for the low-fat, high-starch trend that so dominated the American diet during that era. However, rather than using the new knowledge to promote regaining balance in our diets, the media made much of these disappointing results, spurring the advent of yet another trend, with the famous Atkins Diet. That was but a predecessor to the high-fat diets trending today.

Women in particular were to suffer the ill effects of this extreme change in recommendations, as it is not safe and certainly not a good idea to load up on fatty foods like bacon and butter. Given the fact that a woman's body is limited in its ability to put fat to good use (versus our innate talent for turning it into a muffin top, among other things), there are clear biological reasons why women should not eat fatty foods indiscriminately.

However, many women are now trying out high-fat or "ketogenic" diets, hoping for both quick weight loss and increased health. These diets are based on the principle that if you eat a very low-carb diet or go completely off carbs, you will force your body to burn extra fat, which may or may not result in a smaller waistline or improved athletic prowess.

Concerning brain health, though, there is no clear evidence that high-fat diets support cognition. As of today, there are only five studies on the effects of keto diets on cognition in humans, each one with a fairly small sample. The largest clinical trial, with about 100 patients, was discontinued in 2017 when supplementing with tricaprylin (a ketone source) failed to improve cognition in mild Alzheimer's patients. At the moment, there are no clinical trials in younger people, and no observational studies linking high-fat diets to improved cognitive performance or a reduced risk of Alzheimer's either. So for now, there is no reason to believe that eating more fat than necessary will do your brain any good.

So what should we eat?

Let's be clear that body and brain alike need all kinds of nutrients for health, carbs and fats included. When a diet is advising that you avoid one of these nutrients entirely, think twice. Not only is it unwise, but it could be detrimental to your health in the long term. In fact, we don't really need a "diet." Most diets focus on restricting food or nutrients, which makes them impossible to stick to, not realistic for your life, and lead to crashes and even weight gain. We need a new way of eating and nourishing ourselves that we can comfortably stick with throughout our lives.

In the next chapter, we will explore a dietary plan that is balanced, well-rounded, and meticulously designed to secure meaningful, long-lasting results for women. But first, let's settle the debate over carbs and fats and review what a healthy diet looks like if you're a woman.

GOOD AND BAD CARBS AND FATS

All the evidence points to the fact that what matters is not a focus on "carbs" and "fat" as if they were unique entities, but rather a focus on the *types* of carbs and fats we're eating, as well as their sources. For example, some carbs support female metabolism, while others will derail your insulin levels instead. Likewise, some fats promote brain function, while others can wreak havoc on your brain and your hormones, especially when consumed excessively. In other words, the quality of your diet—and its ability to fulfill your nutritional requirements—is what really makes the difference.

High-fat diets are currently all the hype, so I'll start by dispelling some myths around fat and women's health. First off, there are many kinds of fat, each with its distinct effects not only on the body but also on the brain. Many lines of evidence indicate that the type, rather than the overall amount of fat in the diet, is key when assessing health risks in women.

Put most succinctly, fat is either saturated (as in butter, meat, dairy, and certain oils like coconut oil) or unsaturated. Unsaturated fat can be monounsaturated, as in olives and avocados, or polyunsaturated (PUFAs), as in fish, shellfish, and various nuts and seeds. While nature provides us with versions of these fats we can trust, commercial preparations often tamper with them, for example by hydrogenating unsaturated oils—a procedure used to make trans fats.

Research focused specifically on women reveals that unsaturated fat, especially PUFAs, is very supportive of women's health, showing a reduced risk of dementia, heart disease, cancer, obesity, and diabetes. On the other hand, trans fat is especially bad news, showing the exact opposite effect. Too much saturated fat can also be harmful in excess, mostly when coming from animal sources.

To give you a sense of the magnitude of the problem, the Nurses' Health Study, one of the largest prospective dietary investigations in women, showed that, among over 75,000 participants, those consuming higher levels of trans fat had a 33 percent increased risk of heart disease. Eating more PUFAs had the opposite effect, reducing the risk by over 25 percent. These effects were particularly marked in women under sixty-five, for whom trans fat intake increased the risk of heart attack by as much as 50 percent. These findings indicate that maximizing PUFAs and minimizing trans fat is an excellent first step toward optimal fat consumption. In fact, these studies estimate that, in the context of a typical 1,500-calorie diet, swapping out 3 grams of trans fat for the equivalent amount of unsaturated fat can lower the risk of heart disease in women by up to 67 percent. In concrete terms, that's the equivalent of replacing the average serving of potato chips with a handful of almonds. Likewise, swapping 8 grams of saturated fat (2 ounces of bacon or 1 slice of cheddar cheese) with the same amount of unsaturated fat (4 ounces of salmon) is all you need to do to cut your risk of heart disease in half.

The type of fat you eat has a substantial impact on whether or not you develop Alzheimer's, too. A large body of studies showed that people who consumed 2 grams or more of trans fat per day had twice the risk of dementia as those who ate fewer than 2 grams. Although it may seem like a small amount, most people in these studies ate at least

2 grams a day, with the majority of participants eating more than double that on a regular basis. Similar findings were revealed regarding saturated fat, especially when from red meat and dairy. Those who consumed more than 13 grams per day were almost twice as likely to develop cognitive impairment than those who ate half that amount.

On the contrary, people who consumed at least 2 grams of PUFAs per day had a 70 percent lower risk of Alzheimer's than those who ate less. This is consistent with reports of thousands of dementia-free elderly people showing that a diet poor in PUFAs increases the speed at which the brain ages, while a diet rich in PUFAs protects our brain cells in the long term. If you need more of an incentive, our brain imaging studies show that women whose diets are more abundant in PUFAs in their early-to-late-middle-age years not only have the highest levels of brain activity but also the lowest levels of Alzheimer's plaques. This is in contrast to those whose diets were higher in trans fat and saturated fat showing reduced brain activity and increased brain atrophy instead.

So unsaturated fat is in, and trans fat is definitely out. For saturated fat, moderation is important, as is keeping an eye on the source. Most studies that reported negative effects of saturated fat focused on intake from animal sources. There is increasing evidence that vegetable fat, including both saturated and unsaturated types, is more supportive of women's health through its beneficial effects on our hormones. For example, replacing animal fats like butter with certain vegetable oils like olive oil has been linked to a greatly reduced risk of heart disease, diabetes, and breast cancer in women.

The effects of dietary fat on breast cancer deserve a special mention. There is a general misconception that patients should go on low-carb diets to "starve" the cancer. This idea can be misleading, as it suggests that high-fat diets may be beneficial. For one, the type of cancer needs to be considered. It has long been known that diets high in animal fat can increase the risk of cancer linked to sex hormones, including breast, uterine, and ovarian cancer. In the Nurses' Health Study, women who consumed large amounts of animal products, especially during their early adult years, had three times the risk of developing breast cancer of those who consumed higher amounts of vegetable oils. Red meat and high-fat dairy were once again the major culprits. In the Women's Health Initiative, even though a low-fat diet wasn't the answer, it was noted that post-menopausal women in the low-fat intervention group did seem to tend toward a lower risk of breast cancer and also had better cancer-survival rates.

These effects are probably due to the fact that animal fat can suppress the action of a particular carrier molecule called SHBG (sex hormone binding globulin). SHBG circulates in the blood and has the job of making sure that estrogen levels are kept in check. SHBG not working well can lead to an overproduction of estrogen, though not in a good way, especially for cancer patients. Studies have shown that women with estrogen-receptive cancers who follow high-fat diets tend to have lower SHBG levels and unusually high levels of "bad" estrogens in their bodies.

In the end, we should take a new approach when it comes to our fat consumption. Rather than avoiding fats like the plague or stuffing our face silly with them, let's be more selective. Our goal is to have the advantages of beneficial, healthy fats while minimizing the less healthy ones. In the next chapter, we'll see how to do exactly that.

Now on to carbs. Carbs are currently getting a bad rap, so let's address some concerns you may have, right off the bat. Research shows that if you are a woman, diets that favor carbs over (bad) fats also distinctly favor your health.

If you recall from above, swapping trans and saturated fat for PUFAs leads to much better health outcomes in women. Well, it turns out that replacing even more of those fats with carbohydrates is an excellent idea, significantly reducing a woman's risk of heart attack and stroke later in life. In the context of a 1,500-calorie-per-day diet, simply replacing 3 grams of trans fats with 7 grams of carbs was associated with a 93 percent risk reduction of heart disease in women. That's trading out another serving of potato chips for 1 ounce of brown rice. Additionally, replacing 8 grams of saturated fat with 19 grams of carbs further reduced the risk by another 17 percent. A real-life example of this would be trading three slices of bacon for a small apple. Many other studies have shown that increasing your carb intake while minimizing these fats also reduces the risk of type 2 diabetes, cancer, and dementia.

However, the type of carbs you choose again makes a huge difference. Looking at this more closely, we see that while favoring carbs over fats generally led to improved health outcomes, it is consuming "good carbs" that showed the best results.

You probably already have a hunch of what "good" versus "bad" carbs are. These attributes reflect the effects each of these carbs have on our blood sugar levels. Good, or complex, carbs, have a low-glycemic load, which means they are lower in sugars and higher in fiber. Plus, the sugars are typically natural, rather than refined white sugar. A good example would be a handful of strawberries or a slice of whole-grain bread. This balance of natural sugar and fiber is ideal when it comes to supplying your brain with the fuel it needs, while at the same time stabilizing your blood sugar levels.

On the contrary, bad, or high-glycemic, carbs, contain plenty of sugars (more often than not refined ones) and low to zero fiber. This imbalance triggers spikes in blood sugar levels, making it hard for your body's insulin to metabolize all that sugar. At the same time, bad carbs also stimulate your appetite thanks to the blood sugar "crash" that occurs after you consume them. So even though women's bodies are generally efficient at burning carbs, too many high-glycemic foods can eventually wear out your pancreas. This leads to chronic high blood sugar levels that cause cells to become insulin resistant. Aging and menopause further reduce insulin sensitivity, making these kinds of foods a serious threat to our bodies, brains, and hormones, especially as we pass age forty. As we already discussed, insulin resistance causes inflammation and is a risk factor for metabolic disorders, type 2 diabetes, and heart disease—all of which raise the risk of dementia in turn. Research shows that the higher the amount of sugar in the blood, the higher the risk of dementia, even in people without diabetes. Even though there are meds that help manage high blood sugar and insulin resistance, they don't deliver the benefits that following a healthy diet does.

So there's no sugarcoating anything—literally and figuratively. To optimize our health as women, it's out with the bad carbs and in with the good ones. To be sure there's no mistaking one for the other, foods with a high-glycemic load include anything that's processed, including refined sugar itself and processed grains like white "sandwich" breads, bagels and rolls, all sodas and sweetened drinks, and sugary foods and snacks including commercial candy, cookies, cakes, pastries, and crackers. These foods should be minimized and replaced with low-glycemic foods rich in fiber. We will get better acquainted with the carbs we're looking for in the next chapter. But first, I want to draw your attention to a specific dietary pattern that not only maximizes both the good carbs and the good fats, but also happens to be the only diet scientifically proven to work for women.

THE MEDITERRANEAN DIET: A CLASSIC

Extensive research points to the Mediterranean diet as an excellent example of a dietary regimen exquisitely suited to women's health. It is telling that this diet has been around for thousands of years. Unlike so many other diets, it wasn't concocted by a celebrity chef or popularized by a media frenzy. It is instead a millennia-long culmination of the enduring lifestyle behaviors of a variety of Mediterranean civilizations. From the ancient Egyptians, Greeks, and Romans to the Arabs and Turks, each left their mark on the development of this delightful cuisine. By interacting with and learning a few tricks from one another, these peoples learned to utilize the best food sources of the rich Mediterranean basin to grow and prosper their cultures while at the same time enriching their health. The women of these cultures are excellent examples of these benefits, to this day ranking at the very top of our world's life-expectancy charts.

Some of the most convincing evidence for the Mediterranean diet comes from studies that looked at its effects on telomere lengths. Telomeres are repetitive DNA sequences found at the ends of our chromosomes, their lengths acting as markers of cellular aging. It turns out that, in a study of close to 5,000 healthy women, the greater the adherence to the Mediterranean diet, the longer the telomeres, a positive sign for longevity. In a nutshell, the women who followed the Mediterranean diet were biologically younger than those who didn't.

Perhaps as a result, women who follow a Mediterranean diet are less likely to develop diabetes, obesity, and heart disease, and also have a much-reduced risk of cognitive impairment and Alzheimer's as they age. One example, a large-scale study of over 78,000 women, showed that those who followed a Mediterranean-style diet enjoyed a 24 percent lower risk of heart disease and a 26 percent lower risk of stroke than those who ate a Western diet high in processed foods, meat, sweets, and sugary beverages. Additionally, when the Mediterranean dieters combined healthy eating with regular exercise, they boasted an outstanding 83 percent risk reduction.

Clinical trials also support the Mediterranean diet as a substantial aid in disease prevention. For example, PREDIMED (Prevención con Dieta Mediterránea), the largest trial to date, randomly assigned 772 asymptomatic people at risk for heart disease to follow one of three diets: a Mediterranean diet supplemented with extra-virgin olive oil, a Mediterranean diet supplemented with nuts, or a low-fat diet. Three years later, both Mediterranean diet regimes had reduced the patients' risk of heart attack and stroke, improved blood glucose levels, stabilized blood pressure, and lowered cholesterol levels. The icing on the cake? These patients also had much less cognitive decline than those on the low-fat diet.

Thanks in part to its beneficial effects on the heart, the Mediterranean diet does a whole lot of good for your brain, too. In a series of brain imaging studies gathering hundreds of participants, we found that those who followed a Mediterranean diet had healthier and younger-looking brains than people of the same age who had been eating a Western diet. The brains of the Western dieters seemed to shrink more rapidly, at an estimated rate of five additional years' worth of aging. Even more striking was that although none of the participants had yet to demonstrate any outward sign of cognitive impairment, the Western dieters were already carrying more Alzheimer's plaques than was usual for their age, whereas the Mediterranean dieters showed none. These beneficial effects were more evident in women than in men, but were clear in men as well, consistent with many studies showing a reduced risk of dementia for both genders. Men may be from Mars and women from Venus—but here on Earth both still benefit from eating right.

The Mediterranean diet has also been consistently linked with a reduced risk of breast cancer in women. This is in part thanks to its high fiber content. Where animal fat impairs the action of the SHBG molecule that keeps estrogen in check, fiber promotes its action, properly balancing estrogen in our favor. This is particularly important not only for reducing the risk of breast cancer, but also for alleviating the menopausal symptoms often experienced as a consequence of cancer therapy. The PREDIMED trial mentioned above demonstrated that, in a group of 4,152 women without a prior history of breast cancer, long-term adherence to the Mediterranean diet cut the risk of breast cancer occurrence in half. In other reports, the Women's Healthy Eating and Living Study showed that among 2,198 women treated for early-stage breast cancer, those who consumed a high-fiber diet showed a decreased severity of hot flashes in as little as one year.

In more good news, women who follow the Mediterranean diet seem to experience fewer and milder menopausal symptoms. In an extensive study of 6,040 women age fifty to fifty-five, those who followed the diet had a 20 percent decrease in hot flashes and night sweats. Interestingly, those who ate more fruits, especially strawberries, pineapple, and melon, were even less likely to report any symptoms. (We'll find out why in the next chapter.) On the contrary, women who consumed a Western-style diet were 23 percent more likely to experience both hot flashes and night sweats as they progressed through menopause.

While you probably get the biggest payoff from adopting such a diet early in life, research shows that it is never too late to reap the benefits of a healthy shift toward better choices. A study of over 10,000 women showed that those who began the Mediterranean diet during middle age were much more likely to live past the age of seventy than those who did not eat as healthily—and were able to do so without the now commonplace burden of chronic and mental illnesses.

You may be wondering: What is so exceptional about this diet?

Although it is called the Mediterranean *diet*, it is not a diet in the same sense that deprivation-based weight-loss plans are. It is, in fact, more a lifestyle than a diet, one that includes certain daily practices and perspectives that are sustainable and, in point of fact, nourishing. Additionally, this lifestyle promotes lower stress levels than are usual in Western countries. One clear example of this is the Mediterranean point of view regarding the act of eating itself. Meals aren't grabbed and eaten in passing but are shared with the family, seated at a table where nobody would dream of watching TV with so much beautiful food in front of them.

Then, naturally, the quality of the food is key. In *Brain Food*, I described the Mediterranean diet as "fresh and sun-kissed." I stand by that. The Mediterranean table is a food feast. One day you might find artichokes drizzled with olive oil, or cremini mushrooms sautéed with garlic and parsley. Perhaps it's braised Swiss chard instead, topped with basil and pine nuts, spread over freshly baked bread. The everyday dishes you find on the menu are invariably colorful, fragrant, and vegetable-centric. If you were thinking pizza and pasta—never fear, we get our fill. But it's the vegetables and legumes, the whole grains, fruits, and nuts, all brimming with extra-virgin olive oil, that are the real stars of the meal. Fish and shellfish are also a primary focus, while other forms of lean protein, such as poultry, are eaten in moderation. Red meats and fancy cheeses make appearances on occasion, like for a special Sunday lunch. Meals, often accompanied by a glass of red wine, are finished off with an inky espresso. I would be lying if I said chocolate, cakes, and pastries never crossed our path (hello, gelato!), but a fresh fruit salad is the more likely after-dinner dessert choice.

From a nutritional perspective, the Mediterranean diet is high in fiber and complex carbohydrates, moderate in fats (mostly unsaturated, and of vegetable origins), and plentiful in vitamins and minerals—all of which seem to suit a woman's needs exceptionally well. And frankly, you don't have to move to Italy or Greece to eat like your Southern European counterparts. I've been in New York for half of my adult life and managed to stick to the diet's principles without problems, while at the same time enjoying nutritionally dense foods like avocados and sweet potatoes that were totally new to me. The beauty of the Mediterranean diet is that it's accessible no matter what country you live in, and can be easily adjusted to suit everybody's needs and tastes. The next chapter will help you do just that—and appendix B provides a weekly diet plan with delicious recipes to get you started. All it takes is eight easy steps.

CHAPTER 10

EIGHT STEPS TO A WELL-NOURISHED BRAIN

IN THIS CHAPTER, we'll go over the eight steps to a well-nourished, active, and resilient female brain. Based on results from rigorous research and randomized clinical trials *in women*, this diet is designed to maximize intake of brain-healthy nutrients with a specific focus on keeping our brains young, balancing our hormones, and improving energy and mood, while also reducing the symptoms of menopause, protecting the heart, and supporting the immune system. A list of all needed nutrients and the foods that best provide them is included, along with recommendations for how to best combine them to achieve optimal, lasting health.

STEP 1. MANAGE YOUR CARBS

As mentioned in chapter 9, not all carbs are created equal. These are my three golden rules to eating carbs:

1. Vegetables and fruits are carbs. Vegetables should make up half of your plate at any given meal.
2. Whole grains are in; refined grains (white flour, white pasta, and white bread) are out.
3. Legumes and starches like sweet potatoes are also excellent sources of good carbs.

Eat the Rainbow

When most people think about carbs, they think bread and potatoes. But fruits and vegetables are carbohydrate-rich foods, and both are essential to your health. They are high not only in healthy carbs but also in vitamins, minerals, and a bounty of phytonutrients that help to reduce harmful inflammation throughout the body, and promote the resilience of our brain cells throughout our adult years.

The irony is that most people are overfed in calories yet starved of the vital array of micronutrients that our brains need, most of which are found in common plant foods. Although we are all aware that fruits and vegetables are good for us, surveys by the Centers for Disease Control and Prevention report that only one in ten adults meets the minimum daily federal recommendation for fruits and vegetables. To remediate this, most nutrition experts recommend "eating the rainbow," that is, consuming a wide array of colorful fruits and veggies.

Among them, look for these all-stars: dark leafy greens like spinach, Swiss chard, and kale, and cruciferous vegetables such as broccoli and cauliflower. These veggies are replete with vitamins, minerals, and fiber, along with the disease-fighting nutrients needed to keep your nervous system healthy. Large-scale studies show that people who consume one or two servings of leafy green vegetables each day experience fewer memory problems and less cognitive decline than people who rarely eat these health-packed greens. Get this: Eating a salad a day can keep your brain younger by as much as eleven years! Low-to-medium-glycemic vegetables such as onions, beets, pumpkin, and carrots are also great choices.

Some of you have been told to avoid fruits due to their sugar content. Not so fast. Many fruits are particularly supportive of memory and mental acuity, thanks to their high vitamin and antioxidant content, the latter possessing powerful antiaging properties. If you're concerned about sugar, favor low-glycemic fruits like berries, apples, lemons, oranges, and grapefruit, and eat higher-glycemic fruits like grapes and mango more sparingly. A study of over 16,000 women showed that those who regularly consumed flavonoid-rich berries, such as blueberries and strawberries, had slower rates of cognitive decline as compared with those who didn't eat these berries. Specifically, eating at least one serving of blueberries and two servings of strawberries each week kept these women's brains younger by as much as two and a half years.

Still not quite convinced? Try this on for size: Women who had a higher intake of fruits and vegetables had lower odds of being overweight or obese and far fewer menopausal symptoms—whereas women who had a lower intake of plant foods and higher intakes of meat and processed foods showed more incidence of all those conditions.

Complex Carbs: Fiber Is Your New Best Friend

So what makes a complex carb so . . . complex? Since nutrition labels don't always tell you if the carbohydrate content of a food is simple or complex, here's the skinny. Carbohydrates contain three components: fiber, starch, and sugar. Fiber and starch make up the bulk of complex carbs, while sugar makes a carbohydrate, well, simple. The balance of these nutrients is what determines just how "complex" a carb is or isn't.

For a woman, keeping yourself at your best does take some doing— believe it or not, it all starts with falling in love with fiber. Extensive research shows that fiber is the name of the game in women's diets. Fiber is a type of carbohydrate that the body can't digest. Why is this a good thing? Fiber-rich foods are not only digested more slowly but are also more filling than simple carbs. This comes in handy as an aid to not overeating. They also keep you regular and help control cholesterol. Additionally, fiber has well-known balancing effects on estrogen levels, and plays a vital role in stabilizing blood sugar and insulin levels, which is also crucial to hormonal balance.

Unfortunately, the average fiber consumption in many Western countries hovers at a measly 10 to 15 grams per day, which puts us at the top of the list for the lowest-fiber eaters in the world. Most Americans, for example, get less than half the recommended minimum fiber intake a day. This also explains the extraordinarily high rates of gastrointestinal issues in this country, from constipation and IBS to an increased risk of colon cancer. We can do better than this. Load up on fiber-rich foods to ensure that your brain, body, and hormones are all working at full capacity.

Current guidelines recommend 14 grams of fiber per every 1,000 calories, which means roughly 25 grams of fiber per day for women and 38 grams per day for men. I'm not in total agreement with this. I think that women should consume more fiber (why less than men, anyway?), but you've got to start somewhere, and 25 grams isn't bad. What does that boil down to? One option is a quarter cup of steel-cut oats and three dried prunes for breakfast (7 grams of fiber), a spinach and kale salad with half an avocado for lunch (9 grams), followed by a dinner of minestrone with legumes (12 grams), and brava, you did it! And you still have room to add your favorite protein, or anything else.

Basically, we need all the fiber we can get our hands on. There are two kinds of fiber: soluble and insoluble. Soluble fiber dissolves in water and gastrointestinal fluids during digestion. It turns into a gel-like substance, which is digested by bacteria in the large intestine and has several functions. It reduces fat and cholesterol absorption and slows down the digestion of sugars, while also feeding the good bacteria in the gut. Insoluble fiber is indigestible. It remains more or less unchanged as it goes through the digestive tract, facilitating movement and processing of waste.

Both types are good for you. See table 4 for inspiration, but here's a preview. Soluble fiber comes from spuds and root vegetables, like carrots and beets, and small leafy greens, such as baby spinach and watercress. Other good sources are pumpkin, squash, and most legumes. Insoluble fiber comes from large-leaf vegetables like spinach, kale, and chards; crunchy, leafy veg like radicchio and arugula; and cruciferous vegetables like broccoli and Brussels sprouts. Then there's the sweet potato or yam (preferably eaten with the skin on), and whole grains with their husks still on—all great examples of hydrating, filling fiber. Fruits have a lot of fiber, too! Fun fact: cooked fruits become very soluble and can have a laxative effect.

TABLE 4. FIBER-RICH FOODS (LISTED BY FIBER CONTENT)

	SERVING SIZE	TOTAL FIBER (GRAMS)		SERVING SIZE	TOTAL FIBER (GRAMS)
Fruits			**Vegetables**		
Raspberries	1 cup	8.0	Soybeans, cooked	1 cup	20.6
Prunes	1 cup	7.7	Pumpkin, canned	½ cup	13.0
Blackberries	1 cup	7.6	Artichokes, cooked	1 cup	10.3
Pear	1 medium	5.5	Green peas, boiled	1 cup	9.0
Avocado	½ fruit	5.0	Winter squash, cooked	1 cup	5.7
Mango	1 fruit	5.0	Spinach, cooked	1 cup	5.1
Dates, Medjool	3 pieces	4.8	Broccoli, cooked	1 cup	5.0
Apple, with skin	1 medium	4.5	Brussels sprouts, cooked	1 cup	4.0
Banana	1 medium	3.0	Sweet potato, with skin, baked	1 medium	3.8
Orange	1 medium	3.0	Beets, cooked	1 cup	3.8
Strawberries	1 cup	3.0	Sauerkraut	½ cup	3.4
Kiwi fruit	1 medium	2.2	Kale, cooked	1 cup chopped	2.6
Grains, cereals			**Grains, Nuts, and Seeds**		
Oatmeal, rolled oats, dry	1 cup	8.2	Navy beans, boiled	1 cup	19.0

Pasta, whole-wheat, cooked	1 cup	6.0	Split peas, boiled	1 cup	16.0
Barley, pearled, cooked	1 cup	6.0	Lentils, boiled	1 cup	15.5
Quinoa, cooked	1 cup	5.0	Black beans, boiled	1 cup	15.0
Wheat germ, toasted	1 ounce	4.2	Chickpeas, canned	1 cup	10.6
Brown rice, cooked	1 cup	3.5	Chia seeds	1 ounce	10.0
Psyllium husk	¼ cup	3.0	Flaxseeds	1 ounce	7.2
Bread, whole wheat	1 slice	2.0	Almonds	1 ounce	3.5

Let's Talk About Grains

While most people agree that fruits and vegetables should be key components of a healthy diet, there is some confusion over whether grains should be in there, too. From a women's health perspective, there are many clinical trials and disease-preventative studies showing that a diet rich in whole grains is vital for brain health and Alzheimer's prevention for both women and men. Additionally, observational studies of hundreds of thousands of women report that those who consistently eat whole grains have the lowest risk of heart disease and a much lower risk of type 2 diabetes.

However, today, as many as one in three Americans avoids gluten, the protein found in wheat, barley, and rye, choosing to eliminate the majority of grains and cereals from their diet. As a neuroscientist and nutritionist, I'm frequently asked whether grains are bad for your brain and whether they should be avoided. The answer is: Brain-wise, not really.

Currently, peer-reviewed science shows no conclusive evidence that eating grains increases the risk of cognitive decline or dementia, a topic I discuss in greater detail in *Brain Food*. There are no clinical trials testing gluten as a trigger for cognitive deficits, and no observational studies reporting negative associations between eating grains and cognitive health, apart from those cases related to celiac disease.

One percent of the population suffers from celiac disease, an immune reaction to gluten, and should avoid gluten. While estimates vary, at least another 6 percent of the population seems to have gluten sensitivities rather than allergies, and they need to be careful around gluten as well. But if you do not have an allergy or sensitivity to gluten, it looks like a certain amount of unprocessed whole grains can surely be part of a healthy diet.

On the contrary, unsupervised gluten-free diets can do more harm than good. By "unsupervised" I'm referring to the tendency to shun not only grains but carbs in general, by going on low-carb or no-carb diets. If people were eating enough high-fiber vegetables, fruits, and legumes to make up the difference, that would be one thing—but we know from population-based surveys that this is not the case. The result is more often than not a diet that can be alarmingly low in fiber—a nutritional deficiency that's not good for anyone, and that can have a severe negative impact on a woman's hormonal balance.

On the upside, the gluten-free movement has led many consumers to turn away from processed foods and discover naturally gluten-free grains in their stead. These include rice, amaranth, buckwheat, millet, quinoa, sorghum, and teff, which are perfectly legitimate sources of fiber and brain-energizing glucose.

Beware of the gluten-free products that have hit the market to capitalize on this issue instead! Too many are marketed as healthy alternative foods when they're nothing more than processed junk foods that, while avoiding gluten, contain the usual high sugar and bad fat, along with a slew of artificial additives.

In the end, if you are concerned with maximizing your cognitive health and preventing Alzheimer's, complex carbs—fiber in particular—are an essential component of your diet. I'm all for condemning the standard Western diet loaded with refined carbs and junk food, but legumes and whole grains are good for you—as also exemplified by the fact they are the dietary cornerstones of the longest living populations on Earth. If gluten is a concern for you, make sure you eat plenty of fibrous vegetables, fruits, and legumes to compensate, focus on the naturally gluten-free grains mentioned above, and throw a sweet potato in there once in a while for good measure.

What's for Dessert?

If you, like me, need the occasional treat, I strongly recommend dark chocolate with a cacao content of 70 percent or higher. When consumed in its purest form, dark chocolate remains a powerful superfood with impressive health benefits. For one, it's rich in theobromine, a strong antioxidant known to support cellular aging, along with many powerful flavonols that reduce the risk of heart disease. Clinical trials showed that consuming cacao with a high flavonol content improved attention and memory in healthy adults while reducing inflammation and insulin levels in as little as eight weeks.

Additionally, dark chocolate has a low-glycemic load for a treat, which makes it satisfying without the unwanted sugar crash. As a bonus, dark chocolate contains substances called catechins that are similar to estrogen and can help soften the effects of declining hormone levels. The key here is to focus on high-quality dark chocolate with little to no added sugar. Unfortunately, the vast majority of the chocolate people eat is in the form of milk, white, or "confectionery" chocolate, or other chocolate-flavored candies, each one containing but trace amounts of actual cacao. What they do contain instead are extraordinary amounts of sugar, fat, and additives, which quickly turns what could have been a good idea into a very bad one.

As for sweeteners, raw honey, maple syrup, stevia, coconut sugar, and coconut nectar are much better choices than refined sugars or sugar substitutes. Richer in vitamins and minerals than any of the white powdery stuff, these sweeteners are also gentler on the liver—and don't pound as much at your blood sugar levels.

STEP 2. MEET MS. PHYTOESTROGEN

Estrogen has the honored distinction of being the most ancient of all hormones. Due to this, we find it in both the animal and plant kingdoms, and it can be shared across species. What does that mean exactly? It means that estrogen made from a plant, or phytoestrogen, translates to usable estrogen in our human bodies—but with a milder effect. There are two major types of phytoestrogens: isoflavones, found mostly in soy; and lignans, abundant in seeds, whole grains, and legumes, and in many fruits and vegetables. This makes a plant-based diet an excellent natural estrogen replacement therapy! As a bonus, consuming these foods consistently may help increase sex drive and relieve any pain associated with intercourse after menopause, a quality not many drugs can boast about.

Soy has been attracting attention for years because of the positive effect of isoflavones on menopausal symptoms like hot flashes. Clinical trials indicate that isoflavones can help stabilize estrogen levels, leading to amelioration of hot flashes by up to 45 percent. However, soy has become one of the most controversial foods on the planet. You will find it promoted as a healthy superfood one minute and blacklisted as a cancer-inducing poison the next.

This deserves a double take, since Asian women eat soy regularly and are four times less likely to get breast cancer as their Western counterparts. They are also less likely to suffer from hot flashes, and less prone than American women to develop osteoporosis and heart disease. How can this be?

It gets even more mysterious. Japan has the highest life expectancy of any country, age ninety for women and eighty-four for men, with the world's longest-living women residing in the province of Okinawa. In the Okinawan diet, soy products like tofu and natto (a traditional Japanese food made from fermented soybeans) are classic staple foods. Aside from soy, over 80 percent of their calories comes from vegetables, fruits, and legumes, as well as complex carbohydrates such as whole grains, brown rice, and sweet potatoes. Okinawans consume very little meat, eggs, or dairy, while fresh-caught fish is much more common. While the specific ingredients certainly differ, there are some obvious parallels between this diet and the Mediterranean diet we encountered in the previous chapter. The results are also similar. These Okinawan centenarian women have markedly delayed or entirely avoided chronic diseases such as Alzheimer's, heart disease, and cancer. Though factors other than diet come into play as well, there's a strong indication that when it comes to health, soy, not to mention plant-based foods in general, appear to be playing an important role. So how has soy become a hero in Japan and a villain in the States?

In the Western world, soy first became popular due to the very fact that Okinawan centenarian women largely preferred it over meat in their diet. However, back in the nineties, some studies showed that isoflavones increased the growth of cancer cells in mice that had been genetically modified to develop breast cancer. This raised concerns that isoflavones might provoke breast cancer in women with a genetic predisposition, but many health professionals took a cautionary stance by recommending that all women avoid soy products, just to be safe.

Over the past ten years, however, extensive research has begun to clarify that isoflavones in and of themselves don't increase breast cancer risk in women. Although more research is still needed, a cross-analysis of studies pooling 20,000 breast cancer patients indicated that isoflavones do not increase the odds of breast tumor recurrence, and in some cases can even reduce mortality. Additionally, soy was found to have no negative effects on endometrial, ovarian, or other cancers.

Chemically speaking, the phytoestrogens found in soy are quite unique compounds in that their effect on your body depends on the levels of estrogen already circulating in your bloodstream. For example, if you have a lot of estrogen in your body, as breast cancer patients do, phytoestrogens will act as estrogen blockers (a bit like the drug tamoxifen does). However, if you are a menopausal woman making too little estrogen, phytoestrogens end up filling in those missing estrogens, similar to taking a mild supplement. Findings like these led the American Institute for Cancer Research and the American Cancer Society to revise their position on soy in 2013, concluding that even breast cancer patients can safely consume isoflavone-rich soy foods. However, neither group endorses isoflavone supplements for fear of overconsumption. It is unquestionably safer to absorb isoflavones from actual foods.

That said, not all soy is created equal. As you may remember if you read *Brain Food*, the type of soy you're eating makes a big difference as to whether it will have a negative or positive effect on your health. There's a clue here that may go some way to explaining why our Okinawan sisters are showing benefits when we are not. So what's the scoop on soy?

In part, Asian populations are likely more genetically apt at absorbing soy and less prone to side effects. But also, the soy, tofu, and soy milk–based products eaten in Japan are distinctly different from what we find on most of our supermarket shelves. The Japanese almost exclusively consume soy in its organic form. Not only that, but the soy is often fermented, as is the case for miso, tempeh, and natto. Frankly, this is the only type of soy worth eating. Unfortunately, these products are not always easy to find in the Western world. What is easy to find are soy products that are made up of 90 percent genetically modified soybeans and that are rife with pesticides and preservatives as well. This distinctly bad soy has proliferated in our cafés and supermarkets. The most disparate products are literally everywhere. Soybean oil made from bad soy is routinely added to over 12,000 food products, from common breakfast cereals and energy bars to snacks and pastas. Isolated soy proteins are used as emulsifiers to lend moisture and consistency to lattes and frappés. Soy lecithin, one of the most widely used food additives on the market today, is found in nearly everything, from prepared pastries and bread to infant formulas. As a result, eating too much of this hidden soy is easy to do and causes the exact opposite effect of what the Okinawans have experienced: hormone imbalances in both women and men. Probably inflammation and allergies too.

Mystery solved. If you are interested in eating more soy to boost your estrogens, make sure you eat fermented organic soy, and in small amounts at that. One caveat: soy is a very allergenic food for many, so if concerned, consult with your doctor to get tested for any allergies or intolerances prior to beginning.

How much soy can we safely eat? If we're talking about using isoflavones to relieve menopausal symptoms, we're looking to consume approximately 40 to 50 milligrams of isoflavones per day. This is equivalent to two servings of traditional soy foods, like a scoop of tofu served with a bowl of miso soup or a cup of edamame, an amount that is well within the range eaten in Japan.

If soy is not your thing, or if you can't find the good kind, other nutrients can help boost estrogen, namely, lignans. Lignans are found in a variety of plant foods including flaxseeds, sesame seeds, and chickpeas, along with apricots, apples, yams, and olive oil to name but a few. Table 5 includes even more examples. It is perhaps no surprise that these foods are also excellent sources of fiber, good carbs, and good fats, as well as other very important nutrients we'll discuss in just a moment.

TABLE 5. FOODS HIGH IN PHYTOESTROGEN CONTENT
(***** = HIGH, * = LOW)

SOY PRODUCTS	FRUITS	VEGETABLES	LEGUMES
Soybeans *****	Dried apricots ***	Garlic ***	Chickpeas ****
Soy nuts *****	Peaches ***	Winter squash ***	Hummus ***
Textured veggie protein ****	Dried dates ***	Green beans ***	Mung bean sprouts **
Tofu ****	Strawberries **	Alfalfa sprouts **	Mung beans **
Soy milk ****	Raspberries **	Olive oil **	Lentils **
Soy yogurt ****	Dried prunes **	Collards **	Peanuts **
Tempeh ****	Oranges **	Broccoli **	
Miso paste ****	Blueberries *	Olives **	
Miso soup ****	Watermelon *	Cabbage **	
Soy protein powder ****		Onions **	
Soybean sprouts ***		Yams **	

	NUTS AND SEEDS	CEREALS AND GRAINS	BEVERAGES
	Flaxseeds *****	Flax bread ****	Green tea **
	Sesame seeds ****	Multigrain bread ****	Orange juice **
	Pistachios ***	Wheat bread ***	Black tea **
	Almonds ***	Rye bread **	Coffee **
	Sunflower seeds **	Sesame bread **	Red wine **
	Walnuts **		White wine **
	Cashews **		
	Hazelnuts **		

STEP 3. PROTECT YOUR BRAIN WITH ANTIOXIDANTS

Of all the organs in the body, the brain is the one that suffers most from oxidative stress. This term refers to the production of harmful free radicals in our body and brain and our ability to counteract them. The more free radicals your brain has to harbor, the more damage done.

However, there are solutions. Enter antioxidants, vitamin warriors that are at the ready to fight off free radicals on our behalf. Among the most powerful antioxidants are vitamins C and E, beta-carotene (the precursor to vitamin A), selenium, and a variety of plant-made nutrients like lycopene and anthocyanins, which give tomatoes and cherries their beautiful bright colors. Our brain imaging research shows that a diet rich in these antioxidants is associated with steady brain energy levels and fewer Alzheimer's plaques, especially in women.

Vitamin E is particularly protective against cognitive decline. Large-scale studies in the United States and Europe found that elderly people who consumed a good amount of vitamin E had a nearly 70 percent lower risk of developing dementia as compared with those who consumed little to none. Dementia risk was further reduced by taking vitamin E in combination with vitamin C. Both these vitamins protect brain cells from free radicals and other various toxins, and vitamin E has the added benefit of increasing oxygen delivery to the brain. Vitamin E is also the only vitamin with validated efficacy in reducing hot flashes, possibly because it helps regulate estrogen levels. It is no coincidence that soybeans are a rich source of vitamin E as well as of phytoestrogens.

When antioxidant levels are lower than those of free radicals—due to poor nutrition, toxin exposure, or other factors—oxidation wreaks havoc in the body. The effect? Accelerated aging, damaged or mutated cells, broken-down tissue, the activation of harmful genes within DNA, and an overloaded immune system. Research indicates that a woman's brain may be particularly vulnerable to these negative consequences, especially in the years leading to menopause, causing accelerated cellular aging and impaired metabolism. The Western lifestyle, with its processed foods, reliance on medications, and high exposure to chemicals and environmental pollutants, seems to lay the foundation for the proliferation of free radicals.

Because many of us are exposed to such high rates of oxidative stress from a young age, more than ever we need the power of antioxidants, which means we need to consume high-antioxidant foods. Many of these also double as anti-inflammatory foods, while at the same time having anti-microbial properties! Given that women are particularly sensitive to inflammation and infections, a diet rich in these foods is really key to women's health. Finally, another benefit of consuming these helpful nutrients is that, by quenching oxidation and inflammation, they are effectively protecting our hormones, too.

Doctors are learning that one of the best ways to reduce oxidative stress and inflammation lies not in the medicine cabinet but in the refrigerator. Plant-based foods make up the bulk of the best antioxidant choices available to us. Fruits such as berries, oranges, grapefruits, and apples (all which have a low-glycemic index) are excellent sources of these nutrients. While blueberries receive most of the attention, blackberries and gooseberries pull an even stronger antioxidant punch. Leafy green and cruciferous vegetables (spinach, kale, broccoli, cabbage), as well as onions, carrots, tomatoes, and squash, are also full of these powerhouses. Artichokes top the charts, possessing more antioxidant density than any other fruit or vegetable. Eat the rainbow, remember?

Extra-virgin olive oil and flaxseed oil are loaded with vitamin E while also acting as excellent anti-inflammatories. When it comes to the rare antioxidant mineral selenium, Brazil nuts are by far the best source, but you can also find it in rice, oats, mushrooms, and lentils. Additionally, herbs, spices, and powders like cocoa and coffee have the highest antioxidant potency of all foods. Plant foods to the rescue!

Take a look at table 6 for inspiration (it's true, cranberry juice can work against UTIs!). And to make sure that we reach our daily requirements of these helpful nutrients, chapter 11 reviews selected supplements and appropriate dosages for a variety of uses.

It is, of course, just as important to avoid or limit consumption of foods that cause inflammation. These include mainly refined carbs, such as commercial white bread and pastries; fried foods; soda and sugar-sweetened beverages; processed meat and red meat (beef, pork); margarine, shortening, and lard; and most processed food. More on this in a moment.

TABLE 6. ANTIOXIDANT, ANTI-INFLAMMATORY, AND ANTI-MICROBIAL FOODS (**** = HIGH, * = LOW)

FOOD ITEM	ANTIOXIDANT AND ANTI-INFLAMMATORY STRENGTH	ANTI-MICROBIAL STRENGTH
Apple, golden	*	*
Artichokes (cooked)	*	**
Basil (dried)	**	**
Blueberries (wild)	*	**
Cilantro	*	*
Cinnamon	***	****
Clove	****	****
Cocoa	***	**
Cranberries; cranberry juice (raw, unsweetened)	*	***
Cumin	**	***
Dark chocolate (85% and higher)	**	**
Elderberries (dried)	*	**
Fennel	*	**
Garlic	*	**
Ginger	**	***
Goji berries	*	*
Hibiscus tea	*	*
Indian gooseberry (amla)	****	**
Kidney beans	*	*
Mustard seeds	*	***

Olive oil	**	**
Onions	*	**
Oregano (dried)	****	****
Parsley (dried)	**	*
Pecans	*	-
Peppermint leaves (dried)	****	***
Rosemary (dried)	****	****
Sage (dried)	***	***
Thyme	**	****
Turmeric	***	***
Vanilla beans	***	**

Antioxidant values are expressed in ORAC (oxygen radical absorbance capacity) units, ranging from <5,000 (*) to >15,000 (****). Anti-microbial values are measured by percent of bacterial inhibition, ranging from <25 percent (*) to 75 to 100 percent (****).

STEP 4. CHOOSE THE RIGHT FATS

As mentioned before, both the type and source (rather than the amount) of fats are key when assessing health risks in women. Does the fat you're eating come primarily from fruits, vegetables, and seeds, or from animal sources? If from animal sources, is it from fatty fish like salmon, or is it from fried bacon? Does it come from fresh, home-made food or from a box?

Below, we will review the healthiest sources of fat. In addition, appendix B includes a number of healthy swaps to get you on the right path!

The Debate Is Over: Trans Fat Is a Health Hazard

Whenever someone asks me what the single most important thing to do is to sustain the well-being of their brain, I always, without fail, give the same answer: do not eat processed foods.

First off, processed foods are the richest source of harmful trans fat, the worst type of fat on the planet. Fortunately, in 2018, the FDA prohibited trans fat from the entire food supply. Other countries were not as lucky, though. In Europe, six countries (Austria, Denmark, Hungary, Iceland, Norway, and Switzerland) have set limits that strictly forbid trans fat from being included in food products. However, consumption remains high in those countries where these policies are not in place. Even if trans fats are eventually banned everywhere, most processed foods contain a host of so many other toxic chemicals that it makes your head spin. The list is longer than we have space for here, but modified starches, high-fructose corn syrup, artificial food coloring, gums, and protein isolates are all things that you'll find over and over again if you're reading labels. Did you know that some processed foods contain substances commonly used as flame retardants? Or that french fries from popular fast-food chains are loaded with anti-foaming agents? (Eek.) I hate to tell you this, but these chemicals have it in for us.

The slowness with which safeguards are put in place is troubling given the fact that the consumption of processed food has already been proven to increase the risks of dementia, heart disease, and breast cancer. A recent large-scale study following over 104,000 people for eighteen years found that consuming processed foods led to a 12 percent increase in all kinds of cancer, with an especially high risk of breast cancer for post-menopausal women. According to the World Cancer Research Fund International and the American Institute for Cancer Research, roughly one-third of the most common cancers in our world could be avoided entirely by eliminating or drastically reducing all consumption of processed foods. It is hard to wrap our minds around the fact that something this deadly continues to be commonplace in so many people's daily lives.

As is the case with cancer, processed foods are also at the root of the heart disease epidemic that's currently sweeping so many countries. In 2012, more than 700,000 Americans died of heart disease, stroke, or diabetes. An estimated 45 percent of these deaths were associated with dietary factors—in particular, the intake of too much sodium (a hallmark of processed food) and processed meat. If that weren't enough, the American Diabetes Association states that given their high content of refined sugar, refined flour, and refined oils, processed foods are responsible for damaging insulin levels, thereby increasing the risk of diabetes.

By some measures, processed food accounts for at least half of the American diet, and probably just as much in other Western countries. This doesn't come as a complete shock when we think about the majority of items available in our supermarkets. Walking down the aisles, we are deluged by commercial bread and pastry products; packaged snacks; industrialized confectionery and desserts; sodas and sweetened drinks; sandwiches and wraps and salads all containing cold cuts and processed cheeses. Then there are the ready-made meals featuring processed meats and chicken nuggets; instant noodles and soups; frozen, shelf-stable meals; condiments, spreads, and creamers—all highly processed foods. On the way home, we'll pass a plethora of cafés and drive-throughs, diners and restaurants, each one serving fast food in the name of making our lives easier.

It is indeed inconvenient to come to terms with this, but it's much worse to continue to harm ourselves and our families. At one time, we may have been uncertain as to just how detrimental these foods could be, but now we know better. We need and deserve access to healthy foods that nourish us instead of making us sick.

Omega-3: Your Brain Booster

As mentioned in the previous chapter, polyunsaturated fatty acids, or PUFAs, are particularly good for the brain. PUFAs come in different varieties, the most common being omega-3 and omega-6. While the brain needs both of these fats, omega-3s are anti-inflammatory (which we need more of), whereas omega-6s are more pro-inflammatory (which we need less of). Research has determined that a ratio of 2:1, or twice the amount of omega-6 to the amount of omega-3, is the balance to shoot for. However, the typical Western diet contains twenty to thirty times more omega-6s than omega-3s! Given the repercussions, it is crucial that we tip the balance toward the soothing omega-3s.

Not only are the anti-inflammatory properties of omega-3s brain-beneficial, but they also help women preserve their heart, breast, and bone health, even keeping moods steady and calm. During the reproductive years, diets low in omega-3s have been associated with increased menstrual pain and infertility, as well as an increased risk of premature birth. Low omega-3 levels are also linked with an increased risk of depression in both genders, though women with lower omega-3s have higher rates of depression and also exhibit more severe symptoms than men do. Additionally, omega-3 supplementation during pregnancy seems to lower the risk of postpartum depression.

In a society where beauty continues to be equated with being thin, women trying to lose weight by restricting these essential fatty acids may unknowingly increase their risk of depressive and hormonal symptoms, not to mention unknowingly tamper with their ability to conceive and sustain a pregnancy.

It's time to turn this around and look for these nutritional omega-3 dynamos instead. Well-selected fatty fish (such as salmon, mackerel, lake trout, herring, albacore tuna, anchovies, and sardines) as well as their eggs (caviar, salmon roe, and the like) are our best natural sources of omega-3s. To date, as many as nine large-scale epidemiological studies have concluded that regular fish consumption is crucial for brain health. In these studies, middle-age and older people who consumed fish once or twice a week reduced their risk of Alzheimer's by up to 70 percent.

Moreover, a study of 35,000 women between the ages of thirty-five and sixty-nine determined that the more fatty fish you eat, the later you enter menopause. Legumes like peas and beans come in second. On the other hand, eating refined foods, especially white pasta, white rice, and sugary snacks, hastened the onset of menopause with a considerable swiftness, explaining perhaps why so many women on a typical Western diet enter menopause early and suffer its effects more severely.

One thing to keep in mind is that although fish is recommended for its many health benefits, mercury, a confirmed neurotoxin, is of growing concern. Luckily not all fish are high in mercury contamination. The highest levels of mercury are found in large fish like king mackerel, swordfish, shark, and most types of tuna—so don't eat them more than a few times a month. Sea bass, snapper, cod, and halibut all fall into the mid-range. Mahi-mahi, Spanish mackerel, and canned albacore tuna are also mid-range. The lowest levels of mercury are found in smaller fish and shellfish such as anchovies, cod, clams, crab, sole, flounder, and sardines, not to mention salmon. This fish can be safely consumed a couple of times a week.

If fish isn't an option, as is the case if you have allergies or are vegan or vegetarian, there are other ways to get your omega-3s. Flaxseeds and chia seeds are good alternatives, as are olives and their oil, almonds, avocados, and soybeans. Additionally, sweet peas, tapioca, and cucumber are good sources of phospholipids, complex fats that also contain omega-3s. However, keep in mind that these plant-based foods are rich in ALA (alpha-linolenic acid), a weaker form of omega-3s than those found in fish, which is called DHA (docosahexaenoic acid). DHA is the big winner when it comes to brain health. While ALA can be converted into DHA, unfortunately, a high amount is lost in the process. If you must avoid fish, it may be helpful to take a vegan DHA supplement, as discussed in chapter 11.

Finally, I am sure you've seen the phrase "a good source of omega-3" stamped across many foods at your grocery store. Food manufacturers have figured out that omega-3s sell. But this is not the right way to take in additional omega-3s given that most enriched foods are also processed. Go for the real thing instead.

Monounsaturated Fat: Another Brain Buddy

In addition to eating plenty of omega-3s, studies of thousands of women have shown that a higher intake of monounsaturated fat was associated with better cognitive performance, especially for patients with type 2 diabetes or pre-diabetes.

Where do you find this fat? Foods high in monounsaturated fat include nuts such as almonds, cashews, hazelnuts, pistachios, and Brazil nuts. Fatty fruits like avocados and olives and some oils and nut butters from peanuts, sesame, and sunflower seeds are also good sources. Freshly ground (versus commercially packaged) nut butters consumed in moderation are also nutritional powerhouses, loaded with healthy fats, protein, and fiber, not to mention a variety of antioxidants.

While some doctors recommend cutting down on nuts due to their fat content, a study of over 86,000 women showed that those who consumed nuts frequently had a much lower risk of heart disease and stroke. A handful of nuts, about an ounce, once a week delivers nice results. The trick here is to buy them with the peel still on, or even better, still inside their shell. Not only does this protect these delicate foods from light and heat, keeping them from turning rancid, but it preserves their nutrients, too, giving you a chance to slow down and appreciate (rather than over-eat) them in the process. Refrain from buying pre-shelled, blanched, fla-vored, salted, or seasoned nuts, as these become processed foods all over again. Try a good old-fashioned nutcracker and taste the difference!

Saturated Fat? Go Easy

While not nearly as harmful as trans fat, too much saturated fat can also negatively impact women's brains and overall health, so it's best consumed in moderation. As mentioned above, animal sources of sat-urated fat, such as red meat, dairy, and butter, can be problematic if consumed in excess. The best way to cut back on these foods is by re-placing them with fish, beans, nuts, and oils. According to some stud-ies, replacing 100 calories of fat from cheese with 100 calories of fat from almond butter on a daily basis might reduce risk of heart disease by close to 30 percent. Plants over animals, as much as possible!

However, this doesn't mean trading out your fried chicken for an or-der of fried onion rings! The sources of vegetable fat are just as impor-tant, so say no to refined vegetable oils. For instance, vegetable fats such as margarine are pro-inflammatory processed foods that should be avoided at all costs. Some widely used oils from sunflower seeds, saf-flower, canola, and peanuts can also be pro-inflammatory and should be reduced. Focus on healthier, unrefined, or, even better, extra-virgin vegetable oils such as olive and flaxseed, and more sparingly on avo-cado and coconut oils as well.

Among vegetable oils, coconut oil deserves our consideration. You can't browse social media or your local grocery store without noticing the spotlight on coconut oil. This sweet-flavored tropical staple has been credited with everything from anti-aging and weight-loss prop-erties to supporting the health of the heart. It has even been touted as a way of protecting the brain against Alzheimer's. Since coconut oil began its meteoric rise in the U.S. marketplace more than six years ago, people have been incorporating it into everything from smoothies to "bulletproof coffee." In spite of its rampant popularity as a potential superfood, the American Heart Association recently took a strong stance against it. They advised, "Because coconut oil increases LDL cholesterol, a cause of cardiovascular disease, and has no known off-setting favorable effects, we advise against the use of coconut oil." As I write this very page, an article shared over a half million times runs in *USA Today*, its headline reading, "Coconut Oil Isn't Healthy, It's Never Been Healthy." Jumping on the bandwagon, some went so far as to re-fer to it as "pure poison." In spite of the news, many nutritionists con-tinue to recommend it, and a variety of dieters swear by it.

What's the upshot? Is coconut oil good or bad for you? And more to the point, can it benefit brain health?

For now, the jury's still out. There is very little research on the effects of coconut oil, especially with regard to brain health. What we do know is that about 84 percent of the calories in coconut oil come from saturated fat in the form of medium-chain triglycerides, or MCTs. Some studies show that the body seems to handle these MCTs differ-ently than the longer-chain, unhealthier saturated fat found in dairy and fatty meats. A recent randomized clinical trial divided roughly 100 participants into three groups and assigned each group to con-sume a daily amount of 50 grams (3 to 4 tablespoons) of one of the following fats: extra-virgin olive oil, extra-virgin coconut oil, or butter. After four weeks, the researchers measured each group's blood lipid levels and found that, while the butter group showed a significant in-crease in the concentration of "bad" LDL cholesterol relative to the gold-standard olive oil group, the coconut oil group did not show this increase. While this particular study didn't focus on gender, a large prospective study of 73,000 women found that another specific type of saturated fatty acid found in coconut oil, called lauric acid, didn't ap-pear to raise heart disease risk quite as much as other types of oil, such as the palmitic acid found to a substantial degree in butter. Last, a smaller study showed that a Mediterranean diet enriched with coconut oil was associated with positive effects on cognition in female patients who had been diagnosed with Alzheimer's.

All of this bears the need for further study, but shows some interesting potential in the meantime. So even though coconut oil isn't the magic bullet some claim, when it is used in reasonable amounts, and especially if to replace commercial butter, margarine, or shortening, it looks like it can't hurt. Besides, it's delicious. I often use coconut oil in my cooking, though I err on the safe side, keeping consumption to no more than 1 tablespoon a day.

Now on to another food rich in saturated fat that has generated a lot of buzz over the years: milk. Milk used to be simple. It was made by a cow, and your local dairy delivered it to your doorstep. Today, we are faced with an unfathomable assortment: no-fat, low-fat, whole milk? From cows or goats? With or without lactase? Raw or pasteurized? Almond, soy, coconut, or rice milk? Is that even milk?

From a women's health perspective, findings from the Nurses' Health Study indicate that drinking milk supports hormonal health and fertility, at least in those who tolerate it well. In fact, your average glass of milk (cow's milk, in this case) can be considered a hormonal cocktail of sorts. This makes sense, since cows, being female, produce estrogen in their milk, along with other female hormones as well as some androgens like testosterone. However, this depends on which type of milk you drink. A more careful look at the study reveals that it was only full-fat milk that improved fertility, whereas women who consumed skim or low-fat milk tended to suffer from the exact opposite condition: infertility. It appears that processing milk to remove butterfat not only waters down the texture and taste of the milk, but also radically changes its balance of sex hormones in a way that tips the scales against, instead of toward, hormonal health. Skimming off milk fat whisks away the estrogens, leaving behind a mix of androgens and other hormones such as insulin-like growth factor 1—which may end up increasing your testosterone levels.

On top of that, manufacturers add refined sugar, starches, and additives to skim milk in an attempt to recuperate lost flavor and texture. Whatever health benefits we thought we were achieving by drinking skimmed milk, it's really not worth it in the end, and can even be detrimental. Think about switching to full-fat milk as a nutritional therapy designed to improve hormonal health, especially if you are trying to get pregnant or are approaching menopause. The same goes for unprocessed yogurts and cheeses—full-fat is the way to go. Organic dairy is also something to consider, as we will discuss further.

In closing, an interesting note about dairy concerning bone health. Most of us grew up thinking that milk is important for children to build strong bones, and for the elderly to prevent osteoporosis. Many women have heard that dairy products provide a good source of calcium, which, when combined with vitamin D, helps fight bone loss. As it turns out, you don't need to drink milk or eat dairy to get your calcium: many non-dairy foods are just as good a source. These include various vegetables (spinach, turnips, kale, and beet greens), legumes (soybeans, tofu, beans, and peas), and even seafood (salmon, sardines, and shrimp). A glass of whole milk contains about 280 mg of calcium—as does a cup of cooked spinach, or 3 ounces of sardines. Additionally, plant-based milks generally have about the same amount of calcium as cow's milk, minus the saturated fat.

As for vitamin D, the very best way to get enough of it is to simply spend time outdoors, in sunlight. When your skin is exposed to sunlight, it makes vitamin D from cholesterol. This happens very quickly; about 15 minutes for a very fair-skinned person, and up to a couple of hours for those with darker skin. Vitamin D can also be obtained by consuming fatty fish as well as from egg yolks and wild mushrooms like chanterelles, maitake, and morels.

Too Much, Too Little—How to Get Cholesterol Just Right

Cholesterol plays a crucial part in so many of our bodily functions, from forming healthy cell walls throughout our body to making hormones—so having adequate levels of this fat is especially important. The cholesterol in your blood comes from two sources: your liver and the foods you eat. Your liver makes up to 80 percent of all the cholesterol your body needs, while only 20 percent or so comes from your diet, especially eggs, fish, meat, and dairy.

Whether due to genetic factors or to unhealthy diets, some people end up with high cholesterol, a condition that can increase the risk of both heart disease and dementia. Typically, "high cholesterol" indicates a blood cholesterol level higher than 240 mg/dL. However, research shows that a level of 220 mg/dL is already too high, nearly doubling the risk of dementia later in life.

For other people, the problem isn't having an overabundance of cholesterol but instead having too little. Strict vegetarian or vegan diets may lead to cholesterol deficiencies since plants do not contain cholesterol. This is a concern, given that women with low body fat and low cholesterol levels tend to produce insufficient amounts of sex hormones. This may lead to amenorrhea, when one's menstruation stops, or to early osteoporosis and fractures.

In both cases—too much or too little—it is essential to have your cholesterol levels checked regularly. Low cholesterol is easier to address, whereas high cholesterol can be quite a challenge. A healthy diet is often crucial in this regard.

Traditionally, in order to lower cholesterol levels, your doctor would advise you to reduce the consumption of cholesterol-rich foods, especially eggs. Long-vilified by well-meaning doctors and scientists researching heart disease, eggs now seem to be making a bit of a comeback. So what changed? Eggs were previously associated with heart disease risk as a result of their high cholesterol content. Just one egg yolk has 200 mg of cholesterol—making it one of the richest sources of dietary cholesterol. However, a solid body of subsequent research showed that, for many people, cholesterol in food has a smaller effect on blood levels of total cholesterol than does the mix of trans fat and saturated fat. In other words, these other fats are more of a problem than cholesterol itself. While more work is needed to better understand the connection between dietary fat and heart disease, specifically for eggs, large prospective cohort studies of over 80,000 women and 40,000 men found that one egg per day was not associated with increased heart disease risk in healthy individuals.

Besides, eggs contain several nutrients that are good for both the heart and the brain. Specifically, eggs are packed with nutrients an embryo needs to grow, and the development of a new organism starts from the neural tube, aka the brain. These include protein, zinc, important antioxidants like lutein and zeaxanthin, and choline, a vitamin that supports memory formation. In addition, the fatty acids in an egg, about 5 grams, are mostly monounsaturated and polyunsaturated, which, as we now know, are good for you.

Of course, this doesn't give a green light to daily three-egg omelets. Other studies indicate that, while eating an egg a day is generally safe (I don't need to tell you that's no more than seven eggs per week in total), going much beyond that could indeed increase the risk for heart failure later in life. In my opinion, it's just as important to pay attention to the "trimmings" that come with your eggs. To your heart, scrambled eggs with vegetables on whole-wheat toast is a far different meal from fried eggs with cheese, sausages, ketchup, and buttered white toast.

The APOE-4 Gene: Fine-Tune Your Fat Consumption

The APOE-4 gene is one great example of the impact diet has on genetics, especially when it comes to dietary fat. One of the ways that APOE affects brain health is that it is involved in moving cholesterol through the body. Of all three APOE variants, the E4 variant that's associated with an increased risk of Alzheimer's also happens to be the least efficient at shuttling cholesterol around, possibly leading to an increased accumulation of plaques in the vascular system, reduced circulation, and, in turn, an increased risk of stroke.

As mentioned above, too much saturated fat can increase cholesterol levels, which seems to be the case especially in APOE-4 carriers. Some studies reported a sevenfold increased risk for Alzheimer's in APOE-4 carriers who consumed a diet high in saturated fat as compared with non-carriers who consumed a comparable amount. Our brain imaging studies also showed that a diet high in saturated fat, trans fat, and cholesterol is strongly associated with an elevated Alzheimer's risk in people with the APOE-4 gene, as well as in those with a family history of Alzheimer's.

Overall, emerging data suggests that too much saturated and processed fat in the diet may encourage this genetic predisposition to further activate itself. Here's one thing you can do about it: randomized controlled trials indicate that omega-3s help preserve memory and cognitive performance in APOE-4 carriers. Moreover, while eating omega-3 rich fish is a smart move for brain health in general, the benefits seem particularly powerful for people with the APOE-4 gene. So if you are an APOE-4 carrier, make a point of getting rid of trans fat from your diet, and while you're at it, replace as much saturated fat as you can with PUFAs, too.

STEP 5. FEED YOUR MICROBES

You may have heard by now that a happy tummy equals a happy brain. That's because our gut is home to the trillions of bacteria and other micro-organisms that make up our microbiome. The vast majority of gut bacteria are beneficial to our health—they help us digest food, power up our metabolism, and even produce some essential vitamins. Additionally, gut flora acts as a mighty warrior on behalf of the immune system, defending us against the harmful microbes that cause inflammation. New research reveals that our microbiome is also involved in several aspects of brain health and behavior, especially in our reactions to stress and anxiety, while at the same time supporting brain longevity.

There are several things we can do to return the favor and support our microbiome in turn.

Sticking to a varied diet, limiting processed foods, avoiding prolonged restricted diets, and consuming adequate fiber, all keep our gut going strong. In an extensive study, elderly people who consumed a diet high in fiber and low in animal fat had the healthiest microbiomes. Those whose diets were low in fiber but high in animal fat tended to have fragile microbiomes and weaker immune systems instead. Not having enough variety of good bacteria in the gut was strongly linked with poorer cognitive performance, as well as increased inflammation and frailty. A poor-quality gut microbiome has also been correlated with an increased risk of obesity, heart disease, stroke, and even some cancers.

The good news is that a positive change in your diet will create a positive change in your microbiome, and fairly quickly at that. For example, a study observed favorable changes in the microbiome of obese patients within just one year of following high complex-carbohydrate diets. This also had a protective effect against the development of type 2 diabetes.

In more practical terms, this is what we should feed our gut to keep it healthy:

- *Fiber-rich foods.* Besides promoting insulin sensitivity and hormonal balance, fiber supports digestive health and regularity. Healthy digestion is essential to removing waste, harmful toxins, and bad bacteria—all of which can harm our gut flora. Given the connection between gut health and brain health, a low-fiber diet risks adverse long-term effects on the brain, especially on what we call "brain mood." When your diet is low in fiber (and high in processed meats and other foods), the harmful bacteria in your gut end up outnumbering the good ones. When this happens, these bad guys can hijack your brain—a hostile takeover that leads to our feeling emotional, anxious, depressed, and even forgetful. Women are about twice as likely to have gastrointestinal issues as men, so we've got to pay even more attention to how we handle this. A growing body of research shows that for women, the combination of subpar nutrition and hormonal issues is quite likely to be at the root of many unpleasant problems, especially IBS. Which brings us back to step 1 and the fiber-rich foods listed in table 4.

- *Prebiotics.* These are non-digestible carbohydrates that act as "fertilizer" for good gut bacteria. Garlic, onions, asparagus, bananas, cabbage, leeks, and artichokes are all great sources, as are a variety of legumes—beans and lentils in particular.

- *Probiotics.* These are live bacteria that, upon reaching the intestine, replenish our microbiome's good guys. You can find them in fermented and cultured foods, including yogurt and kefir, and fermented vegetables like sauerkraut and brine-fermented pickles. If yogurt is more appealing to you, choose carefully. Most commercial yogurts are chock-full of artificial colors, sugars, and additives. Instead of delivering any health benefits, these products may end up nourishing the disease-causing bacteria in your gut instead. As mentioned above in step 4, plain, full-fat, probiotic-rich yogurt is the only yogurt worth eating. Probiotic supplements can also be helpful, especially those that contain at least three different strains such as *Lactobacillus acidophilus*, *Lactobacillus rhamnosus*, and *Bifidobacterium.*

STEP 6. ALCOHOL AND COFFEE . . . MAKE WAY FOR SPRING WATER

Coffee and alcohol are both influential when it comes to women's health, and not in the best of ways. Many studies have shown that alcohol in particular can increase the risk of hot flashes and, even more disturbingly, breast cancer in women. Drinking too much alcohol encourages weight gain as well. Past the age of forty, your liver begins to slow down, not processing alcohol as well as it used to. This results in a slower metabolism, in some cases up to 70 percent slower, which in turn raises your cortisol level, the stress hormone. This hormone can famously ruin your sleep, up your weight, and turn the cranky on, three of the things you were trying to avoid when you reached for that drink in the first place. Limiting alcohol intake is especially important for women with the APOE-4 gene, for whom alcohol consumption may pose even greater risks.

That said, for most people, a small glass of wine wouldn't hurt, especially if it's red. Red wine has a good reputation when it comes to protecting our brains thanks to its high levels of resveratrol, a potent antioxidant. Alcohol is a very personal choice, one to be made with care. If you're someone for whom it's advised, a 5-ounce glass of wine once in a while (and no more than once a day) can be good for you.

On to coffee! Many of us feel we can't function without our morning fix, and some research shows that moderate coffee intake may promote a healthy brain. "Moderate," however, refers to less than 300 mg of caffeine a day, which is the equivalent of a single espresso or two small cups of regular coffee (6 to 8 ounces). The type of coffee you drink also matters. Freshly brewed espresso has the highest antioxidant capacity among all beverages, whereas instant coffee is no more than a chemical concoction to be avoided at all costs. Adding things to your coffee, whether tons of sugar or creamer, is also a no-no. Same goes for the extra-large, sugar-enriched "fancy" coffee drinks brimming with bad fats, artificial coloring, and hidden additives. Try fresh full-fat milk instead, and if you really need sweetener, honey and coconut sugar are much healthier choices!

Even if you drink "good" coffee, keep in mind that responses to caffeine are highly individual. Some women break it down faster, making them less prone to its side effects, while others find that caffeine negatively affects their heart rate and sleep quality. If coffee gives you the jitters and keeps you up at night, tea is a great alternative. Just remember that green tea and even more so the new health obsession, matcha tea, contain more antioxidants than black tea, and are better for you and your brain.

Interestingly, women metabolize both alcohol and caffeine differently throughout their menstrual cycle. During the initial follicular phase at the beginning of your period, your body responds faster, requiring less of these beverages to feel their effects. During the luteal phase, which begins the day after ovulation, there's a marked slow-down instead. This can lead some of us to drink too much, making the idea of an extra drink of either beverage more tempting. So be careful.

When it comes to what drink is the healthiest, the best advice I can give you is to drink water, and a lot of it. Water is a crucial element for the brain and the body, male or female (see table 7).

TABLE 7. THE POWER OF WATER

Water is the major component of most body parts: • The brain is up to 80% water. Even mild dehydration can trigger cognitive issues. • The heart is 73% water. Dehydration strains the heart. • The lungs are over 80% water, muscle and kidneys are 79%, and the skin is 64% water.
Water allows the body's cells to grow and reproduce.
Water is key to the metabolism of both the body and the brain. It also helps deliver oxygen, which is key to cellular respiration.
Water increases blood flow to the brain, which is why dehydration can also impair cognitive function.
Water is needed by the brain to make hormones and neurotransmitters.
Water acts as a shock absorber for your brain and spinal cord, and for your baby if you're pregnant.
Water is needed to first dissolve foods into nutrients, and then transport the nutrients to the body and brain.
Water flushes waste out of your body, mainly in urine.
Water forms saliva, which is the first step in digestion.
Water helps regulate body temperature (think hot flashes).
Water lubricates the joints. Even the bones are watery, at 31% water.
Water lubricates your private parts, too, which comes in handy, especially after menopause.

The brain itself is 80 percent water. Every chemical reaction that takes place in the brain depends on water. The brain is so sensitive to dehydration that even a minimal lack of water can cause symptoms like brain fog, fatigue, dizziness, confusion, headache, and most alarmingly, brain shrinkage.

It is important to appreciate how quickly dehydration can occur. Simply going four to six hours without water can cause dehydration, and therefore, those neurological symptoms in turn. The well-known recommendation to drink eight 8-ounce glasses of water a day, or about two liters, is backed by research that shows that this simple practice will not only maintain the proper percentage of bodily fluids in your system, but can also speed up your reaction time and cognitive performance by up to 30 percent.

Just the same, most people don't drink nearly enough of it. According to the Centers for Disease Control, 43 percent of adult Americans drink fewer than four cups a day. Of this group, 36 percent drink one to three cups a day, and 7 percent drink none at all. Instead, the vast majority of Americans consume carbonated soft drinks as their primary source of hydration, followed by "purified" water and beer. (I will clarify why purified water doesn't count as water in a second.) Milk, coffee, fruit juice, and sports beverages come in next. Replacing water with other drinks doesn't deliver, especially if you're opting for beverages that contain bad fats, hard-core sugars, chemical sweeteners, preservatives, and coloring. For women, soda in particular has been associated with an increased risk of ovulatory infertility, and what's bad for your ovaries is bad for the rest of you!

Even those who think they are getting enough water might have to take a closer look. Most people who drink purified water, club soda, and seltzer don't realize that these beverages do not contain any of the hydrating nutrients that true water does: natural minerals and electrolytes. Spring or mineral water is the best way to support hydration, as is naturally sparkling water from a spring. If the cost of drinking mineral water is a concern, consider that a twenty-four-bottle case of Poland Spring is $3.99 at Target. By comparison, a twenty-four-can pack of Diet Coke comes in at over $9. In some cities, tap water can be perfectly safe—in which case I recommend investing in a glass carafe with a good water filter. If your tap water isn't safe and you must drink purified water, consider rehydrating with aloe juice, coconut water, or just plain electrolyte salts.

Before we move to the next step, I want to share one of my favorite brain-healthy tips: Drink a glass of plain warm water first thing in the morning. Warm water is more hydrating than cold water because it has a vasodilating effect, which means it makes your veins pop, promoting absorption. Cold water acts like a vasoconstrictor instead. This simple practice is effective at replenishing your brain with much-needed fluids—and at the same time, it wakes you up and kick-starts your digestion. As an aside, whenever my patients are getting ready to do their brain scans or to get their blood drawn, I always encourage them to drink a couple of glasses of warm water before we start the procedures. And what a difference it makes!

STEP 7. GO ORGANIC AS MUCH AS YOU CAN

Your body's estrogen is not only influenced by the foods you eat—it is also being altered by your environment: what you breathe, absorb, and consume on a regular basis. While natural estrogens can be safe and helpful, there are innumerable man-made chemicals that masquerade as estrogen but in reality are its evil twin. These are known as xeno-estrogens or endocrine disrupting compounds (EDCs). Scientists who study these substances, the Endocrine Society among them, regard EDCs as a serious environmental hazard that have a disruptive effect on hormonal health and thyroid function.

The impact of xenoestrogens on endocrine health continues to be studied but early evidence raises serious concerns. When we're routinely exposed to hormone disruptors, they fool our bodies into believing they are our own estrogens, which then causes a number of imbalances. Studies show that these substances not only wreak havoc on our endocrine system but also are stored in body fat for decades, the highest concentration of the toxins lodging in breast tissue. As you might conclude, this can lead to an increased risk of cancer. Additionally, xenoestrogens have been implicated in a number of disorders of the reproductive system, from "precocious puberty" (a phenomenon by which girls are becoming women at a younger and younger age) to infertility, endometriosis, miscarriages, and even males developing breasts.

On top of this, some pollutants do direct damage to our DNA, leading to all sorts of problems down the line. For example, pesticide exposure has been associated with an increased risk of Alzheimer's, especially in people with the APOE-4 gene. The most common pesticide, DDT, has been outlawed in the United States and Canada since the late 1970s but is still used in other countries. If you have the APOE-4 gene, pay even more attention to this information as well as to your exposure.

The widespread use of these synthetic chemicals in modern life has dramatically changed the chemical makeup of our environment, both inside and outside our bodies. More than eighty thousand different compounds are routinely used in manufacturing, agricultural, and consumer products to combat pests and infections, add convenience, save money, and increase productivity. Estrogen-disrupting compounds such as bisphenol A (BPA), polychlorinated biphenyl (PCB), and phthalates, to name a few, are contained in most plastic products, in the coating on cooking pans and utensils, and in countless additional sources.

Overall, we are constantly exposed to thousands of substances that can seriously mess with our hormones. I have summarized the most common sources in table 8.

TABLE 8. CHEMICALS THAT ARE XENOESTROGENS, AND WHERE THEY'RE FOUND

CATEGORY	WHAT	WHERE
Food additives	Erythrosin (FD&C Red No. 3)	Food dye
	Phenosulfothiazine	Food dye
	Butylated hydroxyanisole (BHA)	Food preservative
Insecticides, pesticides	Atrazine	Weed killer
	Dichlorodiphenyldichloroethylene (DDT), dichlorodiphenyl-dichloroethylene (DDE) dichlorodiphenyldichloroethane (DDD)	Insecticides
	Dieldrin, Endosulfan, Heptachlor, Lindane, Methoxychlor	Insecticides

	Glyphosate	Herbicide
	Nonylphenol and derivatives	Industrial surfactants, emulsifiers for emulsion polymerization, laboratory detergents, pesticides
Industrial products and plastics	Bisphenol A	Plastics
	Phthalates	Plastics, nail polish, hair spray
	Di-2-ethylhexyl phthalate (DEHP)	Plastics
	Polybrominated diphenyl ethers (PBDEs)	Plastics, foams, building materials, electronics, furnishings, motor vehicles
	Polychlorinated biphenyls (PCBs)	Plastics
	Alkylphenol	Cleaning detergents
	Chlorine and chlorine by-products	Cleaning detergents
Skin care	4-Methylbenzylidene camphor (4-MBC), benzophenone	Sunscreen lotions
	Parabens (methylparaben, ethylparaben, propylparaben, and butylparaben)	Cosmetic products, including makeup, moisturizers, hair care products, shaving creams/gels
	Formaldehyde, phenacetin, coal tar, benzene, methylene glycol, ethylene oxide, chromium, cadmium and its compounds, arsenic	Cosmetic products
Building supplies	Pentachlorophenol	General biocide and wood preservative
	Polychlorinated biphenyls (PCBs)	Electrical oils, lubricants, adhesives, paints

As far as our diets are concerned, more than fourteen thousand of these chemicals are used in our food alone. As many as 25 percent of the pesticides routinely sprayed on non-organic fruits and vegetables are known to disrupt the estrogen balance in the body. If you examine the labels of most foods in supermarkets today and know what you're looking for, you will see that chemicals have been added to "pretty up" foods and prolong their shelf life. Commercially raised non-organic dairy and meat products, especially from cattle and sheep, are also very likely to contain contaminants, given that all sorts of chemicals are routinely mixed into the animals' feed to grow them larger, faster. These same chemicals are stored in their fat and muscle, which you consume when you ingest their meat, milk, and any dairy products derived from that milk.

Given that most people eat at least three times a day every day, paying attention to our food choices is a significant first step to avoiding contamination and thereby protecting our bodies, our brains, and our hormones. Although many of you may wonder if it's really necessary, I urge you to choose organic foods as much as you can. While some experts maintain that pesticide levels in conventional food are safe for most people, the National Academy of Sciences has officially called that into question. Recent evidence shows that even low-level pesticide exposure can be significantly more toxic for children (due to their having less developed immune systems), pregnant women (putting added strain on their already taxed organs), and finally, for women in general. Current regulations ensure that organic food is free of pesticides and other harmful substances. Organic crops are generally grown without synthetic pesticides, artificial fertilizers, irradiation (a form of radiation used to kill bacteria), or biotechnology. Animals on organic farms eat organically grown feed, aren't confined as they sometimes are on conventional farms, and are raised without antibiotics or synthetic growth hormones.

Additionally, according to some research, organic food tests at higher nutritional levels than its conventional counterpart. In the absence of pesticides and fertilizers, plants naturally multiply their vitamin, mineral, and phytochemical content, the latter strengthening their resistance to bugs and weeds. As you eat these more resistant plants, you, too, benefit from this same protection.

The only downside is that organic food is generally expensive, an issue that I address at length in *Brain Food*. One way to reduce the cost is to prioritize which foods, due to their inherent vulnerability to pesticides and other contaminants, really need to be purchased organic, and then to just do your best with the rest.

Produce is the highest priority food to buy organic, to avoid pesticide residues. But even within that category, you can cut costs with this loose guideline: if a fruit or vegetable has a peel that you eat, buy organic. If you don't eat the peel of the fruit or vegetable, buying organic is less critical. As a rule of thumb:

- The most contaminated produce, which you should try to always buy organic, includes these fruits: apples, cherries, grapes, nectarines, peaches, pears, and strawberries; and these vegetables: bell peppers, celery, potatoes, spinach, and tomatoes.

- Conventional produce that is safer, and that you don't need to buy organic, includes asparagus, avocados, broccoli, cabbage, cantaloupes, cauliflower, eggplant, honeydew, kiwis, mangos, onions, papayas, pineapple, sweet corn, and sweet peas.

- Other products fall somewhere in between, so just buy them organic whenever possible.

Animal foods are another very high priority for buying organic. Most commercial meats and fish are exposed to antibiotics and unhealthy hormones, among other things, so:

- Reduce your consumption of beef, lamb, and their dairy products, and focus on poultry and eggs, preferably organic and free-range. Chicken, turkey, and duck meats, as well as goat meat and dairy, are safer to consume. Note: organic birds can't be fed poultry litter or arsenic drugs.

- When you eat red meat, look for organic meat that's also labeled "Grass-Fed Approved" or "USDA Process Verified Grass-Fed," which guarantees that the animal was raised on a diet of grass and forage, with access to a pasture. Also, grass-fed beef tends to have a higher concentration of omega-3s.

- "Organic" labels on fish and shellfish are meaningless because there are no government-approved organic standards for seafood. As a rule of thumb, wild-caught fish is healthier and safer than farm-raised fish. Frozen or canned wild-caught fish is cheaper than fresh fish and just as nutritious.

STEP 8. EAT LESS

New research indicates that reducing our caloric intake can boost cognitive capacity, reduce cellular aging, and promote longevity. The strategy behind this practice is based on nearly a century of scientific data showing that stressing our bodies and brains via calorie restriction pushes our cells to grow stronger and more resilient. Just as muscles get stronger the greater the resistance, so do your brain cells strengthen as they resist hunger. Caloric restriction also boosts the brain's antioxidant defense system, which is particularly important for the female brain.

Additionally, caloric restriction can be a great way to lose a few pounds, if you need to. As discussed before, keeping a healthy and stable weight is beneficial for women. Since excess body fat contributes to the development of insulin resistance, diabetes, and heart disease, as well as hot flashes, carefully planned, medically supervised weight loss for women who need to lose weight may help reduce these symptoms (refer to chapter 6 to determine if you need to shed some pounds). Clinical trials have shown that overweight women who lost weight over the course of the study also reported a dramatic reduction, and in some cases a complete elimination, of hot flashes in as little as one year. Additionally, there is strong evidence that being overweight increases the risk of breast cancer post-menopause, while maintaining a healthy weight is an effective way to reduce this risk.

There are different and specific ways to practice caloric restriction, fasting among them, which are all outlined below. I am not advising you to undertake any of these options in the haphazard, experimental way often offered by popularized diets. For example, when it comes to fasting, reactions differ, and frankly, it isn't for everyone. If you are underweight, suffer from hypoglycemia, or have an eating disorder, fasting may not be for you. Same goes if you are experiencing unexplained weight loss, muscle loss, or bone frailty. Be sure to discuss this practice with your doctor before starting.

Caloric Restriction

Caloric restriction, or reducing calories within reason, aims at reducing your habitual caloric intake by 30 to 40 percent. So instead of consuming an average of 1,500 calories a day, one would consume 900 to 1,100 calories per day. A clinical trial of fifty healthy, normal-to-overweight elderly participants showed that those on the calorie-restricted plan had a 20 percent improved memory performance in as little as three months. Those who stuck to the diet more closely also showed markedly improved insulin levels and reduced inflammation.

The 5:2 Diet

This plan involves eating normally five days a week and eating no more than 600 calories a day for the remaining two days of the week. Some studies showed that this regimen is effective at reducing inflammation and insulin resistance and lowering blood pressure, cholesterol, and triglycerides, especially in women who have more weight to lose. For example, in a study of more than 100 overweight and obese women, those who followed the 5:2 diet not only lost weight but also showed a reduced risk of cardiovascular and inflammatory markers after just six months on the diet.

Intermittent Fasting

Intermittent fasting or "time-restricted feeding" can provide many important health benefits, from "rebooting" your metabolism to helping your body burn fat more efficiently—and it doesn't involve counting calories. Of the many intermittent fasting schedules available, overnight fasting is my personal favorite. You allow yourself a twelve-hour break between dinner and breakfast the next morning, during which time you are not eating or snacking, which you shouldn't be doing anyway! This simple practice has been shown to reduce adipose body fat, improve insulin sensitivity, and protect against obesity and diabetes.

Here's how you start: Have dinner early, around 6:00 p.m. or so, and refrain from eating until 6:00 the following morning (drinking water and unsweetened herbal tea is totally fine). This food-free window will achieve for you a reasonably effortless twelve-hour fast since you'll sleep through most of it. If this window of time doesn't work for you, there is some flexibility. Some people prefer to have a later dinner around 8:00 p.m. and refrain from eating until 8:00 a.m. the following day. Find the schedule that works best for you, and when you are ready, try to increase it to fourteen or even sixteen hours if you can.

All that said, intermittent fasting works only in the context of a balanced, nutritionally dense diet. In this case, whatever calories you are consuming best be healthy ones. If you go without eating for fourteen hours as an excuse to then inhale 3,000 calories' worth of pizza in what remains of the day, that will clearly defeat the purpose!

I'd argue that just eating less throughout the day may very well be equally effective. For example, the Okinawa centenarian women have adopted the philosophy of *hara hachi bu*, in which they stop eating when they are 80 percent full—a practice that's been tied to their longevity. As most people in Western countries tend to eat too much to start with, paying more attention to portion size and meal frequency can only help. One efficient way to consume fewer calories and maintain nutritional quality is to increase consumption of low-glycemic fruit, vitamin-rich vegetables, lean protein, and essential fats, while "squeezing out" sugary, fatty, and processed foods. To further optimize a woman's health, it is also important to focus on fiber-rich and estrogenic foods that balance hormonal levels and minimize the risk of chronic diseases, while restoring energy levels throughout the entire body and brain.

Now that we've discussed what foods to put on our plates, let's make it even easier. A detailed protocol, complete with meal plans, recipes, and healthy swaps, is included in appendix B. It is important to note that for many women this diet plan can be just as effective as MHT or antidepressants—and is undoubtedly better tolerated than either. In the next chapter, we'll also discuss select supplements that will further aid in your quest.

To achieve its maximum prevention and disease-combating potential, nutritional optimization for brain health is best initiated well before any cognitive decline begins. That said, a good nutrition can't help but put you at an advantage, "late bloomer" or otherwise! Your quality of life can be enhanced by these practices regardless of your age, genetics, or medical predispositions. In a world that presents the particular challenges reviewed in these chapters, it is a relief to know that the decision to be selective about the food we eat has the power to safeguard, rejuvenate, and replenish us, no matter what.

CHAPTER 11

SUPPLEMENTS FOR WOMEN'S BRAINS

IN WESTERN SOCIETIES, THE GENERAL trend is to rely on pharmaceuticals rather than on nature. Supplements, herbal remedies in particular, are often disregarded as harmless or even bland. Perhaps that's why, when you are at the doctor's office filling out an admission form, you'll find a long section for medication history and a shorter section (if there's one at all) for vitamins and "other." Very few clinicians will actually read the "other" list. Hardly anyone will be interested in how many cups of green tea you drink every day.

But times are changing. The World Health Organization estimates that 80 percent of people worldwide now rely on herbal medicines for some part of their primary health care. During the past few decades, public dissatisfaction with the cost of prescription medications, combined with an interest in returning to natural remedies, has led to a dramatic increase in the use of herbal medicine in industrialized countries. This is quite a turnaround for our highly "drugged" society, where the typical American senior takes an average of eighteen prescriptions per year.

As our approach to health is opening up to integrative practices, herbal preparations are becoming more mainstream, especially as a result of serious improvements in analysis and quality control. Nowadays, the herbalist's arsenal can be an important aid for prevention and management of at least some medical concerns.

But do they work for your *brain*?

Today, more than a quarter of adults in the U.S. age fifty and older take at least one supplement for brain-health reasons. Brain-health supplements—vitamins, minerals, herbal mixtures, nutraceuticals, and nootropic drugs—generated $3 billion in sales globally in 2016 and are projected to reach $5.8 billion by 2023. More and more people are turning to these often heavily advertised remedies to gain an edge at work and in life. Others still take supplements in hopes of preserving memory and fending off dementia.

In 2019, I had the honor to join the Global Council on Brain Health (GCBH), a collaborative of scientists, doctors, and policy experts brought together by AARP. Our first task force focused on supplements for brain health, and whether they are worth your money and trust. After undertaking an evidence review of supplements' potential effectiveness, the GCBH determined it could not endorse any ingredient, product, or supplement formulation designed for brain health. Basically, unless you have a nutritional deficiency or subclinical deficiency, most supplements are a massive waste of money.

As a brain scientist, I am well aware that supplements cannot replace a healthy diet or a healthy lifestyle. This is particularly important as recent research, including my own work, supports the notion that nutritional supplementation is not equivalent to absorbing our nutrients from the whole foods we eat. For example, there is strong evidence that a lifelong diversified diet that includes an abundance of antioxidant-rich foods is superior to gleaning these nutrients from artificial supplements. Too many people shortcut to pills rather than improving their diet to reach their nutritional requirements.

However, if you haven't been eating enough nutrient-dense foods, or if you have a medical condition that limits absorption of some nutrients, supplements can help correct insufficiencies. And if you have any medical concerns that can be resolved with supplements instead of mind-altering medications, it is certainly worth trying the supplements first.

This is particularly the case for women, as some vitamins and herbal products have been proven to help improve mood, sleep, and the discomforts of menopause. Some of these remedies have not only been used for centuries by women all over the world, but have also validated clinical efficacy. For example, not getting enough B vitamins and omega-3s can contribute to depression in women, especially during menopause. Carefully planned doses of these supplements have been associated with positive outcomes in at least some patients with mild depression, as well as with sustained memory, focus, and mental clarity.

The tables below include supplements that are indicated for specific concerns, from memory support and Alzheimer's prevention to stress management and hormonal support. Only supplements with established clinical efficacy are reviewed. You might find that supplements you're already taking are not included in the list, which means they are not as effective, or as scientifically valid, as you were led to believe. In that case, and especially if they don't seem to make much of a difference, toss them.

A word of caution before we start looking into options. Most supplements and herbal remedies carry a low risk of harm, but some can interact with prescription medications or cause unexpected problems. Major interactions are reported in the tables below. Try this website to check for minor to moderate interactions: www.rxlist.com/drug -interaction-checker.htm.

MEMORY SUPPORT AND ALZHEIMER'S PREVENTION

Over two decades of research on risk factors for dementia has yielded promising findings about which nutrients and other dietary components are required for normal physiological functioning of the brain, neuronal protection against cell injury and oxidative stress, and dementia prevention. Epidemiological studies and clinical trials have provided early firm evidence that specific nutrients may be protective against Alzheimer's. These are chiefly B vitamins such as B6, B12, and folate, omega-3 fatty acids, and vitamins C and E.

Obtaining these nutrients from foods is the best choice by far, as supplements don't work for everyone. However, supplements can be helpful if you are low in these nutrients, or if you have concomitant medical conditions that can be ameliorated by these nutrients, improving your memory in turn.

B vitamins are crucial for a healthy nervous system, thanks in part to their balancing effects on homocysteine levels (see chapter 6). Randomized, double-blind, placebo-controlled trials of mild cognitive impairment patients showed that, over a two-year period, high-dose B vitamin supplementation not only maintained memory performance, but at the same time reduced the rate of brain shrinkage when measured via MRI scans. While more research is needed to assess B vitamin effects among individuals without cognitive impairments, it's long been known that our metabolism naturally slows down with age, and absorption of B vitamins, especially B12, may decrease as a result. So, if you are over fifty, it is important that you talk to your doctor about getting tested for possible B vitamin deficiencies and absorption issues as well as homocysteine levels. If you have high homocysteine, B vitamins can help, especially when taken together with omega-3s.

Additionally, as mentioned in chapter 6, if you suffer from gastritis, reduced stomach acid, Crohn's or celiac disease, or take medications for diabetes, acid blockers, or birth control pills, talk to your doctor about having your vitamin B status checked, as all these conditions can negatively impact your B vitamin levels. Vegan and strict vegetarian diets can also lead to B12 deficiencies.

Omega-3 oils are potent anti-inflammatories that support the heart and brain. Although results are not always consistent, for people with low omega-3 levels, supplementation has been associated with reduced brain shrinkage, better memory, and a lower risk of dementia, particularly in APOE-4 carriers. Omega-3s are also helpful to counteract symptoms of low mood and mild depression, especially in women experiencing hormonal changes (see "Mood Support and Mild Depression," below). Vegan and strict vegetarian diets can lead to omega-3 deficiencies, while the typical Western diet can lead to low omega-3 index measures (see chapter 6 for recommended testing).

Additionally, as mentioned in chapter 10, vitamins C and E are strong antioxidants that help boost the immune system, and have been associated with a reduced risk of dementia. These vitamins are particularly important for peri- and post-menopausal women (see "Hormonal Support and Menopausal Symptoms" and "Sleep Support," below), as well as for smokers and ex-smokers, women with high CRP levels (see chapter 6), and those consistently exposed to environmental toxins (see chapter 14).

There is some evidence that ginkgo biloba might also help with age-related cognitive decline. Although the results are not unanimous, some clinical trials showed beneficial effects on attention, memory, and overall cognitive function, especially in patients experiencing reduced blood and oxygen flow to the brain—for example, following a TBI or stroke. However, ginkgo has quite a few contraindications, so be careful (see chart below).

Other supplements, including ginseng, turmeric, and a variety of so-called nootropic drugs, haven't shown consistent efficacy in clinical trials and are not recommended at this time.

TABLE 9. MEMORY SUPPORT AND ALZHEIMER'S PREVENTION

(**** = HIGH; * = LOW)

SUPPLEMENT	INDICATED FOR	EFFICACY	DOSAGE
B vitamins (B6, B12, folate)	• Women of all ages with low blood levels of B vitamins and/or high homocysteine. • Vegans and strict vegetarians.	***	B-complex formula that contains 500 mcg of vitamin B12, 600–800 mcg of folic acid, and 10–50 mg of vitamin B6, taken daily with food. The easiest way is to take one B-complex vitamin, or separate pills, with the closest amounts that you can find. If your plasma levels don't improve after 3–4 weeks of supplementation, talk to your doctor about switching to methylated B vitamins (methylcobalamin and methylfolate).
Omega-3s	• Women of all ages with low blood levels of omega-3s. • Women over 50 or who are post-menopausal, especially APOE-4 carriers. • Vegans and strict vegetarians.	***	If you eat fish: high-purity omega-3 fish oil containing 500–800 mg DHA and 300–500 mg EPA/day, especially if you are 60 or older. If you don't eat fish: 2,000 mg of omega-3 DHA or DHA + EPA/day from DHA-rich high-purity algae oil. For APOE-4 carriers: 800 mg–1.8 g/day of DHA from either high-purity omega-3 fish oil or DHA-rich high-purity algae oil.

Supplement	Who should consider it		Details
Omega-3s (cont'd)			[Warning: Moderate interactions with blood-thinning medications, such as warfarin and heparin. Too much omega-3 can result in bleeding and bruising.]
Vitamins C and E	• Women over 50 or who are peri- or post-menopausal. • Smokers and ex-smokers. • Women exposed to environmental toxins. • Women with high CRP levels.	***	150–200 mg daily of vitamin C for at least 6 months, and 1,000–2,000 IU/day of a mixed tocopherol complex (containing alpha, beta, gamma, and delta tocopherols) for at least 6 months. [Warning: If you have a condition such as heart disease or diabetes, do not take more than 400 IU/day.]
Ginkgo biloba	• Women with a history of TBI, concussion, or stroke (discuss with your doctor).	*	240 mg/day of ginkgo extract for 6 months. [Warning: Moderate interactions with blood thinners, NSAIDs, anti-platelet drugs, anticonvulsants, antidepressants, diabetes medicines, and Saint-John's-wort.]

HORMONAL SUPPORT AND MENOPAUSAL SYMPTOMS

Throughout the centuries, several herbal supplements and more recently vitamins have been used to alleviate hot flashes and night sweats. The most commonly used plants are soy, red clover, and some herbs like black cohosh and Siberian ginseng.

There is increasing evidence that soy isoflavones could be an alternative to MHT, at least for some women. For example, in one study of 60 post-menopausal women, those who received isoflavone supplementation for sixteen weeks had a 50 percent reduction in hot flashes, while those on MHT had a 46 percent reduction. But keep in mind that there are different forms of isoflavones: genistein, daidzein, and glycitein. Isoflavone preparations that provide higher amounts of genistein are considerably more effective in reducing hot flashes. However, these supplements are not effective against night sweats, insomnia, or depression.

If night sweats are disrupting your sleep, you don't want to rely on chance. So instead of searching for a mythical four-leaf clover, seek out red clover. Red clover isoflavones are quite good at easing night sweats. Discuss this with your doctor first though if you are on the birth control pill, MHT, or taking cancer medications, especially tamoxifen.

Whether to use isoflavones is a decision best made in consultation with a physician, considering a woman's diet, age, individual health conditions and risks, other medications and supplements she's already using, and the severity of her menopause symptoms. Isoflavones are commonly well tolerated without any serious side effects. But because they function like estrogen in the body, long-term use may carry risks.

A safer option is found in vitamin E, the only vitamin with proven clinical efficacy in reducing hot flashes, possibly because of its restorative action on estrogen levels. Clinical trials reported a significant decline in the occurrence of hot flashes after four weeks of vitamin E supplementation at a dose of 400 IUs per day. Vitamin E may be particularly important for peri- and post-menopausal women (see "Memory Support and Alzheimer's Prevention"), as well as for smokers and ex-smokers, women with high CRP levels (see chapter 6), and those consistently exposed to environmental toxins (see chapter 14).

Other commonly used herbs are black cohosh and ginseng. Although the effects of black cohosh are not consistent, some studies show that the combination of black cohosh with isoflavones or vitamin E resulted in reduced hot flashes. Likewise, Siberian ginseng is often prescribed in China to help fatigue, headaches, insomnia, and depression during menopause, although there is no strong evidence that it is superior to a placebo. However, many women have told me that these herbs can help ameliorate hot flashes, as well as headaches and palpitations. Ginseng also seems effective at relieving stress and restoring sexual energy, at least in some women. I'd try the other remedies first, but discuss it with your doctor.

Other products, including Saint-John's-wort, evening primrose oil, chaste tree, and wild yam haven't shown efficacy in clinical trials and are not recommended at this time.

TABLE 10. HORMONAL SUPPORT AND MENOPAUSAL SYMPTOMS

(**** = HIGH; * = LOW)

SUPPLE-MENT	INDICATED FOR	EFFICACY	DOSAGE
Vitamin E	• All women, especially those over 50 or who are peri- or post-menopausal. • Smokers and ex-smokers. • Women exposed to environmental toxins. • Women with high CRP levels.	****	400–800 IU/day of a mixed tocopherol complex (containing alpha, beta, gamma, and delta tocopherols). [Warning: If you have a condition such as heart disease or diabetes, do not take more than 400 IU/day.]

Soy isoflavones	• Peri- and post-menopausal women experiencing hot flashes (in the absence of contraindications).	****	40–50 mg/day for 12–16 weeks.
Red clover isoflavones	• Peri- and post-menopausal women experiencing night sweats (in the absence of contraindications).	***	80 mg/day for 12–16 weeks. [Warning: moderate interactions with birth control pills, MHT, and tamoxifen.]
Black cohosh	• Peri- and post-menopausal women experiencing hot flashes (in the absence of contraindications).	*	20–40 mg of a standardized extract taken twice a day, for no more than 6 months in combination with isoflavones or vitamin E. [Warning: Moderate interactions with birth control pills, MHT, and blood pressure medicines.]
Siberian ginseng	• Peri- and post-menopausal women experiencing hot flashes (in the absence of contraindications).	*	400 mg/day of Siberian ginseng standardized to contain 4–5.6 mg andrographolide. [Warning: Do not take with blood-thinning medications (e.g., warfarin and aspirin).]

MOOD SUPPORT AND MILD DEPRESSION

Antidepressants are often prescribed to women over forty, and perhaps too easily. Unless you suffer from severe depression, the recommendations contained in this book, from a healthy diet to exercise and good sleep hygiene, could do wonders to lift your mood. Additionally, here are some clinically validated supplements that may help with mild depression, especially if emotional distress and mood swings are caused by the hormonal fluctuations associated with approaching menopause.

Saint-John's-wort seems particularly promising in alleviating depressive symptoms. Based on clinical trials showing that this herb seems to be about as effective as many antidepressants, the American College of Physicians' guidelines suggest that Saint-John's-wort be considered an option for short-term treatment of mild depression, including for peri- and post-menopausal women. Saint-John's-wort is *not* safe to take with antidepressant medications, and is not recommended for moderate to severe depression. It is, however, safe to take together with the next supplement on the list, omega-3s.

Probably thanks to their anti-inflammatory properties, omega-3s can also help with both hormone-related mood swings and symptoms of mild depression. Several randomized clinical trials reported beneficial effects of combined DHA and EPA supplementation on depressed mood, especially in women.

TABLE 11. MOOD SUPPORT AND MILD DEPRESSION
(**** = HIGH; * = LOW)

SUPPLE-MENT	INDICATED FOR	EFFI-CACY	DOSAGE
Saint-John's-wort	• Women experiencing "the blues" or mild depression, as well as related symptoms such as nervousness, tiredness, and trouble sleeping. • Women experiencing mood changes during perimenopause and post-menopause.	****	300 mg Saint-John's-wort extract (standardized to 0.3%–0.5% hypericin content) 3 times daily for no longer than 3–4 months. [Warning: Do not take together with any of these medications: Xanax, birth control pills, antidepressants, HIV medications, pain medications, and sedatives. Stop using for at least 2 weeks before a surgery.]

| Omega-3s | • Women of all ages with low blood levels of omega-3s.
• Women experiencing mood changes during peri- and post-menopause.
• Vegans and strict vegetarians. | *** | If you eat fish: 950 mg/day of high-purity omega-3 fish oil containing DHA + EPA. If you don't eat fish: 2,000 mg of omega-3 DHA + EPA/day from DHA-rich high-purity algae oil. [Warning: Moderate interactions with blood-thinning medications such as warfarin and heparin. Too much omega-3 can result in bleeding and bruising.] |

SLEEP SUPPORT

Unless you suffer from sleep apnea or another medical condition that disrupts your sleep, the recommendations contained in this book, from a healthy diet to exercise and good sleep hygiene, could do wonders to coax your mind to sleep. Additionally, here are some validated supplements that might help you relax and get a good night's sleep.

Melatonin, a hormone produced by the brain, is probably the most effective. Melatonin helps control sleep cycles. Because sleep and mood are closely connected, supplementing with melatonin can alleviate stress and help you fall asleep. If you're waking up in the middle of the night, try the extended-release preparation. If that doesn't work, try valerian root instead.

Valerian root, a herb commonly used to treat insomnia, anxiety, and stress, can be effective in helping you fall asleep and stay asleep, as it shortens sleep latency and reduces nighttime waking.

But if your sleep is disturbed because of perimenopause or low progesterone (or both), try vitamin C. Clinical trials show that, at doses of 750 mg per day, vitamin C is effective in raising progesterone levels by over 50 percent in as little as three months, which also seems to restore sleep. If vitamin C doesn't help, try progesterone creams. There are different varieties of creams that include bioidentical or natural progesterone. Some clinical trials demonstrate that they all can be effective for hot flashes and disturbed sleep.

Finally, quite a few women take magnesium for sleep support. Magnesium is a mineral essential for nerve and muscle function. Multiple studies have shown that, while magnesium is crucial for sleep, the effects of supplementation are not very consistent. I'd recommend trying the other supplements first.

TABLE 12. SLEEP SUPPORT
(**** = HIGH; * = LOW)

SUPPLE-MENT	INDICATED FOR	EFFICACY	DOSAGE
Melatonin	All women, except patients taking sedative medications.	****	Start with 1 mg at bedtime for no more than 2 weeks. If 1 mg isn't effective, bump it up to 3 mg. The maximum dose is 6 mg. If this is not effective, melatonin isn't the right fit. [Warning: Do not take with sedatives.]
Valerian root	All women, especially those having trouble staying asleep.	***	Drink one cup of valerian tea at bedtime. For pills, the starting dose is 400 mg one hour before bedtime. If you have a tincture, try 2 to 5 droppers full.
Vitamin C	Perimenopausal and post-menopausal women with low progesterone levels.	***	750 mg/day for about 3 months.
Progesterone creams	Perimenopausal and post-menopausal women with low progesterone levels.	***	Rub ¼ teaspoon (about the size of a dime) into your arms where the skin is thin and hairless, for at least 2 weeks.

Magnesium	All women.	*	200 mg of magnesium citrate one hour before bedtime. If 200 mg doesn't work, increase to 400 mg as long as it doesn't cause loose stools. Magnesium creams to rub on the skin are also available.

STRESS AND ANXIETY

Stress has become an unwelcome addition to our daily lives. While it is tempting to declare one stressor more significant than another, our bodies perceive all stress equally. Cortisol levels rise, neurotransmitter levels become erratic, key nutrients are depleted, and hormone levels become difficult to predict. While stress is pervasive, there are ways to mitigate its effects, which are reviewed in chapter 13. Additionally, some supplements have been shown to help alleviate stress and its symptoms.

B vitamins, especially vitamins B12 and B5, are in high demand for support of cell metabolism, for production of hormones, and for a healthy nervous system—by which they help combat the effects of stress. Our metabolism naturally slows down with age, and absorption of B vitamins, especially B12, may decrease as a result. If you are over fifty, it is important that you talk to your doctor about getting tested for possible B vitamin deficiencies as well as absorption issues. Additionally, if you suffer from gastritis, reduced stomach acid, Crohn's or celiac disease, or take medications for diabetes, acid blockers, or birth control pills, talk to your doctor about having your vitamin B status checked. Vegan and strict vegetarian diets can also lead to B12 deficiencies.

Additionally, rhodiola and ashwagandha are adaptogenic herbs with stress-relief properties. Adaptogens are a group of plants that can help your body adapt to physical, chemical, and environmental stress. Clinical trials show that rhodiola helps balance the stress hormone cortisol, while supporting the immune system and balancing blood sugar regulation. If you suffer from stress-related fatigue and ultimate burnout, consider taking rhodiola along with practicing regular exercise and relaxation techniques. Ashwagandha, a herb used for centuries in Ayurvedic medicine, is also a common remedy for stress, especially for stress mixed with mild depression or low mood. While the evidence is not conclusive, some clinical trials showed a 44 percent reduction in stress levels after taking ashwagandha, paralleled by reduced cortisol levels after just sixty days. Ashwagandha may be taken safely along with antidepressants, which is not the case for many other supplements.

Finally, there's some evidence that gamma-aminobutyric acid (GABA) supplements can help promote relaxation, reduce anxiety during times of stress, and even reduce PMS symptoms. GABA tends to be calming without being sedating, so it's fine to take during the day.

TABLE 13. MANAGEMENT OF STRESS AND ANXIETY
(**** = HIGH; * = LOW)

SUPPLEMENT	INDICATED FOR	EFFICACY	DOSAGE
B vitamins	All women under stress, especially if over 50.	****	B-complex that contains at least 50 mcg of vitamin B12 and 100 mg of vitamin B5 (pantothenic acid), taken daily with food.
Rhodiola	All women experiencing stress-related fatigue and burnout.	***	200–400 mg/day, whether in capsules or liquid form.
Ashwagandha	All women experiencing stress mixed with low mood.	*	300 mg per day in tablets; or tea for milder stress levels.
GABA (gamma-aminobutyric acid)	All women experiencing stress-related anxiety mixed with drowsiness.	*	500 mg as needed in times of stress.

METABOLISM SUPPORT AND INSULIN REGULATION

As we age, our metabolism—that calorie-burning engine we rely on to keep our brains active while also keeping extra pounds off—slows down. The years leading to menopause can be marked by a decline in brain and bodily energy, leaving women exhausted and forgetful, but also more prone to developing insulin resistance and weight gain. Our best bet is to turn to two old standbys, diet and exercise (see chapters 10 and 12), and also to seek a little extra help from supplements known to boost metabolism and maintain blood sugar levels.

As mentioned in "Stress and Anxiety," rhodiola is an adaptogenic herb with stress-relief but also fat-burning properties. If you suffer from stress-related weight gain or cravings, taking rhodiola along with regular exercise may help accelerate your weight-loss efforts.

Women with high blood sugar levels may benefit from different supplements, namely berberine and cacao flavonols. Some research suggests that taking 500 mg of berberine 2 to 3 times daily for up to three months might help control blood sugar as effectively as the diabetes medications metformin or rosiglitazone. Berberine, however, is not for everybody. A more gentle approach is found in cacao flavonols, which have been shown to improve markers of cardiovascular health in women with high blood sugar levels and insulin resistance. You can find cacao flavonols as commercial preparations. That said, my favorite way to obtain these healthful nutrients is by consuming 90 to 100 percent raw cacao powder, either as cacao tea (www.lisamosconi .com/recipes/cacao-tea) or simply as a piece of sugar-free 100 percent dark chocolate.

TABLE 14. METABOLISM SUPPORT AND INSULIN REGULATION

(**** = HIGH; * = LOW)

SUPPLE-MENT	INDICATED FOR	EFFICACY	DOSAGE
Rhodiola	Women' experiencing weight gain, especially if stress-related.	****	100 mg/day.
Berberine	Women with high blood sugar levels.	**	The appropriate dose of berberine depends on several factors, such as your age, medical health, and several other conditions. Speak to your doctor. [Warning: Major interactions with immunosuppressants such as cyclosporine.]
Cocoa flavonols	Women with high blood sugar levels and/or insulin resistance.	**	150–200 mg of cocoa flavonols/day, mixed with water or milk. Best if taken in the morning. If well tolerated, increase the dose to 375 mg/day. Do not exceed 900 mg/day. Limit use to 1 to 2 weeks under medical supervision.

CHAPTER 12

WOMEN AND EXERCISE: COULD LESS BE MORE?

WHEN IT COMES TO BEING PHYSICALLY ACTIVE, there's no shortage of good reasons to get a move on. If avoiding heart disease, stroke, and type 2 diabetes aren't motivation enough, relieving depression and anxiety and maintaining a healthy weight also make for convincing arguments. There's another reason, though, one that applies especially to our brains. Exercise causes actual physical changes in the brain that not only act as a safeguard against future dementia, but also invigorate our abilities to think, reason, and remember the here and now. Evidence shows that there are no two ways about it: our brains receive positive benefits every time we don our sneakers and move away from the couch.

The undeniable boon that physical exercise brings to brain function is evident on multiple fronts. First off, physical activity promotes heart health, and what's good for the heart is good for the brain. Aerobic exercise in particular—the kind of exercise that makes your heart beat faster—enhances blood flow and circulation, pumping more oxygen and nutrients to the brain. It is this enhanced blood flow that makes you feel clearheaded post-exercise, while working its magic behind the scenes, slowing plaque buildup deep in your arteries. Plus, when we move our bodies enough, endorphins, our body's natural painkillers, flow freely, automatically lifting our mood. Serotonin is released, relaxing and "happifying" us. The antidepressant effects of exercise have also been linked to a drop in stress hormones, which, let's face it, we all could use.

At the same time, exercise stimulates the production of growth hormones, brain-derived neurotrophic factor (BDNF) among them. BDNF promotes our neurons' abilities to build new connections and acts as a first-aid kit for any brain cells in need of repair. Thanks to that, our brain experiences increased plasticity and connectivity, improving our ability to both make and retain memories. Plus, exercise keeps our DNA young! In several studies, higher levels of exercise have been linked to a good nine fewer years of aging at the cellular level.

Exercise is not only a muscle-building, stress-busting, endorphin-releasing memory enhancer and time reverser—it powers up the immune system, too. Regular exercise turns down inflammation, increasing our defenses against a variety of diseases, not the least of which is Alzheimer's.

YOU GOT TO MOVE IT, MOVE IT

The positive effects of exercise are particularly evident when we peer into the brain via brain scans. When comparing the scans of people who exercise with the scans of those who don't, we catch a glimpse of a very tangible picture of what these improvements look like inside our heads. The parts of the brain that control thinking and memory in the exercising participants not only show heightened activity in the regions responsible for processing and recall, but also an actual physical enlargement of those areas. However strange this sounds, this is a good thing, mind you, as this "plumping up" results in better reasoning and memory performance.

These results are not the only findings. Study after study shows that leading an active lifestyle really keeps your brain younger. On brain scans, as compared to physically active people, the sedentary ones show an acceleration of cellular aging and brain shrinkage, while also exhibiting a much higher number of Alzheimer's plaques. When my colleagues and I looked into this further using brain scans, we found similar results in people who were as young as thirty, forty, and fifty, indicating that a sedentary lifestyle triggers adverse brain changes far ahead of time.

We also have multiple clinical trials reporting that even an activity as simple as brisk walking can slow down brain shrinkage. In one of the most convincing trials to date, 120 sedentary adults were divided into two groups. Half were assigned to a walking program to improve aerobic fitness, and were asked to increase their walking speed and duration until they reached forty minutes of continuous brisk walking, three times a week. ("Brisk walking" means walking as one does when in a hurry, as if late for an appointment.) The other half of the participants were assigned to a toning regime that included yoga and stretching, without brisk walking. A year later, the stretching group showed 1 to 2 percent brain shrinkage, which is considered normal in older adults. The walkers, on the other hand, exhibited a 2 percent *increase* in brain size instead. This increase specifically took place in the memory centers of the brain and produced a measurable improvement in memory performance, rolling back the clock by a good two years.

Overall, clinical trials and observational studies support the concept that exercise improves cognitive function, and in some cases can prevent the onset of cognitive decline later in life. But not only that. Although more evidence is needed to firmly establish causality, research shows that physical activity can counteract many aspects of one's DNA too. Recent breakthroughs indicate that physical activity can make all the difference for people with the aggressive genetic mutations that cause Alzheimer's. In one example of this, among family members carrying the mutations, those who engaged in regular exercise had markedly lowered levels of Alzheimer's plaques as compared with those who exercised less or not at all. Very similar results are shown in people with the APOE-4 gene and those with a family history of dementia: those who exercise are better off than those who don't.

These discoveries have upended previous historical misconceptions that our lifestyle had too little power to mitigate the onset and progression of diseases like Alzheimer's. Thanks to the later research, it is now acknowledged that not only is keeping your body moving a crucial component of leading a brain-healthy life, but it also has the effect of "turning back the clock" and reducing genetic risk. Today, lack of physical activity is currently listed as one of the top risk factors for

Alzheimer's, ranked even higher than conditions such as diabetes, obesity, or hypertension.

WOMEN AND EXERCISE: MOTIVATORS, BARRIERS, AND REMEMBERING TO HAVE FUN

Current statistics show that most of us aren't on the move nearly as much as we need to be. According to the Centers for Disease Control, less than 40 percent of adults engage in even two and a half hours of physical activity per week. Twenty percent don't do any formal exercise at all. Worse still, when the data was broken down by gender, it turned out that women were less likely than men to exercise, at any age.

At first glance, this might seem peculiar. Looking more deeply though, this stat belies historical sociocultural clues about the world in which we live. First, a look backward. In the United States, which is generally thought of as a "progressive" country, female students did not even have access to physical education in schools until 1823. Even then, it took several more decades for girls to be allowed to exercise in proper workout clothes instead of in their skirts and stockings, which clearly inhibited any real physical "education."

Although exercise is now more strongly encouraged than ever before in modern history, women still exercise less than men, and the divergence begins at a relatively young age. A study of over 9,000 American schoolchildren found that not only do females tend to exercise less than their male counterparts, but the disparities grow wider once high school ends. Once this period of soccer games, track practices, and cheerleading is over, 73 percent of males remain active, while only 62 percent of females do. For women of color, this drop-off in exercising is even starker. Of the 70 percent who were physically active in their teens, only 45 percent remain active into their twenties.

Getting married and starting a family seem to play a big part in this. Likely due to gender roles in parenthood, as well as to the roles attributed to marital status, married women with children often end up further hampered from exercising. While both parents tend to exercise less than their child-free counterparts, mothers also tend to eat less healthily and gain more weight than women without children. In comparison, the average father's body mass doesn't generally differ from that of men without children. Although the "dad bod" may exist, it isn't nearly as prevalent or dramatic as what's happening to their spouses.

Fortunately, some moms manage to catch a break once their children are old enough to start kindergarten, succeeding in accessing more time to exercise. For many women, however, that much coveted "me time" can coincide with their ovaries getting ready to slow down and close up shop—and when you can't sleep and are not feeling at your best, hitting the gym is probably the last thing on your mind. Of course, this part of the equation doesn't affect only those of us who are moms. In the years leading up to menopause, and even more so post-menopause, the drop in hormones can trigger fatigue, slow our metabolism, promote achy joints, and reduce stamina, all combining to make the couch appear far more inviting than, well, getting off it. This is independent of how active most women were in the past.

Perhaps as a result, recent statistics report that as a whole, women in midlife are by far the largest demographic to exercise inconsistently. This deeper drop-off in physical activity unfortunately comes at the same time that we need it more than ever.

Thankfully, there is something each and every one of us can do to turn this around. Let's shift our gaze back to brain health in particular. New research shows that the beneficial effects of exercise on our brain as females are as evident in our twenties as they are in the middle-age and post-menopausal years. When it comes to our brain, the payoff doesn't flag, no matter our age. One study of 9,000 women showed that, although exercising in the teenage years was particularly brain-protective in the long term, being physically active reduced the risk of cognitive impairment for women of all ages. Another study of close to 200 women who were followed for as long as forty-four years showed that a higher level of cardiovascular fitness at midlife was associated with very low rates of future dementia, whereas over 30 percent of those with the lowest level of cardiovascular fitness developed dementia later in life.

Exercise has even been shown to improve cognitive deficits in women with a diagnosis of dementia. One such study reported that, in women already diagnosed with cognitive impairment, walking for only thirty minutes three times a week improved complex information processing within just a few months. Further, there seems to be the glimmer of an advantage for females in this department. Encouraging findings reveal that exercise seems to lower the risk of cognitive decline and Alzheimer's more in women than in men!

Without a doubt, exercise is as critical to our health as mammograms and annual checkups are. It becomes even more crucial once women hit fifty and want to counteract a number of menopause-related effects as well as lean-muscle loss. It's time to use this knowledge to our advantage.

A POWER COUPLE: EXERCISE FOR WOMEN

Women have demonstrated beyond a shadow of a doubt that we can do whatever we put our minds to. For our purposes today, the question becomes whether there's a fitness formula that has shown superior results with regard to our long-term physical and cognitive well-being. We are all struggling to find enough time to devote to ourselves. How can we put our energies to their best use, exercising smart rather than hard? Are there certain kinds of exercise and physical activities that work best for us as women?

The typical clichés around exercise are that his idea of getting in shape is pumping iron, while she'd rather pull out the yoga mat. These are indeed stereotypes—there are plenty of women who rave about their latest triathlon and many men who are amazing yogis. However, there are real physiological differences between the sexes that may cause different responses to exercise. As we've acknowledged in previous chapters, not only do women and men differ in the way they age, metabolize medications, and assimilate food—they also have different reactions to their workouts. A substantial contributing factor to these differences depends on something called "muscle fiber type" and how our sex hormones affect it.

There are two types of muscle fibers: Type I fibers, which are great for long, sustained activity; and Type II fibers, which are well-suited to shorter, intense activity. While we all possess both types, men have a higher percentage of Type II fibers. Combined with higher testosterone levels, this makes them excel at "explosive performance," or short, intense bursts of effort, like sprinting or high-intensity interval training (HIIT).

Women, on the other hand, tend to have a higher proportion of Type I muscle fibers, more sugar-burning estrogen, as well as greater capillary density. This combo allows us to circulate more blood throughout our muscle tissue, and to use our glucose more efficiently for sustained energy, allowing us to go longer, stronger. This makes us better at endurance training. Or to put it simply, quick, instant, kill-yourself type workouts aren't always the answer. Most women need to exercise for longer periods at lower intensity to boost metabolism and optimize aerobic fitness.

SORRY, MR. HARE

New research bets on the tortoise of the classic fable, suggesting that slow and steady does, in fact, win the race, provided the tortoise is female. For the average woman, low-to-moderate-intensity exercise is generally better than exercise that favors intense bursts of effort.

In the exercise world, low-to-moderate-intensity exercise is anything that ups your heart rate and makes you sweat lightly rather than profusely. You can carry on a conversation, albeit a little breathily, but you couldn't belt out a tune if you tried. In comparison, during high-intensity exercise such as a spin class, you can get out a few words here and there, but not carry on a full conversation.

We're putting our money on the tortoise.

What's the problem with high-intensity exercise?

There can be a few problems. First off, high-intensity exercise increases one hormone in particular: cortisol. Cortisol promotes stress, while at the same time increasing inflammation and exacerbating the risk of joint, muscle, and heart issues. It also performs the so-called pregnenolone steal, a hormonal sleight of hand that promotes hot flashes, anxiety, and even the potential for depression. By not taking cortisol into consideration, high-intensity regimes can create more trouble than they're worth, especially for peri-menopausal and post-menopausal women. High-intensity exercise is also reliant on one's sleep being sound, which, as we know, is not always the case for many women. Sleep is not only paramount for recovering from intense physical training, but it's also essential in preventing sarcopenia, or muscle-wasting. If you lack shut-eye, neither you nor your muscles will have the time they need to recover adequately post-workout. Finally, the impact of high-intensity exercise can be taxing for older women, causing muscle and joint pain, and risking fractures as well.

This is not to say that women should lift lighter dumbbells or ditch the chin-ups. Obviously, there are plenty of women who can do all of that and much more. If you are used to high-intensity exercise, good for you! But if you aren't, don't worry. As a rule of thumb, several studies have shown that low-to-moderate-intensity exercise optimizes metabolic performance in women, especially when sustained over time. Both the American College of Sports Medicine and the American Heart Association recommend exercising three to five days a week, then adjusting the duration of the workout based on your age and overall health, including your fitness level, personal goals, risks, and medications. Menopausal status is also a big factor to consider, whether you're adjusting your current routine or starting a new one.

Below you'll find a science-backed take on how to do this, employing exercise to maximize your cardiovascular and cognitive fitness while hacking your metabolism at the same time.

FROM YOUR TWENTIES TO MENOPAUSE

When it comes to women and exercise, the higher our estrogen levels, the greater the benefits. Since this hormone runs higher between adolescence and menopause, from a cardio point of view, pushing yourself a bit harder during this time might be a smart investment. The payoffs will show up not only in your day-to-day well-being but also in terms of your future mental and physical health.

During these decades we should strive for a moderate (rather than low-to-moderate) intensity. The best available evidence we have at this time points to pairing moderate-intensity aerobic exercise with resistance training (yes, pick up those weights!). Body-weight exercises like push-ups and pull-ups, as well as knee raises, planks, lunges, and squats, also help build muscle tone while improving your core strength and balance. Aerobic exercise of sufficient intensity, especially when coupled with improved muscle strength, provides the best one-two punch on behalf of your cognitive performance.

Typically, for women in this age range, forty-five-to-sixty-minute sessions three to five times a week are recommended. Research shows that this specific session length is particularly effective at improving both brain fitness and cardiovascular strength, slowing down the aging process as we go. These workouts simultaneously strike a delicate balance between glucose and fat utilization, while at the same time boosting hormonal levels. Findings from the Nurses' Health Study showed that this formula offers the biggest window of opportunity for optimal ovulatory fertility—and the longer your ovaries are fertile, the later you go through menopause.

And if you're wondering if one type of exercise might be better than another, there is no universal rule. Remember, no more one-size-fits-all thinking allowed! Not all exercise is created equal—the fit is a personal one. The best exercise program for your pal may not be right for you. Lucky for us, we have plenty of options. Here are some ideas:

- Walking stairs for 15 minutes.
- Walking two miles in 30 minutes.
- Biking five miles in 30 minutes.
- Swimming laps for 20 minutes.
- Taking an aqua gym class for 30 minutes.

- Running a mile and a half in 15 minutes.

- Doing water aerobics for 30 minutes.

- Playing pick-up basketball, softball, volleyball, doubles tennis, etc., for 20 minutes.

- Jumping rope for 10 minutes.

While doing these exercises at a moderate pace won't make you struggle to catch your breath, it is important to push yourself enough to feel your heart rate ratchet up a notch. You should be moving at a rate that is faster than usual and that gets your blood flowing, bringing color to your cheeks. The key is to make sure that you exercise consistently enough to get the payoff you deserve.

Experts also insist that a workout aimed at optimizing metabolism in women should focus on "periodizing" their training program. This refers to the intensity and repetition with which you train. In more practical terms:

- Interval training: regularly incorporate aerobic workouts that are longer duration, lower intensity with some aerobic workouts that are shorter duration, moderate intensity. For example, let's say you're on an elliptical machine. You can keep the resistance steady while changing your pace—faster for 1 minute; moderate for 4; repeat. Then, pull a switcheroo, maintaining your pace while changing your resistance instead: higher resistance for 1 minute; moderate for 4; repeat.

- Cross-training: training in different types of exercise avoids overtaxing specific regions of the body while at the same time not allowing the body to get bored with moving the same muscles in the same patterns over and over again. This also helps reduce muscle and bone stress, preventing soreness and potential injuries.

- Don't overdo it! Adjust the frequency and intensity of your workouts based on your body's needs, the amount of stress you're under that day, and your overall health. Listen to your body. Your goal is to feel energized afterward, not exhausted or light-headed.

AROUND AND AFTER MENOPAUSE

The benefits of being physically active throughout our lives are well proven and well known. However, it is less understood how much perimenopause and menopause can alter a woman's response to exercise—an essential factor that is overlooked by most mainstream workout regimes. When it comes to exercise for the menopause-age woman, we're met with a dearth of information. Women over fifty are rarely the subjects of exercise-related research, and reliable data on women in their seventies or older is especially scant, as if they aren't supposed to be physically active in the first place.

This lack of knowledge has led to several myths around aging and exercise. Many women in this age group are looking to change this, but all too often find themselves patronized, told that "there's only so much you can do at your age." This is a blanket misconception. Women are perfectly capable of working out at all ages. The key is to find the exercise that suits you.

Another recurrent myth is that the older you get, the harder you have to exercise to stay in shape. On the contrary, the key to the "less is more" concept is less intensity but more frequency. Two of the most extensive exercise interventions on post-menopausal women to date, the Dose-Response to Exercise in Women Aged 45–75 Years (DREW) and the Australian Longitudinal Study on Women's Health trials, concluded that an average of five days a week of thirty-minute, low-to-moderate-intensity physical activity was associated with a decreased risk of heart disease, diabetes, obesity, and even cancer. An unexpected yet striking finding was that increasing the intensity of the workouts did not improve its benefits, but rather, diminished the returns. "Slow and steady wins the race" is never more true than post-menopause.

Interestingly, in some studies, tweaking one's activity to these specs produced a hormonal improvement so pronounced that it alone dramatically decreased both the number and severity of menopausal hot flashes! In one study of 3,500 women, those who exercised for a minimum of thirty minutes a few times a week were 28 percent less likely to have severe hot flashes than those who exercised less. Active women were also 17 percent less likely to feel sad or depressed while at the same time resisting weight gain and not risking obesity. Once we find a fitness formula that we enjoy, these impressive benefits become the icing on the cake.

For those of you who experience menopause like a kick in the pants and suddenly decide it's time to get fit, *whoa, Nellie*. Throwing yourselves into pounding away at the gym is probably not the way to go. Strive to build a good foundation for your newfound goals instead, pacing yourself as you find the combination of exercise that suits your needs and inclinations, while delivering the goods.

Keep in mind that even women who have exercised regularly throughout their lives can experience reduced stamina and weight gain as they transition into menopause. In a changing hormonal environment, exercise regimes that worked in the past may or may not have the same effect or offer the same results. However, many women, especially those with a history of enjoying these workouts, can become frustrated and even upset when confronted with having to consider slowing down. With all the buzz around boot camps, boxing, Zumba, and HIIT, not "hupping to" these trendy workouts can make us feel "lesser" or older than we actually are. Watch out for all the hype and the various myths attached to these trends. They are perpetuated by one thing that has little to do with reality—it's called marketing. They're trying to play on the vulnerable you that wants a flat belly and wants it now. Fortunately, they've underestimated us. With each turn of the page, we arm ourselves with the strategies that work—rather than being tempted by the mirages that threaten to bench us instead.

What are we then to do?

For women ages fifty to seventy, and for younger women going through early menopause, the goal is to exercise three to five days per week, but at thirty to forty-five minutes a clip. For women over seventy, daily sessions of at least fifteen minutes each are recommended.

Keep an open mind as you consider different forms of exercise—many that seem too gentle at first glance can be particularly beneficial in keeping your body and brain pointed in the right direction while your energy levels increase. Some examples of properly paced exercise are:

- Briskly walking at a speed of at least 2.5 miles per hour.
- Taking a bike ride at a speed of 7 to 10 miles per hour.
- Gentle swimming.
- Joining a gentle aqua gym class.
- Doing yoga or Pilates.
- Playing golf.
- Hopping on the elliptical machine at a slow but steady stride.
- Doing mind-body exercises such as hatha yoga, tai chi, or resistance training.
- A variety of group fitness classes will do the trick, as well as many kinds of dancing.

If you are new to exercising, I would recommend the speed-walking regime described at the beginning of this chapter. Start by walking twenty minutes a day. Do so at a speed slightly faster than your normal pace, as if you were in a hurry. Little by little, increase your walking speed and duration. Once you are comfortable speed-walking for twenty minutes, bring it up to twenty-five. Once you are comfortable with twenty-five, crank it up to thirty. Do this until you reach forty minutes of brisk nonstop walking at least three times per week. If you are over seventy or have injuries, fifteen minutes a day is perfectly fine.

Especially if you're suffering from hot flashes, anxiety, and poor sleep, it might be helpful to consider exercises that incorporate the power of deep breathing and functional strength such as yoga and Pilates. For best results, yoga should be done in tandem with other forms of physical activity, not in place of them. However, if yoga is the only type of exercise you're currently doing, focus on a practice that includes enough movement to make your heart beat faster, such as Kundalini. Pilates can be quite challenging as well. These practices promote grounding and hormonal balance while reinforcing and toning your entire core. When our core is in shape, it feels as if our entire body pulls itself together, elongating our height, strengthening our posture, and "youthifying" our movement and gait. If you love your cardio and want to keep it as part of your workouts, consider switching to a lower-intensity choice until menopausal symptoms are no longer a big issue.

Last, with an eye on proper form, weight lifting and resistance training are particularly helpful in building stronger muscles and bones. In fact, one of the most obvious and sought-after benefits of exercise is that it increases bone density. When we strengthen our muscles, we strengthen our bones. A combination of strength training and low-impact activities like walking can help offset the decline of bone density, preventing osteoporosis. It also reduces back pain, especially when it comes to the lower back. Take a look at table 15 for a list of exercises that can help build and maintain bone density and mass if you're post-menopausal. Keep in mind that non-impact exercise alone does not help strengthen bones, so it is best to combine it with weight-bearing exercise.

TABLE 15. EXERCISES THAT CAN HELP IN BUILDING AND MAINTAINING BONE DENSITY AND MASS

TYPE OF EXERCISE	EXAMPLES	BEST FOR WOMEN WHO
Weight-bearing, high-impact exercises	High-impact aerobics, running, jogging, jumping rope, stair climbing, dancing, and sports like tennis, basketball, volleyball, or gymnastics	Don't have low bone mass or frail bones (osteoporosis, osteoarthritis)

Weight-bearing, low-impact exercises	Walking (treadmill/outside), elliptical training machines, stair-step machines, and low-impact aerobics	Have low bone mass or frail bones (osteoporosis, osteoarthritis)
Weight or strength training, or resistance training exercises	Lifting light to moderate weights and using elastic bands or weight machines, calisthenics (using simple functional movements such as squatting or lifting own body weight)	All women
Non-weight-bearing, non-impact activities	Gentle cycling, swimming, stretching, and flexibility exercises	All women
Non-impact exercises	Exercises that help balance and posture (yoga, Pilates, tai chi)	All women

THE GYM IS OPTIONAL. MOVING YOUR BODY IS NOT.

There are subtle but important differences between exercise and physical activity. Exercise is an intentionally planned, structured, repetitive movement intended to improve or maintain physical fitness. Physical activity refers to any movement of the body that consumes energy.

While it's crystal clear that exercise is good for you, emerging research indicates that just keeping physically active significantly contributes to your cognitive performance too, reducing the risk of dementia later in life. The simple truth is, you can't overcome twenty-three hours of inactivity with one hour of exercise. What you do during the other twenty-three hours of the day when you're not at the gym matters just as much, if not even more.

This concept introduces the Mediterranean lifestyle (similar in its approach to the Mediterranean diet), a way of life that's been associated with a much lower risk of pretty much every disease under the sun, dementia first and foremost. So what does "keeping active" mean in a Mediterranean sense? First off, instead of jogging or heading to the gym at designated times of the day, these cultures engage in a great deal of leisurely physical activity that happens regularly on a daily basis, like walking and riding bikes. You won't find many locals sweating it out at the gym. However, you will find them covering miles as they run errands and do chores throughout the day, outside and at home, before topping it all off with a stroll after dinner, or on Sundays, with friends and family. Believe it or not, as far as your brain is concerned, doing activities that require a certain amount of movement, such as taking the stairs, carrying groceries, straightening up, mopping the floors, raking leaves or taking a stroll in the park, is just as welcome as an actual workout. Especially if these activities are done with enough zest to break a light sweat, this is a clear thumbs-up that you've succeeded in activating both your body and your brain.

Several studies show that engaging in regular physical activity, including all sorts of activities you can do in street clothes, for roughly four hours a week lowers your risk of dementia later in life by a good 35 percent. By comparison, engaging in more strenuous exercise reduced the risk by 45 percent, making the two fairly comparable. This is good news for those who don't have the extra time or resources to hit the gym regularly, or at all. There are many shades of gray between being a professional athlete and a professional couch potato. If you fall somewhere in between, you might just find yourself more "Mediterranean" than you thought! The important thing is to forgo the couch and move that precious body of yours every excuse you get.

I've heard it said that the modern, urban woman here in the States has two modes: sitting or spinning—with little in between! As it turns out, your brain actually prefers a gentler, more "everyday" variety of movement, and the slow, steady burn it delivers. This fact reiterates that, for women in particular, it's not about intensity as much as frequency and consistency. I encourage you to experiment with everyday movement as an integral part of your overall well-being, rather than fixating on time spent inside a gym. If you feel like your life leaves you no time for things like walking to the store or taking the stairs instead of the elevator, it's time to step back and see what can be done. Strangely, the stress and fatigue we struggle with in modern life typically have as much to do with what we aren't doing as with doing too much.

The cognitive bonus we experience when we get enough physical activity reminds us that our brains don't operate in isolation. What you do with your body has a direct and vital impact on your mental faculties. Sitting still all day turns out to be dangerous. So it's best not to dither too long about what form of exercise or activity to do. Find something you enjoy, then get up and do it. Weave a walk, a stroll, or a bike ride into your weekly habits. Pick up a vacuum cleaner and dance with it as you houseclean.

Your mind is a powerful thing. Flex that too! Exercise it in making the wise decisions that will keep it that way.

CHAPTER 13

BE MINDFUL: DE-STRESS, SLEEP, AND BALANCE

MILLIONS OF US ARE LIVING in a near-constant state of stress. Women in particular strain to accept this as an inevitable consequence of our modern, fast-paced lives and the roles we've taken on as partners, mothers, and caregivers. Welcoming these multiple roles and their expectations has placed many of us between a rock and a hard place.

Today, underacknowledged Wonder Woman expectations paired with misleading misinformation about how to manage our health and hormones have led to a full-blown crisis. Confronted with a clashing array of crash diets and boot camps, sleeping pills, antidepressants, and plastic surgery, women often turn to supposed health solutions that are not, in actuality, healthy at all. Unable to imagine how our situation might improve, we bend over backward trying to improve ourselves instead. Many women overwork themselves to that end while still feeling unappreciated both at their jobs and at home. Others struggle to keep balance within an equation that possesses none. Eventually, something gives and the physical symptoms of these accumulated stressors can get the best of us.

It is no wonder that women are suffering considerably higher levels of stress than men. Official figures report that the discrepancy occurs primarily in women ages twenty-five to fifty-four, and peaks between thirty-five and forty-four, when many of us are juggling career ladders and the brunt of familial responsibilities simultaneously. Since the latter often includes caring for children and elderly parents at the same time, many women are shouldering what could be considered a minimum of two full-time jobs at once, often without recognition of the fact, and without extra support. As bad timing would have it, all of this coincides with hormonal shifts that require women to take more care of themselves rather than less. Instead, with work and family obligations at an all-time high, we are left with absolutely no time for self-care.

When our systems are taxed beyond their means for years if not decades at a time, there is a toll, emotionally, psychologically, and physically. We may find ourselves short-tempered, jumpy, and frazzled, losing our patience, stamina, and calm. Sometimes we feel empty or depressed, or find that we can't think straight. Feeling worn down and worn out can often lead to a sluggish mental state, in which we end up losing our keys, spacing on a colleague's name, or wrestling with that word on the tip of our tongue. So many of us soldier on blindly, feeling there is no other choice. Perhaps we think if only these outside stressors would subside, our internal stress could do the same. The trouble is, stress can lead to serious medical problems, so it's best not to ignore it, no matter how noble the cause.

Perhaps more than any other health risk, stress is the silent killer our society has yet to acknowledge fully. Those of us in the health field already recognize it as a major contributing factor in all leading causes of death, including heart disease, cancer, lung disease, and Alzheimer's. Especially for women, research shows that prolonged periods of stress, and the subsequent surge in cortisol levels, decreases overall cell function while sending our hormonal levels plummeting, which can accelerate neuronal aging and aggravate the symptoms of menopause. It is perhaps our tendency to take care of others, even when under stress, that puts women at higher risk of suffering from "caregiver burden." From a medical perspective, there is evidence that women's brains are more vulnerable to long-term stress than men's. For example, a recent study of more than 2,000 middle-aged people showed that if you lead a high-stress life, you could experience memory loss and brain shrinkage before you even turn fifty. According to these studies, the adverse effects of high stress and high cortisol are harsher in the female brain than in the male's.

A main reason stress has such a powerful impact on well-being is because it is activated in the brain. Let's examine how this process works, why stress affects us the way it does, and how to get rid of it! We will discuss scientifically validated strategies proven to work for women for keeping stress in check while at the same time improving restful sleep. Reducing stress in our everyday life is vital for maintaining our overall health, as it can improve mood, boost immune function, and promote longevity.

STRESS MESSES WITH OUR STATE OF MIND

Unlike the symptoms that occur once stress becomes chronic, the initial response is an innocent one, an expression of the brain's natural instinct to protect us. Our stress response has been exquisitely honed over millions of years as a protective mechanism, beginning with our ancestors having to deal with their fair share of threats, like saber-toothed tigers and famines. Today, the tigers have been replaced by an onslaught of "mental monsters" instead. Where there were once moments of quiet in our lives, we are now daily plagued by the modern "convenience" of making ourselves accessible 24/7—whether it be to view and review the global live-streamed headlines of the day, or the day and night notifications we receive via email, messaging, phone alerts, alarms, and nonstop social media prompts. We are virtually bombarded by incessant interruptions that require our reaction, many of them urgent, most at least pressing. Anxiety mounts as we navigate headlines reflecting a challenging sociopolitical territory often charged with violence, looming health crises, and climate disasters.

Although none of this includes a saber-toothed tiger, our bodies respond as if it does: with hypertension, strokes, ulcers, heart attacks, and hormonal crashes. Evolutionarily, our stress response was intended to warn us of immediate danger, and as such was a response or state that we would discharge as soon as we had physically confronted that danger. But the chronic stress we experience today is often experienced while commuting, working at a desk, texting in bed, or otherwise inside our heads. As we "sit with it," its repercussions can ravage our physical, emotional, and cognitive health.

Gender Differences in the Stressed-Out Brain

The way men and women respond to stress can be somewhat different. You are probably familiar with the term "fight-or-flight," referring to a primordial hormonal response to either attack or flee oncoming potential danger. As discussed, given that the preponderance of medical research is based solely on males, this was the case for fight-or-flight as well. Until 1995, women constituted as little as 17 percent of participants in studies focused on the behavioral and psychological effects of stress. But there's a new theory in town that focuses on a "female" response to stress.

As scientists finally turned their attention to stress-related differences between the genders, it soon became clear that, while both sexes shared the capacity for fight-or-flight, females seemed to show an alternate reaction. Women often proved more cerebral rather than physical in their stress response to danger. This uniquely female response to stress is called "tend-and-befriend."

This response likely evolved ages ago, when our ancestors lived in hunter-gatherer communities. Back then, it was normal for men to go hunting (and deal with those tigers) and for women to stay behind, harvesting and taking care of the family. Given that fighting or fleeing is not so easy when you are pregnant, nursing, or caring for your children, females developed their own brand of responding to danger when it arrived. In such moments, they became even more protective of their children (*tend*ing to them) while banding together with other women (*befriend*ing) to increase everyone's likelihood of survival. This teamwork also benefited them day to day, not only guaranteeing extra protection and support in raising their offspring, but also providing a more efficient way to gather and share resources such as food. Still today, this primal impulse to form tight, stable alliances may very well be behind our current tendencies to seek out friends to talk, vent, and share our stories.

This difference is due in part to our hormones. Three hormones in particular play a crucial role in the stress response: cortisol, adrenaline, and the "love hormone," oxytocin. When stress strikes, cortisol and adrenaline raise your blood pressure and sugar levels, which might prompt you to land a punch . . . or turn tail and run. That happens in both men and women. However, in women, as cortisol and adrenaline flood the bloodstream, the brain steps in with a shot of oxytocin. Oxytocin is a hormone that promotes nurturing, loving emotions. Scientists suspect that the additional release of oxytocin may be behind women's impulse to "tend" to their loved ones and "befriend," finding comfort in their peers.

Brain imaging studies further confirm this theory by showing that men and women tend to activate different parts of their brains when faced with stress. Women tend to have particularly strong activity throughout the limbic system, the part of the brain primarily involved in emotions, while men tend to activate their frontal cortex, the area in charge of reason. Women under stress also show increased "functional connectivity," a phenomenon by which different areas of the brain become simultaneously activated and work together. The very same areas of a man's brain show the opposite effect, a disengagement between these regions. In other words, when women are stressed, both social and emotional areas of the brain go on alert, perhaps reflecting the tendency to reach out and connect, while men may be more likely to withdraw.

The Caregiver Burden

There are over 65 million people in America alone serving as caregivers for their ill or disabled relatives. Women account for over 60 percent of these caregivers. (Who among us, I wonder, is not being taken into account in this percentage?) The rates are even higher for Hispanic and African American women. There is a steep physiological-emotional strain that accumulates with caregiving, now acknowledged as the "caregiver burden."

Research indicates that caregiver burden can severely tax caregivers' health, while simultaneously compromising their immune response to stress, limiting their ability to cope and heal. At the same time, this type of stress is known to exacerbate existing chronic health conditions, which is quite a problem given that, due to the demands on their time, caregivers are less likely to engage in preventative health behaviors than non-caregivers, such as sleeping and eating properly, exercising, or resting when necessary. As a result, they are not only managing higher levels of stress but do so at a health deficit in comparison with the rest of the nation, sometimes resulting in an increased risk for heart disease, stroke, depression, and even premature mortality. To make matters worse, caregivers tend to have a higher risk of developing Alzheimer's themselves. We surmise that this is most likely due to the multi-stressors inherent in this commitment, paired with the lack of caregiving to the caregivers themselves.

In keeping with the fact that the effects of shouldering stress have a more severe impact on a woman's health than a man's, according to the National Alliance for Caregiving, female caregivers experience a twofold higher level of this burden than male caregivers. This fact might have to do with more than our biology, however. For example, unlike sons, the daughters of Alzheimer's patients tend to provide more routine assistance (such as changing diapers, cooking, and cleaning), while simultaneously experiencing more guilt for not managing more. Also, female caregivers are less likely to receive support from their spouses, and are instead more likely to quit their jobs to care for their parents. In contrast, male caregivers are more likely to ask for help from other family members, most often their sisters or wives.

In other words, it is not only the sheer number of women acting as caregivers that is of concern but also the fact that they tend to offer fuller assistance, to do so alone, and to even surrender jobs in the process. Nearly 19 percent of all female Alzheimer's caregivers end up quitting work to manage their caregiving commitment or end up losing their jobs because of these duties—either event ending in financial crisis and an additional emotional toll.

An ironic timing also rounds out this picture, since typically it is middle-aged women who become the primary caregivers for their parents or loved ones. These women are often approaching menopause or are already dealing with it amid these competing pressures, and are therefore managing stress, inside and out, and on all fronts. Their bodies are paying the price.

My goal in writing this book is not only to acknowledge what women are going through but to provide relief and solutions. Stress-management strategies are the vital first line of defense against stress for all women. While it's perfectly natural to experience stress from time to time, it shouldn't be a daily visitor in your life. It is paramount that each one of us assesses how to minimize stress in our lives. It is then nothing short of vital to deploy whatever strategies are necessary to make a change, because the simple truth is, you can't pour from an empty cup. You can't help others unless you help yourself too. Personally, I repeat this to myself many times a day: I must make time for myself to de-stress and recharge. If you too recognize this need in your life, I've outlined simple steps that you can begin taking today. While I cannot promise instantaneous bliss, these tools will help you manage your stress more effectively so that you can take care of yourself more genuinely. Doing this is a proven way to add years to your life, and much happier ones at that.

R&R for the Mind
We may not have much control over many of the sources of stress in our lives, but we do control how we respond to stress. Three key lifestyle factors are crucial in this respect: diet, exercise, and relaxation. If you eat the balanced diet detailed in chapter 10, while strategically supplementing with the vitamins and herbs proven to reduce anxiety and boost energy in chapter 11, and engage in consistent physical activities as described in chapter 12, you're already on your way. Now as for relaxation, which is something as fundamental to your well-being as

food, water, and physical activity, there are many ways to go about it, depending on what your stressors are.

MAKE TIME FOR FRIENDS

Many women under stress tend to withdraw and cut back on their social life. If research is any indication, we should be doing the opposite, spending time with family and friends on a regular basis. On top of helping women de-stress, having a sense of purpose and social connection has been associated with a longer life span and a reduced risk of dementia. "Social connection" doesn't mean how many followers you have on Facebook, though those networks can be wonderful, too—it means real personal relationships with people who show up when you need them. Several studies agree that even if your social ties are not very extended, having a family you love is enough to protect your brain, provided you connect with them happily and as often as possible.

And if you're more of an introvert and need solitude to recharge—do your very best to book in some unstructured time for yourself. By "unstructured" I mean that you're not on a schedule, you're not checking your calendar, and you're not wondering how somebody else is doing. Just use the time to do whatever comes to your mind.

PULL THE PLUG

Regularly "unplugging" is particularly important when your stress is work or relationship-based. Studies indicate that deliberately detaching from work-related communication during non-work time is positively associated with employee recovery and health. Moreover, research has now proved that time spent on cell phones, tablets, and computers does minimize our ability to sleep. Whether you're surfing the Web, playing a video game, or using your phone to knock out a few emails, you're inadvertently preventing yourself from a restful night. The blue light that screens emit restrains the body's production of melatonin, the hormone that controls your sleep-wake cycle, or circadian rhythm. Reduced melatonin makes it harder to fall and stay asleep, while also increasing cortisol levels. Cortisol is great at waking you up and keeping you up while messing with your hormonal balance, too.

To make sure technology isn't making you even more stressed out, give yourself at least thirty minutes of screen-free transition time before hitting the hay. A small ritual like putting your cell phone to charge in another room at night or switching it to airplane mode can cue immediate relief. Even better, consider periodic breaks from electronics and social media, designating an e-free weekend or a twelve-to-twenty-four-hour detox. Start a challenge with family and friends and enjoy the results!

Green Time Over Screen Time

There is an emerging body of science indicating that natural settings hold restorative powers for the mind and the body. Those of us who are city dwellers spend far less time in nature than is good for us. Lack of outdoor time is linked to higher levels of stress, depression, and anxiety. So it's safe to say that we would all benefit from bringing a little more nature into our lives. Make a point of enjoying a day at the beach, going for a hike, or doing something as simple as taking a stroll in the park, phone-free. You could also get creative and bring the outside, in, introducing plants, flowers, and water elements to your office or home.

Mind and Body: BFFs

Even those people who do shut down their phones and venture outside regularly can suffer from persistent stress. Then it's time to reach for mind-body techniques like meditation, mindfulness training, or yoga. While rigorous research in this field has only just begun, the available evidence indicates that relaxation techniques perform target-reduction on the harmful consequences stress has on the brain. At the same time, they promote hormonal balance. This is especially important for women who suffer from hot flashes but have limited pharmaceutical options, such as cancer patients and women with a history of heart disease, liver disease, or endometriosis. Additionally, mind-body techniques can be helpful to women choosing to navigate menopause naturally, without any help from medications.

These time-tested relaxation techniques might also give caregivers an opportunity to take a breather while calming their loved ones. Since anxiety and panic attacks often afflict patients with dementia, especially in the early stages of the disease when they first come to grips with declining cognitive capabilities, sharing a mindfulness practice with whoever is in your care gives you both a moment's peace amid an otherwise stressful day. And let's not forget the positive effect that deep breathing and mindfulness can have on both parents and children, especially when started at a young age. For instance, we always encourage our four-year-old daughter to take three deep belly breaths if she is feeling upset or overwhelmed, and encourage open discussion about how she is feeling and her emotions. This simple practice really made an enormous difference during the so-called terrible threes.

Meditation

For millennia, cultures worldwide have used meditation as a way to cultivate physical, mental, and spiritual well-being. We have since begun to study how these practices also protect the brain from stress overload. Emerging research suggests that meditation not only reduces stress and anxiety but also has a positive influence on neuroplasticity. This refers to the brain's ability to adapt and change, thereby restoring and repairing itself. Breathing techniques, in particular, have been associated with reducing the brain shrinkage that can happen over time and reversing gene expression responsible for stress-induced symptoms. Practicing slow, deep breaths lowers a racing heart, melting stress into calm, while also pulling back on the reins of the inflammation that would have ensued otherwise.

There are many different forms of meditation available to try. For those of you with ants in your pants, there is even something called a "walking meditation," or a "doing the dishes" meditation, so keep an open mind as you find the practice that suits you best. Each of the alternatives below can be effective at reducing stress while subsequently improving multiple aspects of your health at the same time.

Transcendental Meditation (TM) has become a popular choice. You sit for a set number of minutes twice a day while reciting a personalized mantra. This mantra is given to you by a teacher and isn't meant to be shared with anyone. Those who practice TM report settling into a state of deep relaxation, often leading to a feeling of inner calm or peace. In clinical studies, TM was indeed shown to lower blood pressure as well as the risk of heart disease. In one example, a randomized controlled trial of 201 men and women with coronary heart disease showed a 48 percent reduction in their risk for mortality and a 24 percent reduction in the risk of heart attacks and strokes after just a few years of regularly practicing TM. If you're interested in learning more, the David Lynch Foundation is a great place to start: www.davidlynch foundation.org.

Mindfulness meditation, a Buddhist-based breathing practice that has been studied quite extensively, involves focusing on what's around you on a moment-to-moment basis. Mindfulness-Based Stress Reduction (MBSR), a technique that focuses on the breath for up to forty minutes at a time, was found to be beneficial to lowering stress in Alzheimer's patients and their caregivers. Additionally, MBSR seems to help relieve the symptoms of menopause. In a randomized trial of 110 late perimenopausal and early post-menopausal women, there was a 15 percent reduction of hot flashes and night sweats in the group that received MBSR as compared with a group that did not. The MBSR group also showed durable improvement in quality of life and sleep, along with lower anxiety and perceived stress.

Another great option is Kirtan Kriya (KK), a singing meditation that comes from the Kundalini yoga tradition. KK prescribes practicing the specific sounds "Saa Taa Naa Maa" accompanied by mudras, elegant finger positions, for just twelve minutes a day. This short but sweet practice has been shown to reduce inflammation while improving memory, sleep, and overall well-being in people with average cognition as well as in patients with mild cognitive impairment. In one study, participants experienced improved mental clarity and up to a 50 percent increase in memory skills within eight weeks.

Currently, KK is the only meditation that's been specifically tested in patients with a dementia diagnosis. Moreover, KK has the added benefit of having been explicitly tested on women. A pilot study by the Alzheimer's Research & Prevention Foundation (ARPF) investigated the cognitive impact of KK on 161 women at risk for Alzheimer's, including some experiencing forgetfulness, some with a diagnosis of mild cognitive impairment, and others under pressure due to their caregiving roles. After two to four months of training, those who practiced every day showed increased blood flow to several parts of the brain, as well as improvement in their overall cognitive function. Wouldn't it be wonderful if a better memory was ours merely by singing for twelve minutes each morning?

If you are new to meditation, I would recommend starting with KK. It's easy and free. Just follow the guidelines in table 16—and check out the ARPF website for additional information: alzheimersprevention .org/research/12-minute-memory-exercise. You can also practice KK to music, if that helps. Several playlists are available on Spotify, YouTube, and other channels. If you do it on your own, I suggest using an app like Insight Timer, which lets you set intervals with gentle sounds that indicate it's time to transition your chanting.

TABLE 16. HOW TO PRACTICE KIRTAN KRIYA

Courtesy of the ARPF

Sit in Easy Pose on the floor or on a chair or couch. Easy Pose is a simple cross-legged position. But if you're new to yoga, sit however is most comfortable for you.
Keep the back of your neck straight and your chin slightly down. You almost feel like the top of your head is being pulled up by a cord. Sit up straight and allow your body to be in alignment.
Rest your hands on your knees with your palms facing upward.

While chanting the sounds *saa taa naa maa*, touch your thumb to your index finger (saying *Saa*), thumb to middle finger (saying *Taa*), thumb to the ring finger (saying *Naa*), and thumb to the pinkie finger (saying *Maa*).

For a 12-minute practice, here is the sequence:
- Chant out loud for 2 minutes.
- Chant in a whisper for 2 minutes.
- Chant in silence for 4 minutes.
- Chant in a whisper for 2 more minutes.
- Chant out loud for 2 more minutes.

Inhale and stretch your arms up. Exhale, lower your arms, and relax for a moment.

Yoga

Yoga is a mind-body practice originating from ancient Indian philosophies. Various styles of yoga typically combine physical postures and movement, breathing techniques, and meditation or relaxation. While so far there is little evidence that yoga helps fend off full-blown dementia, a randomized clinical trial of Kundalini yoga provided promising evidence of short- and long-term benefits in patients with mild cognitive impairment after just twelve weeks of treatment. Moreover, five separate studies showed that women who practice yoga had reduced symptoms of stress and insomnia. Other encouraging results are in from clinical trials that evaluated the effects of yoga and meditation on breast cancer survivors. A study of 40 breast cancer patients showed that a twelve-week intervention combining traditional hatha yoga with meditation significantly lowered menopausal symptoms in the patients, including those on chemotherapies. After twelve weeks, the patients reported an overall improved quality of life, including fewer hot flashes, fewer urogenital symptoms, as well as less fatigue.

Acupuncture

Acupuncture is a pillar of the practice of traditional Chinese medicine (TCM) in which a practitioner stimulates specific points on the body associated with the body's "meridians," or energy channels, to treat disease and the pain they produce. The insertion of fine needles into the skin stimulates various systems and organs of the body to reduce ailments and symptoms. Relative to our focus, studies have shown a reduced frequency and severity of hot flashes in post-menopausal women, however less so than that achieved by MHT. Just the same, it poses a med-free alternative to those women seeking one. One of my best friends described acupuncture, when practiced by a highly educated practitioner, as "almost freakin' magic."

"HELLO, MOON"

Restless nights, obsessive thoughts, and counting sheep. Ring any bells?

Well, it's a fact: women have a harder time sleeping than men do. The National Sleep Foundation's Women and Sleep Poll found that women have more difficulty not only falling asleep but staying asleep as well. It is no wonder then that they also experience more daytime sleepiness, especially in the years to either side of menopause. Menopausal night sweats persistently wake women up in the middle of the night, making for poor sleep if you're lucky, and insomnia if you're not. And let's not forget the many years of lost sleep taking care of children. A friend just sent me this, which made me smile: "Moms do not sleep. Moms hover in a state of semi-consciousness, waiting for someone to need something." So true, no matter how young or how old your children are.

That said, chronic sleep disturbance is a big problem. It triggers not only low mood and potentially depression but cognitive troubles as well. Essentially, when we sleep, the brain is processing information and coming up with solutions to complex problems. Anyone who's experienced sleep difficulties, let alone insomnia, knows how hard it is to function properly after even a few nights of missed sleep. While a good night's rest is a non-negotiable ingredient for the brain's memory consolidation and learning, poor sleep makes quick work of degrading these essential abilities. There's also the way that we process emotional information. The tired brain remembers negative experiences and negative facts, and it forgets the positive ones, which in and of itself can trigger mood swings and depressive feelings.

Basically, lack of sleep is a more serious problem than one might think. With so many people typically suffering from it, we begin to rationalize that it's "doable"—since, for many of us, it has become the norm. But an emerging body of evidence shows long-term ill effects, many of them fairly grave. Among a long list of heavy hitters, an increased risk of cognitive decline and dementia has made an appearance. Recent studies demonstrate that sleep is the only moment the brain has during an otherwise too-busy day to get to the "housekeeping" essential to relieving itself from harmful toxins. Both too little sleep and fragmented sleep have been linked to the increased accumulation of Alzheimer's plaques in the brains of otherwise seemingly healthy people, along with poorer cognitive function.

Sleep Goes in Cycles

When you draw back the curtains, sleep is quite the spectacle. Even though any heavy sleeper you've observed may seem to be doing nothing more than working on his snore, deep sleep is not as simple as it appears. In actuality, an intricate succession of sleep stages is in the works. Of course, the first stage is managing to fall asleep in the first place! Once we've achieved that, we drift through the "light sleep" of the second stage. It's during this moment that the brain prepares to shut itself down, much like our computers do when put to sleep. During the third and fourth stages, your brain finally enters a deep, "slow wave" sleep. It's during this stage that the brain gets to tend to its housework, washing away the day's waste along with harmful toxins such as Alzheimer's plaques. After a while, this restorative phase is interrupted by the rapid eye movement (REM) stage, cuing dream time. When REM is over, this five-step cycle begins all over again, giving your brain additional chances to heal and repair.

But when you're not getting enough sleep in the first place, or waking up throughout the night—especially in the middle of precious slow-wave sleep—this vital process is compromised, hobbling your brain's overall performance, as well as the successful removal of Alzheimer's plaques. When something regularly obstructs our nightly slow-wave sleep, a substantial buildup of Alzheimer's plaques can result.

Consequently, sleep hygiene (doing what's necessary to put a stop to this) is not a maybe—but a must. While studies continue to waffle as to exactly how long we should sleep (perhaps due to the collapsing of a one-size-fits-all approach), for now, shooting for seven to eight hours per night is probably a safe bet for most people, with a minimum of six for those sixty-five or older.

Curiously, the crucial slow-wave sleep stage is typically a bit longer in women than in men. So why aren't we reaping the benefits? Because we're generally not getting it! If that weren't enough, sleep apnea has also become a problem for women over fifty, affecting over half of all post-menopausal women. Typically considered a "male issue," sleep apnea is a potentially dangerous sleep disorder that interrupts a person's breathing during sleep, sometimes hundreds of times a night. Additionally, these interruptions in breathing can lead to the brain not getting enough oxygen. So if you snore loudly and feel dull after a full night's sleep, sleep apnea could be the culprit.

Thinking Clearly Means Prioritizing Sleep

Fortunately, we've got some solutions to support our sleepy brains.

For sleep apnea, interventions range from lifestyle changes to CPAP therapy and surgery. If you are concerned you might suffer from it, talk to your doctor or visit the National Sleep Foundation website for more information. For those of you who don't have sleep apnea and still can't sleep, you're up next.

In the United States, doctors tend to hand out sleeping pills like candy at Halloween. I am not a fan of sleeping pills, and neither should you be. These meds are not always the best solution, mainly because they are not as helpful as pharmaceutical companies would have us believe. In fact, the average sleeping pill adds a maximum of forty minutes of sleep to your night while potentially bestowing multiple side effects instead. If you're tired of staring at your clock, forgo the meds and look to these suggestions before hitting the hay:

- Practice a "wind down" time with electronic devices (no texting, TV, streaming, or email) for at least thirty minutes before bed. Once you regularly embrace, rather than resist, this practice, it not only reduces stress but also allows your body to access melatonin to re-acclimate itself to falling and staying asleep.

- Consider keeping smartphones, TVs, and electronics in general out of the bedroom. Your bedroom should be a place of sleep.

- Make sure your bedroom isn't too warm. Part of the initiation of sleep is a slight drop in body temperature. If the room is too warm, you can't lose that body heat, which means it is more difficult to go to sleep.

- Minimize light coming into the bedroom. If you don't want to get up early, the bedroom should be dark.

- For many women, ambience is important. If this is you, create a comfortable environment by dimming the lights or lighting a few candles around the room. Putting some calming music on and perhaps burning essential oils like lavender oil can really help one unwind.

- The mind and body practices described above should also help you sleep. For example, there are some really nice guided sleep meditations available on iTunes and on the internet (some of my favorites are by Jon Kabat-Zinn).

- Aiming to go to bed and wake up at the same time each day promotes regular sleep habits. Your body likes relying on a rhythm when it comes to sleep. Try to reassure it this way.

- If you wake up in the middle of the night, don't panic. Do something relaxing, like a sleep meditation, or listen to calming music to allow your brain to fall back asleep. *Do not* check your cell phone or watch TV instead.

- If you have to get up in the night, use a soft amber-colored night-light rather than turning on overhead lights.

- Some doctors recommend using a wearable sleep tracking device, which can be helpful to become more aware of your sleep patterns and make adjustments accordingly. But once you have a better sense of your typical sleep pattern, take it off. There's no particular need to have these devices on at night when we're bombarding ourselves with technology all day as it is.

- Low-adrenaline physical activity such as a light tidying up or a non-exerting yoga can relax your brain.

- The healthy diet outlined in chapter 10, with the right combination of supplements, is also crucial for recharging and restoring our endlessly active brains. Look into this combo as an alternative to OTC and prescription sleep meds.

- Nutritionists know a thing or two about sleep; here's a little trick. The same foods that help bolster mood also help you sleep. Mood and sleep have an ally in common: the amino acid tryptophan. The brain needs tryptophan to make serotonin (which calms you down) as well as melatonin (which makes you fall asleep). There are two key steps to ensure you're consuming enough tryptophan to do the trick. First off, make a dinner including foods rich in tryptophan. These include milk, yogurt, fish, shellfish, and chicken. Plant-based foods such as chia, raw cacao, rice, oats, soybeans, prunes, and sesame and pumpkin seeds also score high in tryptophan. Second, eat some select carbohydrates with these tryptophan-rich foods to help increase their absorption. Salmon served with brown rice hits the mark. Or try a dessert of yogurt drizzled with cacao after dinner. (There's a reason why warm milk and honey has survived the centuries as a bedtime favorite.)

- Another trick is to eat foods that contain melatonin, the hormone that makes you sleep. Among these, pistachios are the real star. These flavorful nuts are simply off the charts as the most melatonin-rich food on the planet. Eating a whole handful of pistachios is equivalent to taking a melatonin supplement, which is clearly preferable, as pistachios are also a great source of tryptophan, fiber, and vitamin B6 (and they're tasty). Wheat, barley, and oats are also high in melatonin, as are grapes, cherries, and strawberries.

- Pay attention to your B vitamins, especially B6 and B12. Too little of these vitamins may promote insomnia. You can quickly fix this by eating the right foods (preferably fish, eggs, and milk for B12, and green leafy veggies like spinach and cabbage for B6) and taking B supplements when needed.

- For some of us, it's more about what to avoid instead. Caffeine and alcohol can keep you awake and intrude upon REM sleep. Alcohol may help you fall asleep, but it can also cause you to wake up in the middle of the night. Avoid these beverages after 2:00 p.m. for a while and see what happens.

- If you haven't yet stopped smoking, avoid any smoking or nicotine for at least four hours before bedtime.

- Sleep recommendations for women would not be complete without bringing up progesterone. Like estrogen, progesterone bottoms out during menopause. Progesterone has anxiety-reducing effects on the brain, so its waning can lead to sleep difficulties. If this is you, it's time to boost your progesterone levels. Studies have found that the supplements described in chapter 11 can prove quite effective.

- Beware of OTC sleep aids, especially those with added painkillers. They can tax the liver considerably over time, along with other concerning side effects we will cover in the next chapter. Using sedative medications like benzodiazepines or Benadryl (by far one of the top meds used by women) are not advised either. Discontinuing sedative medications when not clinically indicated also deserves consideration, under your doctor's supervision.

In the end, every woman experiences sleep and stress differently. But the basic premise of optimizing both is the same: take the time to listen to yourself, search for the root causes of your symptoms, implement gradual changes, and give yourself enough time to receive the results. Be persistent and consistent. Taking this approach can genuinely help you in the long term. Reaching for medications that often do no more than mask your symptoms can give an illusion of better sleep in exchange for any actual improvement. Tweaking your way to a stress-free day and a sound night's sleep is well worth your time, as is finding ways to relax and de-stress for the long haul. Your present and future well-being rely on it.

CHAPTER 14

MORE WAYS TO PROTECT YOUR BRAIN

As we approach the end of the book, I want to draw your attention to some additional lifestyle practices known to protect our brains and improve mental clarity. In addition to the foods we eat, how often we move our bodies, how much stress we have in our lives, and how soundly we sleep, other well-established disease-prevention activities chiefly include how often we challenge ourselves intellectually and even how content we are with our careers. We will review those first, and then go over a few more tricks to quench inflammation, boost hormonal health, and protect our brains for the years to come.

I also want to underline that, while each of the practices we've discussed supports brain health, when combined with one another on a regular basis, they become greater than the sum of their parts. The extent to which we are able to incorporate all these healthy habits into our everyday lives determines just how healthy and durable our brains are, and will become.

ENGAGE YOUR INTELLECT

It's long been recognized that intellectually exercising one's brain helps keep it active, improving cognitive function while lowering the risk of dementia later in life. Experts believe that continuing education, satisfying occupations, and intellectual engagement all help stave off cognitive deterioration by boosting our brain's "cognitive reserve." This is an interesting concept that has received a lot of attention especially in the field of brain aging. Just like a nice car with a powerful engine upshifts seamlessly into gear to avoid an obstacle, a brain in top form shifts and swerves to cope with its many mental challenges. The more you use your brain cells, the stronger the connections between those cells become, and the faster your brain is able to respond to external and internal signals. In other words, a well-stimulated brain is a more flexible brain, with a greater reserve capacity. Consistent engagement in tasks and activities that stimulate your brain in a variety of ways pumps up this cognitive reserve, enhancing the brain's ability to protect itself from harm, while also warding off unwanted age-related changes.

Multiple lines of evidence link various forms of intellectual activity with improved mental capacities. A study following 9,000 people for fifteen years found that those with a higher education or those partaking in reflective and cerebral activities throughout their lives had a larger cognitive reserve to offset brain aging, maintaining cognitive fitness over time. Another study of over 400 seniors showed that those who regularly engaged in intellectual activities had a 54 percent reduced risk of cognitive decline as compared with those who did not.

Brain imaging studies also revealed that lifelong participation in cognitive activities, such as reading books and newspapers, writing, playing music, or joining a chess or card club, had the power to slow down and perhaps even prevent Alzheimer's plaques. Particularly impressive is evidence that even in patients carrying mutations that cause Alzheimer's, a higher educational level was associated with a delayed onset of any cognitive decline.

How does all this matter to women's health? Because, historically, lack of access to education or to more intellectually active lifestyles has penalized women more than men. It's a fact that while women over the ages have been able to participate in activities such as reading books, doing arts and crafts, and attending to certain social activities, they have had fewer opportunities to achieve an education or have access to high-level occupational attainments. Since recreational activities are typically performed less rigorously or consistently, they may have less of a protective effect on the brain than formal education or a stable occupation.

Fortunately, as indicated by the most recent census, times are changing, and finally, educational attainment in many countries is now just as high, and in some cases even higher, for women than for men. As discussed, there has also been a shift in occupational engagement, with more women beginning to take on higher-level positions and other roles that used to be men-only prerogatives or dominated by "boys' clubs." One can only hope that this trend will eventually add up to lowered rates of Alzheimer's for females in the future, especially as we succeed in finding a balance between working more . . . and stressing less.

Since getting an education or finding a great job isn't always within our control, we can take it upon ourselves to stimulate our minds in a variety of other ways, too.

So many people are interested in "brain games," so let's discuss those first. In recent years, there has been an explosion of computer-based cognitive-training software, all claiming to improve your memory while bumping up your IQ a few points. Whether these tools have any appreciable impact on cognition is, however, controversial. Basically, there are two types of cognitive training. There are tests that are scientifically validated and tests that claim to be backed by science but aren't.

In particular, there is increasing evidence that commercial Web-based cognitive training programs are just not worth your money. In the past, companies such as Lumosity have received some heat regarding the true effectiveness of their programs, including a $2 million fine from the Federal Trade Commission (FTC) for misleading advertising. However, some users do report improved performance over time. Are the benefits real, or are they just an illusion?

A recent randomized controlled trial may have solved this mystery. The study looked at 128 participants divided into those playing standard video games and those playing Lumosity brain-specific games. They played these games five times a week for half an hour. After ten weeks, the researchers found that all participants scored higher over time. However, it was the process of repeatedly taking the tests that improved scoring—not the tests themselves. In other words, the so-called practice effect can easily be mistaken for an actual improvement. But in reality, cognitive training did not improve brain activity, choice behavior, or cognitive performance. That's certainly not what anyone had signed up for.

As for scientifically validated cognitive training, while these tools certainly don't hurt, there is no clear evidence that they achieve all that they promise either. The two major trials to evaluate the effects of this sort of training, the Advanced Cognitive Training for Independent and Vital Elderly (ACTIVE) and the Iowa Healthy and Active Minds Study (IHAMS), have both shown some improvement in attention and processing speed, but not in memory skills. None of the interventions slowed down the development of dementia either. Overall, large-scale analysis of these trials and others concluded that cognitive training has only limited or modest effects. Whether these effects can be extrapolated to show broader, longer-lasting benefits remains unclear.

While we wait for more effective cognitive training software to be developed, the best advice I can give you is to engage in activities that do have proven efficacy against cognitive aging and dementia, and are also fun. These include things like reading a book, going to the theater, or playing traditional, off-line games with friends and family. The key is to really engage in activities that make you *learn new things*. You need to challenge your brain. For example, if you are a chess player, playing more chess won't help you nearly as much as learning to play a different game will. If you're used to easy, breezy novels, try to pick up something more substantive, like a good classic book. You get the gist. Make those neurons fire!

Here are some of the top evidence-backed mind gymnastics known to help build cognitive reserve and delay cognitive decline:

- Read the newspaper regularly.
- Learn a new language or brush up on a language you used to speak.

- Take up new hobbies.

- Learn how to play a musical instrument or return to an instrument you used to play.

- Regularly listen to music, selecting more stimulating music during the day and more calming music in the evening. Give classical music a try; studies show it might particularly enhance your mental acuity. For many patients with dementia, memory of music is not lost to the disease. Music is therefore an effective caregiving tool that, by tapping into deep memories, can bring patients with dementia joy and relief, enabling them to feel like themselves again, at least for a little while.

- Watch a documentary.

- Join a book club or cultural group.

- Be social. Loneliness and a lack of stimulation have both been linked to depression and an increased risk of cognitive decline. So make social time a priority within your weekly schedule. No, I don't mean Facebook. I mean remain active in your community, be it your church, your political party, or your yoga group.

- Play games. Bingo, bridge, cards, board games—these games can be proper brain teasers, while at the same time providing a good excuse to hang out with your friends and family.

MORE BRAIN-HEALTHY TRICKS

In closing, I want to go over a few more brain-healthy practices that are really important to taking care of our brains. These practices are also based on the principle that you can't control everything in your life, but you can control what you put in your body, and therefore, directly or indirectly, in your brain. The most important tricks include reducing exposure to environmental toxins, chiefly cigarette smoking and plastics; rethinking your medicine cabinet; and, believe it or not, taking good care of your teeth!

The Smoking Gun

As mentioned throughout the book, smoking is a major health hazard. Historically, since it was once considered more socially acceptable for men to smoke, males cornered the market. But in the 1920s and '30s, in a mistaken act of "liberation," women jumped on the bandwagon. The gender gap has been narrowing ever since. Statistics show that as of ten years ago, men had only a 6 percent lead over female smokers, while today we may be neck and neck.

There are well-known behavioral differences between male and female smokers. Men typically smoke to reinforce the effects of nicotine itself, whereas women smoke to relieve stress, or unfortunately, just out of habit. These differences originate once again in the somewhat different architecture of our brains. Brain imaging studies show that smoking activates different parts of the brain depending on gender. In men, it stimulates the striatum, a part of the brain that reinforces the drug effect of cigarettes—while in women, it activates rapid responses in the putamen, an area associated with habit formation. The result? For decades, men have had better luck quitting by using medications and nicotine blockers such as patches.

Although strides have been made in helping people quit, smoking continues to be a major health issue. Cigarette smoking is still responsible for more than 480,000 deaths nationwide each year. Further, smoking causes 90 percent of all lung cancer deaths and 80 percent of all chronic obstructive pulmonary disease deaths, while more than doubling the risk of getting heart disease or having a stroke.

Let's not mince words. Smoking is a bad idea no matter how you slice it. For women, in addition to deteriorating the systems and functions with which you're already undoubtedly familiar, smoking attacks your ovaries, your hormones, and specifically, the finely tuned female mind. The toxins in tobacco actively reduce estrogen levels in a woman's body, speeding up the ticking of your biological clock. This reduction sabotages the hormonal balance that preserves your fertility, triggering early menopause and all the symptoms that can come with it.

The 93,000-person Women's Health Initiative showed that those who smoked even as few as one hundred cigarettes or more in their entire lives had a 14 percent greater risk of infertility and a 26 percent greater risk of going through menopause before they turned fifty. In the Study of Women's Health Across the Nation, smokers had 60 percent more hot flashes than non-smokers, and they had the nasty kind, which persisted for over six years. Additionally, smoking can block the efficacy of interventions targeted at lessening hot flashes in breast cancer patients. Speaking of which, we are all too aware by now that smoking increases the risk of the cancer in the first place.

So if you're under the impression that smoking calms you, offers you a social crutch, or makes for a nice accessory, you might want to re-evaluate, examining its costs. Some think smoking might even make a woman appear more attractive, while in effect it's doing the opposite, accelerating the aging process. This, as it wreaks havoc through our insides, eventually shows up on the outside, too.

Unfortunately, there's more. Emerging evidence shows that smoking increases the risk of Alzheimer's for both women and men, likely due to its causing inflammation and oxidative stress. Smoking is also correlated with a higher risk of heart disease in women, whereas quitting, or at least substantially reducing the frequency with which you smoke, diminishes this risk. Abstinence from smoking is particularly important for women with the APOE-4 gene, for whom smoking may pose even steeper risks.

If you are a smoker or a past smoker (even if that was in high school!), it is crucial that you focus on increasing the antioxidant foods in your diet, engage in regular moderate-intensity exercise, reduce stress, and minimize the amount of pollutants in your environment. Supplementation with antioxidant vitamins is also helpful to combat the long-term effects of smoking on your systems (see chapter 11).

Go Green

Speaking of toxins, let's talk about other common products that contain estrogen-disruptive chemicals, or xenoestrogens. In chapter 10, we talked about how these pollutants are hiding in our foods, but environmental pollution is just as big a deal in this regard.

In 2015, diseases caused by pollution were responsible for an estimated 9 million premature deaths in the United States—and 16 percent of all deaths worldwide! Outdoor air pollution causes three times more deaths than AIDS, tuberculosis, and malaria combined; and fifteen times more than all wars and other forms of violence.

Unfortunately, we don't have much control over the environment, but one thing we can certainly do is be careful with our personal choices. In fact, household products turn out to be a huge part of the problem.

Unless specifically indicated, most food and beverage containers, toiletry bottles, and disposable plates and utensils contain chemicals such as BPA, which can get into your food easily when the containers are scratched or heated. For example, BPA leaks into your food whenever you microwave frozen food or stored food in plastic containers, or when your plastic wrap suctions into the food you're heating. This also applies to plastic water bottles heated if left in a car, out in the sun, or used for warm beverages. Coffee in plastic cups, burgers in Styrofoam, veggies in steaming bags, noodles in a take-out carton? Sayonara to all of that. When ordering in, it is safer to favor cold food, like sushi. If you order hot food, take it out of the containers immediately. Use glass, ceramic, porcelain, enamel-covered metal, or stainless-steel pots, pans, and containers for heating up, cooking, serving, or storing food at home.

And don't put plastic in your dishwasher! Heat, plastic, and water are a very bad mix. If the manufacturer says the plastic is dishwasher safe, place it on the top rack, away from the heating source. And don't select cycles that use high wash or dry temperatures, such as the "sanitize" cycle.

Further, many commercial household cleaners contain caustic chemicals like ammonia, and are often loaded with synthetic fragrances to mask the smell. These fragrances can contain phthalates, with severe repercussions on your hormones. So why risk it, especially when cleaning with more natural products is actually cheaper! Get rid of Windex and "all-purpose" cleaners—distilled white vinegar and *olio di gomito* (elbow grease) is where's at.

And did you know xenoestrogens might be hiding in your mascara too? Commercial cosmetics and skin-care products contain many chemicals that make us look, feel, and smell nice . . . while at the same time disrupting our hormones and, at certain exposure levels, even contributing to cancer development. Same goes for your toothpaste, deodorant, and anything else you put in and on your body. The skin is the largest organ of the body, and over 60 percent of what you put on your skin is absorbed into your bloodstream. By paying more attention to your choices, you will not only dramatically decontaminate your immediate environment, but also help reduce our collective carbon footprint on our beautiful planet.

Personally, I am a big fan of the "clean beauty" movement and have been using organic skin-care and makeup products for years. It may take some research to find the right ones for your own skin type, but the benefits far outweigh the efforts. To find out whether specific cosmetic products are safe, visit the Skin Deep website of the Environmental Working Group (EWG): www.ewg.org/skindeep. Products are given a hazard score based on the ingredients' links to cancer, allergies, and other issues. Meanwhile, to get you started, try using coconut oil to remove your makeup at night. You just take a few drops and slather it all over your eyes, face, and lips. Then rub it off with a soft cloth. It's magic!

Mind Your Meds

While you're cleaning out your kitchen and your beauty case, let's take a look at your medicine cabinet, too. Did you know that your chances of experiencing cognitive changes could depend on what's in there? While there are no firm conclusions that prescription drugs may cause cognitive decline and dementia, certain medications could increase our risk significantly. Toxic reactions to medications can also mimic the symptoms of dementia, which makes for quite a disconcerting experience.

In particular, common medicines for depression, asthma, and allergies may be riskier than meets the eye. These drugs are known as "anticholinergics." This means that they function by blocking a brain chemical called acetylcholine, which is crucial for memory formation. By doing so, they achieve the exact opposite of those drugs used to treat Alzheimer's, like Aricept, which work to increase the absorption of acetylcholine instead.

The drugs that showed more consistent adverse effects on memory and dementia risk were the common allergy drug Benadryl, the motion sickness remedy Dramamine, and the antidepressant Paxil. Both Benadryl and Dramamine are also commonly used by people suffering from insomnia as an alternative to sleeping pills. In a study of over 3,000 older adults, those who took any of these drugs for several years were four times more likely to develop mild cognitive impairment or dementia than those who never took the medicines.

Additionally, long-term use of benzodiazepines, a class of drugs used to treat insomnia, anxiety, and sometimes epilepsy, has also been linked to an increased Alzheimer's risk. Ambien, the most widely prescribed sleep medication that created so much trouble for women, is one of those benzodiazepines. A study of 7,184 older adults found that those who had used benzodiazepines for more than three consecutive months had an almost 50 percent higher risk of Alzheimer's over the following six years. This is also an indication of how long these meds may affect your system given that shorter-term use did not raise the risk of Alzheimer's. This data reinforces what most clinicians have known for quite some time: benzodiazepines should not be the first line of treatment, especially for sleep.

For any of these medications, occasional use is unlikely to cause dementia. However, prolonged use may increase your long-term risk. If you are taking prescription medications and/or OTC drugs (or have taken them for months or years in the past) and are experiencing challenges with memory, thinking, or concentration, ask your doctor to review the full list of your medications to explore whether any of them might be causing the symptoms. This is also a good reminder that we should all feel empowered to have a conversation with our doctors about the risks and benefits of any drugs prescribed to us. The good news is that if a particular medication is the source of your cognitive changes, you will likely experience an improvement or even a reversal of symptoms after ceasing to use the drug.

Caution, though: it is important that you do not stop, start, or change your medication regimen without consulting your doctor.

Brush Away!

When you're done inspecting your medicine cabinet, take a moment to look at yourself in the mirror. A big smile, please. How are your teeth doing? And your gums?

Oral hygiene is one critical component of brain health that is often completely overlooked. Periodontal disease in particular, a gum disease that may cause loosening or loss of teeth, is currently in the spotlight. In addition to its harmful effects in the mouth, it does a number on the brain as well. Though more evidence is needed, there seems to be an association between periodontal disease and an increased risk of brain inflammation and Alzheimer's plaques. Since periodontitis is a reasonably easy infection to treat, do not leave it unattended.

Recommendations for proper oral hygiene include:

- Regular dental cleanings.
- Brushing after every meal and at least twice a day.
- Flossing every day.
- If your dentist advises you to see a periodontist, take the advice seriously.
- While you're at it, check your toothpaste. Does the ingredient list contain titanium? Other harmful chemicals? If so, toss it.

ARRIVEDERCI, FOR NOW

I'm not fond of goodbyes. Thankfully, in my native tongue, we do not say goodbye at all. Loosely translated, "arrivederci" means "until we meet again." But before we do, I want to be certain that you turn the last pages inspired to blaze a happy, healthy trail ahead. With the strategies you've gathered in hand, I send you off serene in the knowledge that you're headed for a straight-up Rinascimento.

I'm often asked to share my thoughts on "aging gracefully." This expression is dear to my heart since it's precisely what I wish for my family and friends, the patients I care for, and for those of you I meet through the pages of this book. That's what I wish for myself, too. The gracefulness of age extends far beyond style, of course; it's also the wisdom, intelligence, and thoughtfulness that come from a vibrant and resilient brain.

The concept of aging gracefully is, however, out of step with the youth-obsessed, results-oriented culture of the day. We live in a time that has stigmatized aging. Where many cultures have and still do admire and respect the benefits of maturing, what I see around us is a culture that dreads and avoids aging at every turn.

Where growing older is shunned, there arise endless options for looking younger, sparing no expense for medications, cosmetic surgery, or the free option of flat-out denial. Nowhere is this standard applied more harshly than it is against women. As men age, they are considered to be like a fine wine that increases in value. Instead, women are treated like milk—met with suspicion after a hypothetical "sell-by" date. As soon as a woman turns forty, ads start popping up about anti-aging tricks, tips to stay in shape, and ways to look good "anyway." Before we attend to the health of our mind and body, it's our exterior appearance we are urged to focus on.

Are we buying this bill of goods? Do we need to subjugate our well-being in the name of the conventions and customs that hobble us? Could our smarts be the emphasis on the covers of magazines, instead of attention to wrinkles and waistlines?

While one could argue that these questions apply to what both women and men confront in various ways today, it's this book's goal to focus on women's health, and our brain health in particular. However clear it's becoming that our brains possess singularly remarkable gifts, as women, our strengths come with risks that have been left unresearched and unsupported. For the many reasons discussed throughout *The XX Brain*, there are vulnerabilities attributed to this indispensable organ that are currently twice or more as common in women. These hazards hail in the form of Alzheimer's and dementia, as well as depression and anxiety, among others. We acknowledge that this is the result of factors both biological and societal in nature, derived from our evolution, our history, and our society, as well as from the present-day powers that be. In spite of the gravity of these risks, many don't exist because they're biologically unavoidable; they exist due to misinformation and neglect.

For me, I am not having it. I'm not having it for myself, nor for my mother—and I'm certainly not having it for my daughter. If you've made it this far, I'm guessing you might feel the same. We're not alone. As a devoted researcher in the field, I am working diligently alongside my global colleagues to reassess, reinvigorate, and level the field of women's brain health, offering select screening procedures and interventions geared explicitly to the female physiology. In doing so, we intend to provide women with the care they merit as a fundamental human right.

The marvel of the female mind and the way it interlaces with its body's many missions offers rich research territory. It deserves the curiosity, attention, and care necessary to establish an entirely new and updated standard in women's health care. Given women's ever-increasing contributions to society at large, the welfare of everyone's future lies in our unflagging commitment to fulfilling this task. Ours is a moment that trembles with a great degree of change. Let's put our foot down, appraise what's lacking, and take what we need to clear these hurdles, a move that's long overdue.

Seeing this through requires a series of shifts, and perhaps like the toppling of dominoes, it begins with those first actions we ourselves take before rippling through society. For the part that's ours to do, I offer a means to an end via the research, recognition, and game plan laid out for you in this book. Together and individually, we can extricate ourselves from these current confines and their subsequent risks.

The primary means available to an individual is not legislation, research, or a magic pill. When it comes to brain health, prevention is everything. Although we are making advances every day to treat diseases once thought unavoidable, preventative strategies rather than pharmaceuticals show the boldest success in the field thus far. Intervening with these strategies in advance, and capitalizing on the windows of opportunity that pop up amid our hormonal ebb and flow, form the basis of this approach.

Typically, women's health care involves some form of hormonal therapy, whether MHT, birth control, or anti-estrogen treatment. Every medication has potential risks and benefits. As women, we need to be aware of both sides of the coin to make smart, informed decisions that honor both our present and future health. At the same time, we merit options that have been thoroughly researched and carefully developed with respect for the health and well-being of our bodies and minds.

The female-sensitive interventions you now have in hand are at the very heart (and head) of this enfranchisement. They are tailored to safeguard the sophisticated workings of a woman's mind, navigating the lifetime of hormonal evolution that defines our gender. Science reveals that a woman's brain functions in accord with her body's rigorous journey, alert to the manifold hormonal map of female adolescence, pregnancy, and menopause. We finally have a lifestyle program that respects these select criteria as women, fine-tuned to promote our cognitive health while enhancing our overall vitality and sense of self. By adequately assessing pharma and non-pharma options, optimizing diet and exercise, downgrading stress and upgrading sleep, while enriching our lives with the social, cultural, and intellectual offerings that fuel our minds as much as heal them, we can build the foundations on which to thrive, not just in the flower of youth but also in the strength of age.

To do this, we must reprioritize.

As the proverb says, "Eat half, walk double, laugh triple, and love without measure." I don't know any scientist who would argue with that. But this is not achieved overnight or with the attitude of finding a temporary fix. Although you may come across articles, apps, and dietary tricks claiming to "change your brain" in a matter of weeks, our work goes deeper and asks patience and persistence. Genuine change takes between three and six months to occur and lasts only as long as you continue to actively care for yourself. This is a forever plan, not just a quick fix. As with anything of excellence, it takes discipline, consistency, and commitment. The difference is, with this quality of investment in yourself, the benefits will last a lifetime—impacting not only you but also everyone you love.

In the end, we are indeed the sum of our parts. Perhaps it's time to take a tip from our XX brain itself and tend and befriend: our brains, our bodies, ourselves, and one another. There is a mounting awareness around the things that need to change in the field of women's health care and concerning women's well-being overall. Now is the time to draw the line, express our needs, and address them.

I look forward to seeing the female mind and all that it achieves fully celebrated, duly appreciated, equally compensated, and downright admired. Until we meet again, know that I'm joining in with you as we pioneer the kind of care that women require and that women can provide.

WHERE TO FIND HELP

FIND A DOCTOR

Choosing your doctor is a very important decision, one that is best made when you are in a good place rather than sick or facing an emergency. Not only do you want a doctor who is competent and well trained in the specific types of health issues you have, but you also want a doctor who takes the time necessary to listen to and address your health problems or questions.

A doctor who knows you (or your loved one) and is familiar with your (or your loved one's) health concerns is always a good starting point. However, your longtime family physician may not necessarily be the best person to go to for a diagnosis, because he or she is unlikely to be trained in the specific issues we are discussing. If you have a family doctor you know and trust, you may want to ask him or her for a referral to a doctor who specializes in diagnosing Alzheimer's disease and/or menopausal issues, or for help finding one.

Find an Alzheimer's Doctor

There are a number of things you can do to help ensure you're seeing the right doctor:

- Call the doctor's office to speak with an office manager or staff person who can provide details about the doctor's credentials, office policies, and payment procedures.

- Ask friends, family, and associates about their experiences.

- Check to see what board certifications the doctor has; these indicate that the doctor has passed critical examinations ("boards") that are developed by professional medical associations to test skills in a particular area of medicine.

- Find out how many of the doctor's patients are in your age range and if he/she has experience with your specific concerns.

Seek out a physician whose specialty is clinical neurology, psychiatry, or geriatrics, a branch of medicine concerned with diseases and problems of older age. These types of doctors are generally well trained in the diagnosis of Alzheimer's and other dementias. Neurologists are doctors who specialize in conditions of the nervous system, including the brain. Neurologists may sub-specialize in various areas, so it is important to consult with a neurologist who has experience diagnosing and treating Alzheimer's disease.

Psychiatrists are medical doctors who specialize in disorders of the mind. Some, but not all, specialize in dementia and cognitive aging. Geriatric psychiatrists are sub-specialists who are primarily concerned with disorders affecting older people. You want your doctor to be a member of the American Medical Association, the premier medical professional organization for doctors and specialists. Primary care physicians, including general practitioners as well as doctors who are board-certified in family practice or internal medicine, may also be able to diagnose Alzheimer's especially those who are board certified in geriatrics.

Other types of doctors who might specialize in or have experience with Alzheimer's include neuropsychologists and neuropsychiatrists.

Use the following options to find an Alzheimer's specialist near you:

- Your local Alzheimer's Association chapter can provide a list of Alzheimer's and other dementia specialists in your area: www.alz.org/local_resources/find_your _local_chapter.

- The National Institute on Aging supports about thirty multidisciplinary Alzheimer's disease centers across the country. These are premier medical research institutions that have dedicated research programs to the study of Alzheimer's. Most of these centers also provide diagnosis, treatment, and support services for people with Alzheimer's disease and their families. Find a center near you: www.nia.nih.gov/health /alzheimers-disease-research-centers.

- If you belong to a managed care plan, you may need to locate qualified physicians through your plan. Contact your health plan's administrator or the plan's physician directory to determine your options.

- You can also ask friends and associates, including your own doctor, for recommendations. Seriously, word of mouth sometimes is a great way to find the right doctor.

Find an Endocrinologist (aka a "Hormone Doctor")

The American Association of Clinical Endocrinologists (AACE) members are physicians treating patients with endocrine disorders as at least 50 percent of their practice. The "Find an Endocrinologist" tool allows you to search AACE members by location and endocrine area of focus: https://www.empoweryourhealth.org/.

Neuroendocrinologists (hormone and brain doctors) are not as easy to locate. Consider reaching out to the AACE or the Endocrine Society for referrals: www.endocrine.org/topics/neuroendocrinology.

Endocrinologists are, however, unlikely to specialize or have expertise in dementia. The best solution is to work with a neurologist or other Alzheimer's expert and an endocrinologist where the two are willing to collaborate.

WHERE TO TURN FOR CLINICAL TRIALS

There are several active clinical trials for Alzheimer's that many patients just don't get to learn about. Online registries that allow people to be contacted about trial opportunities in their area are incredibly helpful in this respect. The shared goal of these registries is to build a large pool of potential participants for therapeutic prevention trials. Most registries include people with or without a diagnosis of Alzheimer's, which is important, as some ongoing clinical trials focus on those at risk for the disease. Some registries also educate members about the disease; others establish active patient communities. Most sites ask for minimal information at sign-up, usually name, email address, birth year, and zip code. After registering, people may choose to complete more detailed health questionnaires in order to be matched to trials.

Here is a list of registries:

- *Alzheimer's Association TrialMatch:* www.alz.org /alzheimers-dementia/research_progress/clinical -trials/about-clinical-trials.

    This clinical study–matching service aims to help people in the United States find an Alzheimer's trial they can join. Registrants complete a health questionnaire online or over the phone, and then receive emails alerting them to studies for which they may qualify.

- *Alzheimer's Prevention Registry:* www.endalznow.org.

    Registrants receive emails about Alzheimer's-prevention research, can browse open studies in their region, and may choose to be contacted with offers to participate in particular studies.

- *Brain Health Registry:* www.brainhealth registry.org.

    Registrants fill out health and lifestyle questionnaires and take cognitive tests online, which they can repeat every three to six months. Participants whose questionnaire and testing data indicate they may be candidates for research are notified and invited to participate in studies and clinical trials.

- *Dominantly Inherited Alzheimer Network (DIAN)*:
  https://dian.wustl.edu.

  > This is an international registry for drug trials in autosomal-dominant Alzheimer's disease, the rare form of Alzheimer's caused by genetic mutations. People eighteen or older who have a family history of early-onset Alzheimer's are invited to register. The staff helps determine if the patient's family history is due to genetic mutations. If so, they are eligible to screen for the DIAN observational study or therapeutic intervention trials.

HOW TO BE PART OF OUR STUDIES

The mission of the Women's Brain Initiative (WBI) at Weill Cornell Medical College in New York City is to discover sex-based molecular targets and precision therapies to prevent, delay, and manage Alzheimer's disease. The WBI, which I have the honor of directing, represents a major commitment to understand how sex differences affect brain aging and risk of Alzheimer's disease.

Our current brain-imaging research addresses the connections between sex hormones, brain aging, and Alzheimer's risk. If you are interested in participating in the WBI, consult our website for more information: https://neurology.weill.cornell.edu/research-clinical-trials/womens-brain-initiative.

SUPPORT COMMUNITIES

Support and advocacy groups can help you connect with other patients and families, and they can provide valuable services. Many develop patient-centered information and are the driving force behind research for better treatments and possible cures. They can direct you to research, resources, and services. Many organizations also have experts who serve as medical advisers or provide lists of doctors and clinics, as well as information on legal and financial planning. Visit a group's website or contact them to learn about the services they offer.

- *Alzheimer's Association:* www.alz.org; www
  .alzconnected.org.
- *Alzheimer's & Related Dementias Disease Education &
  Referral Center (ADEAR):* www.nia.nih.gov/alzheimers.
- *Alzheimer's Foundation of America:* www.alzfdn.org.
- *CaringKind:* 24/7 helpline: 646-744-2900; https://
  caringkindnyc.org/caregivertips.
- *For APOE-4 carriers:* www.apoe4.info/wp.
- *Office on Women's Health:* www.womenshealth.gov.
- *North American Menopause Society (NAMS):* www
  .menopause.org.

FAQ: MEDICAL INSURANCE COVERAGE

Some insurance and managed care plans will cover the costs of a diagnostic assessment for Alzheimer's. This includes medical exams and lab tests, and in some cases cognitive testing. Testing for menopause is also typically covered, whereas brain scans are not. Check with your health plan's administrator to understand the policies and procedures.

Medicare, the government's health-insurance program for people sixty-five and up, and Medicaid, the joint federal-state medical-assistance program for people with limited income or assets, typically reimburse doctors for a diagnostic assessment and certain medical tests needed to determine if a patient has Alzheimer's disease—provided your doctor accepts these plans as payment. Hormonal tests are commonly covered. Talk to your doctor or doctor's staff about what is covered.

Medicare and Medicaid are complicated, but do not worry, there is help available. Call the Medicare Helpline to get your questions answered: https://medicarehelpline.com/. You can also read more online here:

- *Centers for Medicare and Medicaid Services:*
  www.cms.gov.

- *The official U.S. Government Site for Medicare:* www .medicare.gov.

- *MedlinePlus, National Institutes of Health:* www.nlm.nih.gov/medlineplus/medicare.html.

It might be helpful to know that Medicare now covers care-planning services for people recently diagnosed with cognitive impairment, including Alzheimer's disease and other dementias. Care planning allows individuals and their caregivers to learn about medical and non-medical treatments, clinical trials, and services available in the community, and additional information and support that can contribute to a higher quality of life. Under this new coverage, physicians, physicians' assistants, nurse practitioners, clinical nurse specialists, and certified nurse midwives can provide detailed care planning that includes

- evaluating cognition and function
- measuring neuropsychiatric symptoms
- medication reconciliation
- evaluating safety (including driving ability)
- identifying caregivers and caregiver needs
- identifying and assessing care directives
- planning for palliative care needs
- referrals to community services for both the beneficiary and his or her caregiver

Talk to your health-care provider about care-planning services. If your provider is not familiar with Medicare coverage of care planning, the Alzheimer's Association can provide more information: www.alz .org/careplanning.

DIET PLAN AND RECIPES

DIETARY RECOMMENDATIONS

Research shows that the best diet for women is rich in fiber, healthy carbs, essential fats, lean protein, and a variety of vitamins and minerals. It is a flexible diet, prevalently plant based with moderate amounts of fish and smaller amounts of meat, eggs, and dairy. You can eat a little bit of everything, as long as it's from the right sources, in the right amounts (see portion size, below), and, whenever possible, in its peak season. Eating produce when it's in season guarantees maximum freshness and nutrition—and it's cheaper. Overall, and regardless of seasons, at least half of the food on your plate should be plant based.

It is also important to emphasize the need to eat regular, scheduled meals, not skipping meals, and being aware of what and when you are eating. Always eat breakfast, lunch, and dinner—and squeeze in two small snacks if you are hungry, or when exercising.

TYPICAL DAY

Breakfast	Herbal tea (no sugar) Choice of: • Yogurt with fresh fruit and/or whole grains (muesli, oats, wheat germ) • Oatmeal or muesli with fresh fruit, nuts, and seeds • Eggs with toast and/or avocado • Smoothie with fruit, vegetables, and nut or seed butter

Morning tea	Cup of coffee or tea (no sugar)
	Choice of:
	• Green juice
	• Handful of nuts
	• Fresh fruit
	• Dark chocolate
Lunch	Green salad vegetables with dressing
	Whole-grain bread, brown rice, spelt, or rye biscuits
	Choice of:
	• Legume dish or soup
	• Tofu dish
	• Vegetarian burger
	• Fish (poached, roasted, grilled, or canned)
	• Eggs (no more than 2–3 times per week)
Afternoon tea	Choice of:
	• Handful of almonds
	• Dried fruit
	• Seaweed snack
	• Edamame
	• Glass of milk or nut milk
Dinner	Cooked vegetables (steamed, roasted, pureed, or soup)
	Green salad vegetables with dressing
	Choice of:
	• Fish or shellfish (poached, roasted, grilled, or canned)
	• Legumes dish or soup
	• Vegetarian burger
	• Poultry (grilled or roasted)
	• Cheese (no more than 1–2 times per week)
	• Red meat (no more than 1–2 times per week)

TYPICAL WEEK

Here is a typical week's worth of healthy menus. Accompanying recipes (for the items in italics) are found at the end of this appendix.

MONDAY	
Breakfast	Cup of green tea; plain yogurt with muesli; blueberries
Morning tea	Green juice (celery, cucumber, spinach, green apple, lemon, ginger)

Lunch	Mixed greens and tomato salad with balsamic–flaxseed oil vinaigrette; *Spiced Chickpeas*
Afternoon tea	Two dried or fresh apricots
Dinner	Mixed lettuce and onion salad with EVOO; steamed green beans; *Dijon Salmon Steak*; brown rice

TUESDAY	
Breakfast	Cup of rooibos tea with a dash of milk; oatmeal with milk and raw honey; fresh raspberries
Morning tea	Handful of tamari-roasted almonds
Lunch	*Coconut-Lime Tofu with Mixed Vegetables*; steamed brown rice
Afternoon tea	Seaweed snack
Dinner	*Must-Have Green Salad* with olives and feta cheese; roasted turkey breast; grilled zucchini and bell peppers

WEDNESDAY	
Breakfast	Cup of rose tea; multigrain toast with raw honey and coconut oil; baked pear with cinnamon
Morning tea	Beet juice (red beet, carrots, apple, ginger, lemon)
Lunch	*Lentil Soup*; two rye biscuits; small apple
Afternoon tea	Edamame
Dinner	*Vellutata di Broccoli*; *Veggie Burgers*; watercress salad with cherry tomatoes with lemon-vinaigrette dressing

THURSDAY	
Breakfast	Cup of black tea with a dash of milk; *Breakfast Egg Muffins* with avocado; slice of toast
Morning tea	Cappuccino
Lunch	*Niçoise Salad*; whole-wheat crispbread
Afternoon tea	Dark chocolate–covered goji berries; almonds
Dinner	*Zucchini Infornati*; *Broccoli Puree*; grilled chicken breast

FRIDAY	
Breakfast	Cup of Earl Grey tea; muesli with roasted hazelnuts, raisins, and almond milk; blueberries or blackberries
Morning tea	Apple
Lunch	*Glory Bowl*
Afternoon tea	Hummus with carrots and celery sticks
Dinner	*Sweet Greens Soup; Almond-Encrusted Fish Fillet;* basmati brown rice

SATURDAY	
Breakfast	Cup of lemon ginger tea; *Avocado Toast;* two dried prunes
Morning tea	½ grapefruit
Lunch	Simple green salad with EVOO; *Pasta Primavera*
Afternoon tea	Carrot juice
Dinner	*Sweet Potatoes with Figs and Goat Cheese Salad*

SUNDAY	
Breakfast	Cup of rooibos tea with a dash of milk; *BB Breakfast Smoothie*
Morning tea	Sesame honey bar
Lunch	*Spring Frittata* with avocado; spinach salad
Afternoon tea	Apple with raw almond butter
Dinner	*Slow-Roast Lemon Chicken; Roasted Vegetables with Sea Salt and Thyme;* slice of sourdough bread

PORTION CONTROL

There is no such thing as an all-you-can-eat diet. At the same time, no matter what you've heard in the news, stuffing yourself silly with only one food type at a time won't make you lose weight and most certainly won't help your mental performance. No, not even kale. A healthy diet is varied and filling, and recommends a specific number of servings per day. But just what counts as a serving?

Arm yourself with a food scale, and let's take a look at the appropriate portion size for the foods that are part of our female-brain-boosting diet:

FOOD GROUP	1 SERVING
Vegetables	1 cup cooked vegetables
	2 cups raw vegetables
	1 cup vegetable juice
	2 cups vegetable soup
Fruits	1 cup fruit
	½ cup fruit juice
	¼ avocado
	5 olives
Grains	½ cup cooked rice or cereal
	1 cup cooked pasta
	1 slice bread
	1 cup cooked oatmeal
	½ cup muesli or granola
Potatoes	½ small potato
Legumes	½ cup cooked legumes (1 cup if main meal)
	¼ cup hummus
Nuts and seeds	1 tablespoon nut or seed butter
	handful of unsalted nuts/seeds as a snack, or ¼ cup as part of a vegetarian meal
	1 cup nut milk
Oils	1 tablespoon
Meat and poultry	2 oz cooked meat or poultry
	1 egg or 2 egg whites
Fish and seafood	3 oz cooked fish or seafood
Dairy	½ cup milk or nut milk
	1 cup yogurt
	1½ oz dry cheese
	2 oz fresh or cottage cheese
	1 teaspoon butter

Sweets and sweeteners	1 oz dark chocolate
	1 teaspoon honey, maple syrup, coconut sugar

ANOTHER WAY TO THINK ABOUT IT:

- A serving of vegetables or potatoes is about the size of a small fist.

- A serving of cooked meat, poultry, or fish is about the size of the palm of your hand.

- A serving of butter is about the size of your fingertip (from the last joint all the way up to the tip of your finger).

- A serving of dry cheese is about the length and width of your index finger.

- A serving of fresh cheese is about half the size of the palm of your hand, in all directions.

- A serving of fruit is a handful of berries, 2 pieces of a small fruit (apricots, mandarins), one piece of a medium-size fruit (orange, apple, pear), half of a large fruit (grapefruit), 2 slices of a very large fruit (melon, pineapple, watermelon), or 2 small pieces of dried fruit (apricots, prunes, dates).

- A serving of dark chocolate is the length and width of your little finger.

HEALTHY SWAPS

SWAP THIS . . .	. . . FOR THIS
Iceberg lettuce	Mixed greens, baby spinach, baby kale
Commercial salad dressing	Extra-virgin olive oil, plain yogurt, fresh herbs mix; or extra-virgin olive oil, lemon juice, balsamic vinegar mix
Canola oil, vegetable oil	Extra-virgin olive oil
Salad croutons	Mixed nuts

Commercial pickles	Raw pickles, sauerkraut
Banana	Berries, apples, citrus fruit
Commercial fruit juice	Fruit-infused water and/or juice your own fruit (add sparkling water for extra fizz)
Breakfast cereal (Corn Flakes, Rice Krispies, Cheerios, etc.)	Oatmeal, muesli, organic rice flakes
Instant oats	Steel-cut oats
White pasta	Whole-wheat pasta
White rice	Brown rice, wild rice, red rice
White potato	Sweet potato
Frozen pizza	Brick-oven pizza at a restaurant, no more than once a week
Conventionally raised beef	Grass-fed organic beef
Conventionally raised chicken	Cage-free organic chicken
Conventional eggs	Cage-free organic eggs
Egg-white omelet	Whole-egg omelet (limit to 1–2 eggs)
Bacon	Turkey bacon
Burger bun	Whole-wheat bread
Burger and fries	Turkey burger with sweet potato fries
Chicken nuggets	Grilled chicken
Mayonnaise	Avocado-based mayo, hummus, Greek yogurt with lemon mix
Ketchup	Fresh salsa
Commercial butter, margarine, buttery spreads	Organic grass-fed butter, ghee butter, avocado
Canned tuna	Albacore tuna, preferably in glass
Commercial tuna salad	Make it yourself: albacore tuna, celery, onion, herbs, and avocado-based mayo
Roasted or flavored nuts	Raw nuts (roast them yourself)
Commercial peanut butter	Natural peanut butter or, even better, almond butter
Frappuccino, frozen coffee drinks	Iced coffee—add milk yourself
Processed cheese	Real cheese
Fat-free or low-fat yogurt	Plain full-fat yogurt (best if organic)

Chips and dips	Carrots and celery sticks with hummus
Tortilla chips with commercial salsa	Sliced cucumber with guacamole
Milk chocolate, candy	Dark chocolate; nut and fruit power bites from my website
Ice cream, frozen yogurt	Yogurt parfait with fresh fruit, nuts, and honey (or artisanal ice cream, of course!)
Splenda, artificial sweeteners	Stevia, honey, maple syrup

BRAIN-HEALTHY RECIPES

Recipes are listed in alphabetical order. More recipes can be found in my book *Brain Food* and on my website: www.lisamosconi.com.

Almond-Encrusted Fish Fillet

Prep: 10 minutes

Cook: 10 minutes

Ready in: 20 minutes

Ingredients (serves 2):

8 ounces cod fillet

1 egg (best if cage-free organic)

½ cup almonds

1 tablespoon coconut oil

sea salt to taste

Directions:

Rinse the cod and pat dry with a paper towel. Set it aside.

In a large shallow bowl, beat the egg.

Using a food processor, chop the almonds finely and pour onto a separate plate.

Dip the cod first in the egg (both sides), allowing excess to drip off. Then dredge it in almond crumbs to coat.

Heat the coconut oil in a large nonstick pan over medium-high heat. Add cod in a single layer. Cook without moving for about 5 minutes until the crust is golden on the bottom. Flip over and cook another 5 minutes until the other side is golden and the fish is cooked through. Season with the sea salt to taste and serve immediately. It pairs nicely with a simple green salad.

Avocado Toast

Prep: <5 minutes
Cook: <5 minutes
Ready in: <10 minutes

Recipe available at www.lisamosconi.com/recipes/avocado-toast.

BB (Blueberries & Banana) Breakfast Smoothie

Prep: <5 minutes
Cook: n.a.
Ready in: <5 minutes

Ingredients (serves 2):

1 cup blueberries (fresh or frozen)

1 ripe banana

1 cup baby spinach

2 tablespoons almond butter

1 tablespoon raw cacao

1 tablespoon hemp seeds

2–3 cups almond milk

Ice (optional)

Directions:

Put all the ingredients in a blender and process until smooth. Pour into glasses and serve.

Breakfast Egg Muffins

Prep: 5 minutes
Cook: 20 minutes
Ready in: 25 minutes

Ingredients (serves 6):

10 large eggs (best if cage-free, organic)

⅓ cup whole milk

1 cup grated Parmesan cheese

1 cup sliced mushrooms

1 cup cherry tomatoes, halved

sea salt or Herbamare to taste

1 tablespoon fresh minced chives

Directions:

Preheat the oven to 375 degrees F (180 degrees C).

In a large mixing bowl, combine the eggs and milk and whisk well.

Stir in the grated cheese, mushrooms, tomatoes, and a pinch of salt.

Divide the mixture evenly among 12 greased muffin cups or a silicon muffin tray. Sprinkle with the fresh chives.

Bake for 20 minutes or until centers are set and muffins are beginning to brown. Let cool for 5 minutes before serving.

Broccoli Puree

Prep: 5 minutes
Cook: n.a.
Ready in: 5 minutes

Ingredients (serves 4):

4 cups broccoli florets, steamed

1 garlic clove

2 tablespoons olive oil

2 tablespoons hemp seeds

sea salt and pepper to taste

Directions:

Place all the ingredients (except salt and pepper) and 2 tablespoons of warm water in a high-speed blender. Mix for 1 minute.

Add sea salt and pepper to taste. Transfer to a serving bowl and serve immediately.

Coconut-Lime Tofu with Mixed Vegetables

Prep: 40 minutes
Cook: 15 minutes
Ready in: 55 minutes

Ingredients (serves 6):

1 (14-ounce) package water-packed extra-firm tofu, drained

3 green onions, cut into 1-inch pieces

3 garlic cloves, sliced

1 tablespoon grated ginger root

4 small baby bok choy, quartered lengthwise

1 red bell pepper, sliced

1 cup snow peas, trimmed

2 tablespoons coconut oil

1 tablespoon sesame seeds

For the marinade:

½ cup coconut cream

juice of 1 lime

1 teaspoon raw honey

2 tablespoons dry sherry

2 tablespoons sesame oil

2 tablespoons Nama Shoyu or tamari sauce

Directions:

Cut the tofu into ½-inch squares. Place the tofu on several layers of paper towels, and cover with additional paper towels. Let it stand 10 minutes, pressing down occasionally.

In a ziplock bag, mix the ingredients for the marinade. Add the tofu and coat to cover. Refrigerate for at least 30 minutes. In the meantime, chop up all the veggies.

Heat a large wok or skillet over high heat. Add 1 tablespoon of coconut oil to the pan and swirl to coat.

Add the tofu to the pan. Stir-fry for about 8 minutes, turning to brown on all sides. Remove the tofu from the pan and place it in a medium bowl.

Add the onions, garlic, and ginger to the pan. Stir-fry for 1 minute. Remove it from the pan and add it to the tofu.

Add the remaining 1 tablespoon of coconut oil to the pan and swirl to coat. Add the bok choy, bell pepper, and snow peas. Stir-fry for 4–5 minutes. Stir in the tofu mixture.

Sprinkle with sesame seeds. Serve with brown rice or other rice.

Dijon Salmon Steak

Prep: 5 minutes
Cook: 15 minutes
Ready in: 20 minutes

Ingredients (serves 4):

4 salmon steaks (4 ounces each)

2 tablespoons Dijon mustard

sea salt and pepper to taste

Directions:

Preheat the oven to 400 degrees F (200 degrees C). Line a shallow baking pan with parchment paper.

Place the salmon on the parchment paper. Spread a thin layer of mustard on the top of each steak, and season with sea salt and pepper to taste.

Bake for 15 minutes, or until the salmon flakes easily with a fork.

Glory Bowl

Prep: 30 minutes
Cook: approx. 15 minutes
Ready in: 45 minutes

Ingredients (serves 4):

For the bowl:

½ cup (3 large leaves) baby kale, finely chopped

½ cup carrots, peeled and chopped

½ cup red beets, peeled and chopped

½ cup broccoli, chopped

¼ cup almonds, slivered

1 cup cooked wild rice

½ cup cooked quinoa

½ cup firm tofu, drained, chopped, and cubed

For the dressing:

2 small garlic cloves, chopped

2-inch piece fresh ginger root, peeled and minced

2 tablespoons tamari sauce or Nama Shoyu sauce

juice of ½ lemon

2 tablespoons organic tahini

1 tablespoon extra-virgin coconut oil

2 tablespoons water

Directions:

For the bowl:

Combine the kale, carrots, beets, and broccoli and steam over medium heat to desired texture (about 10 minutes).

Over medium heat, toast the almonds in a skillet (1 minute).

Combine the steamed vegetables and toasted almonds with the cooked grains and tofu. Distribute in serving bowls.

For the dressing:

Combine all the dressing ingredients in a food processor or high-speed blender. Blend until creamy.

Dress the bowl contents with the sauce; toss, serve, and enjoy.

Lentil Soup

Prep: 5 minutes
Cook: 35 minutes
Ready in: 40 minutes

Ingredients (serves 4):

2 cups organic red lentils

4 cups water

1 tablespoon extra-virgin coconut oil

1 teaspoon ground turmeric

1 teaspoon ground cumin

1 yellow onion, chopped

3 garlic cloves, minced

1-inch piece fresh ginger root, grated

1 organic carrot, peeled and finely chopped

2 organic celery stems, finely chopped

½ teaspoon dried rosemary leaves

6 cups vegetable stock

sea salt to taste

Directions:

Soak the lentils in the water either overnight or for no less than 5 hours (soaked legumes are easier to digest and will not cause bloating). Drain and set aside.

Heat the oil in a large, heavy saucepan over medium heat. Add the turmeric and cumin and stir for 1 minute.

Add the onion and cook, stirring frequently, until golden and soft, about 5 minutes. Add the garlic and ginger and cook for 2 minutes.

Add carrots, celery, lentils, and rosemary. Stir to combine. Add the stock and bring to a boil. Reduce the heat to a simmer. Season with sea salt to taste. Cover and cook for 25 minutes or until the lentils are cooked but not mushy.

Must-Have Green Salad

Prep: 15 minutes
Cook: n.a.
Ready in: 15 minutes

Ingredients (serves 4):

For the salad:

1 cup mixed greens, chopped

1 cup baby spinach, chopped

1 cup baby kale, chopped

8 scallions, sliced (white part only)

4–5 radishes, thinly sliced

1 baby fennel, thinly sliced

¼ cup Kalamata olives, chopped

½ cup fresh sauerkraut or pickled cabbage

1 ripe avocado, peeled, pitted, and cubed

For the dressing:

1 tablespoon flaxseed oil

juice of ½ lemon

1 tablespoon apple cider vinegar

Directions:

Chopping takes the most time. Using a food processor with a chopping option cuts the preparation time in half.

Add all veggies to a large bowl and mix.

In a blender, add all ingredients for the dressing and blend until well combined. Pour over the salad and toss until coated. Serve immediately.

Niçoise Salad

Prep: 45 minutes
Cook: 10 minutes
Ready in: 55 minutes

Ingredients (serves 4):

For the salad:

1 pound red-skinned potatoes, sliced ⅓ inch thick

4 large eggs (best if cage-free, organic)

10 ounces haricots verts or thin green beans, trimmed

8 cherry tomatoes, halved

1 head Boston lettuce

6 radishes, trimmed and quartered

2 jars or cans Italian or Spanish tuna packed in olive oil, drained

½ cup Kalamata olives, halved

For the dressing:

1 shallot, minced

¼ cup white wine vinegar

2 tablespoons old-fashioned Dijon mustard

1 tablespoon fresh thyme, chopped

½ cup extra-virgin olive oil

Salt and pepper to taste

Directions:

Put the potatoes in a medium saucepan. Cover with cold water. Bring to a simmer over medium-high heat and cook until fork-tender, about 5 minutes. Drain and transfer to a medium bowl and let cool.

Use the same saucepan to boil the eggs. Place the eggs in the saucepan and cover with cold water. Bring to a simmer over medium-high heat, then cover, remove from the heat, and let stand 7–8 minutes. Drain, then run under cold water to cool. Peel under cold running water. Quarter the eggs.

Meanwhile, bring a separate saucepan of salted water to a boil. Add the haricots verts and cook until crisp-tender and bright green, 2–4 minutes. Drain immediately and pat dry.

To make the dressing: Whisk the shallot, vinegar, mustard, and thyme in a bowl. Whisk in the olive oil in a slow, steady stream until emulsified. Add salt and pepper to taste.

In a small bowl, mix the potatoes and cherry tomatoes. Add about ¼ of the dressing and toss. Divide the lettuce among 4 plates. Arrange the tomatoes, potatoes, haricots verts, eggs, radishes, and tuna on top. Drizzle with the dressing and top with the olives.

Pasta Primavera

Prep: 10 minutes

Cook: 20 minutes

Ready in: 30 minutes

Ingredients (serves 4):

1 cup broccoli florets

4 asparagus spears

½ pound whole-wheat penne

4 tablespoons extra-virgin olive oil

2 garlic cloves, minced

1 zucchini, diced

2 tomatoes, seeded and diced

¼ cup organic heavy cream

½ cup peas, fresh or frozen

½ cup grated Parmesan cheese

handful of chopped basil leaves

sea salt to taste

Directions:

Get a large pot of water boiling, about 8 cups. Boil the broccoli for 1 minute. Add the asparagus and boil another minute. Drain under cold water and set aside.

In the same pot you boiled the vegetables in, cook your pasta al dente. Feel free to start over and boil fresh cold water; I use the water the veggies were cooked in and just add a handful of sea salt.

While the pasta is cooking (typically 10–12 minutes), in a large sauté pan, heat the olive oil over medium-high heat. When the oil is hot, add the garlic and zucchini and sauté 1 minute. Add the diced tomatoes and sauté another 2 minutes, stirring often.

Pour in the water the vegetables coated in and turn the heat to high to bring it to a boil. Add the cream and toss in all the vegetables, including the peas. Stir to combine.

Turn the heat down until the cream-broth mixture is just simmering, not boiling.

Add the Parmesan cheese and stir to combine.

As soon as the pasta is done, drain it under cold water and mix it into the sauce. Stir to combine. Add the basil, and sea salt to taste, if needed. Serve immediately.

Roasted Vegetables with Sea Salt and Thyme

Prep: 15 minutes
Cook: 45 minutes
Ready in: 60 minutes

Ingredients (serves 4–6):

4 medium carrots, peeled

2 parsnips, peeled and cut in half lengthwise

1 large potato, cut in thick lengthwise pieces

1 large red onion, chopped

2 tablespoons coconut oil

3–4 sprigs fresh thyme

3–4 sprigs rosemary

1 teaspoon ground cumin

sea salt and pepper to taste

Directions:

Preheat the oven to 350 degrees F (180 degrees C). Line a large baking tray with parchment paper.

Place cut vegetables in a large bowl. Pour the coconut oil over the veggies. Sprinkle with thyme, rosemary, cumin, and sea salt and pepper to taste. Gently mix to coat well.

Place the veggies on the baking tray and spread them around to allow them to cook evenly. Put them in the oven and roast for about 45 minutes or until they are cooked through and golden.

Remove from the oven and serve immediately. They will keep for up to 4 days refrigerated.

Slow-Roast Lemon Chicken

Prep: 10 minutes

Cook: 3 hours

Ready in: 3 hours and 25 minutes

Ingredients (serves 6):

1 whole organic, free-range chicken

1 large onion, chopped

6 garlic cloves, crushed

4 sprigs fresh rosemary

small bunch of fresh sage

3 tablespoons extra-virgin olive oil

juice of 1 lemon

3 tablespoons Bragg Liquid Aminos or tamari sauce

sea salt to taste

Directions:

Preheat the oven to 300 degrees F (150 degrees C).

Rinse the chicken and place it in a French oven, breast side down. Scatter the onion and garlic cloves around the pot, as well as inside the chicken. Insert the rosemary and sage inside the chicken. Pour the olive oil and lemon juice over the chicken. Drizzle it with Bragg Liquid Aminos. Cover with the lid.

Put the pot in the oven and cook for 3 hours. Every hour, baste the chicken with its juice.

For the last 10 minutes, or once the chicken is cooked through, switch to broiler mode to brown and crisp the skin. Sprinkle sea salt over the chicken skin (optional). Allow to cool for 15 minutes.

Spiced Chickpeas

Prep: 10 minutes
Cook: 20 minutes
Ready in: 30 minutes

Ingredients (serves 4):

2 tablespoons extra-virgin coconut oil

1 red onion, peeled and finely diced

4 garlic cloves, peeled and finely minced

1 tablespoon garam masala

1 teaspoon turmeric

1 teaspoon cinnamon

2-inch piece fresh ginger root, grated

3 cups organic chickpeas, cooked, drained, and rinsed in a
colander

2 tablespoons raw honey

sea salt to taste

Directions:

Heat the oil in a cast-iron skillet or large saucepan over medium heat. Add the diced onion and garlic. Sauté until the onion and garlic look partly translucent and slightly browned around the edges, about 3–4 minutes.

Stir in the garam masala, turmeric, cinnamon, and grated ginger, and cook for 1–2 minutes, or until very fragrant.

Add the chickpeas. Sauté for 10 minutes, until the chickpeas start to brown. Lower the heat, stir in the honey, and sauté for 2–3 minutes. Remove from the heat, and add sea salt to taste.

Spring Frittata

Prep: 15 minutes
Cook: 20–25 minutes
Ready in: 35–40 minutes

Ingredients (serves 6):

3 tablespoons extra-virgin olive oil

1 medium onion, sliced

3 garlic cloves, minced

3 cups baby spinach

1 cup sweet peas (pre-steamed)

½ cup edamame (shelled, pre-steamed)

8 eggs (best if cage-free, organic)

¼ cup whole milk

½ cup grated Parmesan cheese

sea salt and pepper to taste

Directions:

Preheat the oven to 350 degrees F (180 degrees C).

While you wait for the oven to reach temperature, heat 2 tablespoons of the olive oil in a large ovenproof (preferably cast-iron) skillet. Sauté the onion until soft, about 5 minutes. Add the minced garlic and cook for another 4 minutes.

Add the spinach, sweet peas, and edamame. Sauté for 2–3 minutes, or until the spinach is soft. Remove from the heat and set aside.

In a large bowl, beat the eggs and milk until well combined. Add the grated cheese and mix well. Stir in the veggies until well combined.

Warm up the remaining 1 tablespoon of olive oil in the same skillet and pour in the egg-and-veggies mixture. Cook for 5 minutes, or until the eggs look set around the edges.

Transfer the skillet to the oven and cook for 10 minutes. The top should have a lightly golden color. Sprinkle with sea salt and pepper to taste. Serve warm.

Sweet Greens Soup

Prep: 10 minutes

Cook: 20 minutes

Ready in: 30 minutes

Ingredients (serves 6):

10 ounces broccoli florets

10 ounces frozen sweet peas

2 large green squash, peel on, chopped

1 bunch lacinato kale (10–12 leaves), chopped, stems removed

4 cups vegetable broth

2 garlic cloves, minced

1 teaspoon ginger root, grated

crème fraîche or sour cream, 1 tablespoon per person (optional)

toasted pumpkin seeds (optional)

Directions:

Add the broccoli, sweet peas, squash, and kale to a large, heavy soup pot. Cover with the vegetable broth.

Bring to a boil, then cover and simmer 10–12 minutes, until the vegetables are just about tender. Add the garlic and ginger and simmer for another 10 minutes, until the kale is tender and the soup is fragrant.

Puree with a high-speed immersion blender until smooth.

Serve topped with a dollop of crème fraîche or sour cream and a few pumpkin seeds.

Sweet Potatoes with Figs and Goat Cheese Salad

Prep: 10 minutes

Cook: 15 minutes

Ready in: 25 minutes

Ingredients (serves 4):

3 cups water

2 large sweet potatoes, cut lengthwise into ½-inch slices

1 tablespoon extra-virgin olive oil

¼ cup maple syrup

2 tablespoons balsamic vinegar

4 scallions, thinly sliced (white part only)

5 dried figs, quartered

4 cups baby spinach

2 ounces goat cheese, crumbled (best if creamy)

Directions:

Preheat a grill or grill pan to high heat.

Bring a large pot filled with 3 cups of water to a boil over high heat. When the water is boiling, blanch the sweet potatoes until tender, 2–3 minutes. Let cool and pat dry.

Brush the grill or grill pan with the olive oil. When the oil is sizzling, add the sweet potatoes in a single layer and grill until charred, about 5 minutes per side.

In a small bowl, whisk together the maple syrup and balsamic vinegar. Add the scallions and figs.

Divide the baby spinach between four plates. Distribute the sweet potatoes over the spinach. Drizzle the dressing over the sweet potatoes and spinach and sprinkle with the crumbled goat cheese.

Serve warm.

Veggie Burgers

Prep: 15 minutes
Cook: 15 minutes
Ready in: 30 minutes

Ingredients (serves 2):

2 tablespoons extra-virgin olive oil

1 medium onion, finely chopped

1 carrot, finely chopped

1 cup cauliflower rice

1 cup cooked lentils

¼ cup sunflower seeds, coarsely chopped

1 cup steamed brown rice

1 tomato, sliced

Directions:

Drain the lentils completely.

Heat 1 tablespoon of the oil in a large skillet over medium heat. Add the onion, carrot, and cauliflower rice, and cook for 5–6 minutes or until soft. Remove from the heat and set aside.

In a medium bowl, mix the lentils, sunflower seeds, and brown rice. Add the cooked veggies and the mix to combine. Use your hands or a burger patty press to make 4 small burgers. Set aside.

In the same skillet, add the remaining oil and heat. Add the burgers and cook until browned, about 3–4 minutes per side.

Transfer the burgers to a plate. Serve the patties on whole-wheat toast if you like. Top with sliced tomatoes.

Vellutata di Broccoli (Velvety Broccoli Soup)

Prep: 10 minutes

Cook: 20 minutes

Ready in: 30 minutes

Ingredients (serves 4):

2 tablespoons extra-virgin olive oil

1 medium white onion, sliced

2 garlic cloves, chopped

3 cups broccoli florets, chopped (stem removed)

1 cup organic sweet peas (feel free to use frozen sweet peas)

1 medium yellow potato, chopped (with the peel on)

6 cups vegetable stock

sea salt and pepper to taste

Directions:

In a medium-size saucepan, heat the oil over medium heat. Add the onion and cook for 5–7 minutes until translucent. Add the garlic and cook until fragrant.

Add the broccoli, peas, potato, and stock. Bring to a boil and cook for 10 minutes.

Remove from heat. With a handheld immersion blender, puree until smooth. Pour back into the saucepan and cook 5 more minutes.

Add sea salt and pepper to taste. Serve immediately with a drizzle of olive oil.

Zucchini Infornati (In the Oven)

Prep: 10 minutes

Cook: 45 minutes

Ready in: 55 minutes

Ingredients (serves 4):

2 large yellow squash, diced

2 large green squash, diced

2 medium red onions, sliced into thin rings

½ cup grated Parmesan cheese

1 teaspoon thyme

⅓ cup whole-grain bread crumbs

2 tablespoons unsalted butter

1 tablespoon extra-virgin olive oil

Directions:

Preheat the oven to 350 degrees F (180 degrees C).

Combine the squash, onions, cheese, thyme, and bread crumbs in a bowl with the butter cut into chunks.

Place the mixture in a baking dish and sprinkle it with olive oil. I sprinkle a little more Parmesan cheese on top at this point.

Bake for 45 minutes, or until the vegetables are cooked through and the top is lightly browned.

ACKNOWLEDGMENTS

Several years ago, just moments before giving a talk at an international conference on Alzheimer's disease, I was about to take the microphone when a woman approached the podium. After the briefest of introductions, she got straight to the point: "How do you feel about the increased risk of Alzheimer's in women?"

Her question stopped me in my tracks. Setting down my slides, we launched a conversation there and then that would dramatically shift the trajectory of my work ahead. As serendipity would have it, she was none other than Dr. Roberta Diaz Brinton, a bold opinion leader in the field. Dr. Brinton had been focusing on how hormonal changes were potentially linked to Alzheimer's in women for decades, and is the ultimate authority on the topic. Within a matter of minutes, she not only convinced me to follow in her steps, but she also took me under her mighty wing, giving me every opportunity to carry out the most exciting piece of research I've ever partaken.

Robbie dearest, you are the brightest of all stars. Every woman is incredibly fortunate to have you on her side, and so am I. This book is a testament to your strength and kindness, both.

My deepest appreciation goes to all my colleagues, students, and collaborators present and past, and to all the scientists who are devoting their time and efforts to understanding the many ways that women's brains are, and aren't, different from men's. My work and career were made immeasurably richer by participating in this quest. Science is often conducted alone in the day-to-day, but never solo in the big picture; everything in this book incorporates the hard work of many teams around the world.

That said, no team is dearer to my heart than my own at the Weill Cornell Women's Brain Initiative. From study coordination to seeing patients, from data processing to statistical analysis, my colleagues and collaborators are all so exceptionally dedicated, hardworking, and just plain brilliant. A special thank-you to Dr. Matthew Fink, who gave me the opportunity to launch the Women's Brain Initiative in the first place and has been tirelessly supporting our cause; Dr. Richard Isaacson, the Sherlock Holmes of Alzheimer's prevention; and our colleagues in Radiology, who remain an incredible source of inspiration.

Beyond citations, it would be daunting to try to express gratitude to every researcher who's helped build the field and inspired me to write this book. Thank you all. Dr. Alberto Pupi, you are my best role model for a scientist, mentor, and teacher. Dr. Dharma and Kirti at the Alzheimer's Prevention Research Foundation, thank you for being so generous in sharing your knowledge of meditation.

None of our research would even be imaginable without the generous support from the National Institutes of Health/National Institute on Aging, Maria Shriver's Women's Alzheimer's Movement, the Cure Alzheimer's Fund, Harold W. McGraw III and Nancy G. McGraw, and many other benefactors.

At the same time, no research at all would be possible if it weren't for our research participants, who must remain anonymous, but you all know who you are. Thank you for informing, inspiring, and making our work possible.

For the book in particular, I couldn't be more grateful to Maria Shriver for writing the foreword. Maria is a formidable force in many arenas: as a journalist, an author, and the former First Lady of California, to name but a few. But nothing rivals her unfaltering commitment to preventing Alzheimer's and empowering women with the knowledge and wisdom we need to shine bright.

Speaking of other shining stars on Maria's team, Sandy Gleysteen, thank you for making this and so much more become reality—you are the bestest.

Heartfelt thanks to my brilliant editor, Caroline Sutton, and my powerhouse literary agent, Katinka Matson, for giving me the opportunity to write this book in the first place. I am truly grateful for your tremendous support and expertise in transforming rigorous science into concepts that can reach and help the greatest number of people, today and in the future.

Finally, my research is only one part of my life, and would be impossible without the love and support of my friends and family all over the world. I love you guys so much. A huge grazie, merci, and thank-you to Susan Verrilli Dutilh, who was once again by my side every step and every page of this book. *Sorellina*, you are a true example of grace, strength, and persistence in the face of some pretty crazy hardships.

I write for, from, and within my beautiful family, whose support also makes it not just possible but even more worthwhile. Mamma e papa', vi voglio un mare di bene. Momo, thank you for always being there for us. And deep within our little hothouse, Kevin and Lily, I love you more than anyone has ever loved anyone.

NOTES

All references accessed as of April 2019.

Introduction: Reclaiming Women's Health

page xix **the most common form of dementia**: Alzheimer's disease facts and figures. *Alzheimers Dement* 2016;12:459–509.

page xix **One of the most startling facts**: www.alz.org/media/HomeOffice /Facts%20and%20Figures/facts-and-figures.pdf.

page xx **to avoid risks to the fetus**: Kinney L, et al. *Ann Intern Med* 1981;95: 495–99.

page xxii **dosages are rarely adjusted by sex**: Yang X, et al. *Genome Res* 2006;16:995–1004.

page xxii **the first "female Viagra"**: https://www.accessdata.fda.gov/drugsatfda _docs/label/2015/022526REMS.pdf.

page xxiii **a greater risk of dementia**: Cheng HT, et al. *J Am Geriatr Soc* 2017;65:2488–95.

page xxiii **discharged mid–heart attack**: Pope JH, et al. *N Engl J Med* 2000;342: 1163–70.

page xxiv **influenced by emotional distress**: http://nationalpainreport.com /women-in-pain-report-significant-gender-bias-8824696.html.

Chapter 1: The Inner Workings of the Female Brain

page 3 **brain function as well**: McEwen B. *J Appl Physiol* 2001;91:2785–801.

page 4 **driver of women's brain health**: Brinton RD, et al. *Nat Rev Endocrinol* 2015; 11:393–405.

page 5 **sexual differentiation of the brain**: Nugent BM, et al. *Horm Metab Res* 2012;44:577–86.

page 5 **mood, sleep, and even appetite**: Nishizawa S., et al. *Proc Natl Acad Sci USA* 1997;94:5308–13.

page 6 **depending upon gender**: Rahman A, et al. *Frontiers Res Topics* 2019;in press; Ferretti MT, et al. *Nat Rev Neurol* 2018;14:457–69.

page 6 **better interconnected**: Ingalhalikar M, et al. *Proc Natl Acad Sci USA* 2014;111:823–8.

page 6 **having a family**: Rogan MT, LeDoux JE. *Cell* 1996;85:469–75.

page 8 **a key protective element**: Mosconi L, et al. *Neurology* 2017;89: 1382–90; Mosconi L, et al. *PLoS One* 2017;12:e0185926.

page 8 **accelerate the aging process**: Lin J, et al. *Brain Res* 2011;1379: 224–32.

page 10 **a major hallmark of Alzheimer's**: Mosconi L, et al. *PLoS One* 2018;13: e0207885.

page 10 **not in old age**: Sperling RA, et al. *Nat Rev Neurol* 2013;9:54–8.

page 10 **genetic, medical, and lifestyle events**: Kivimaki M, et al. *Lancet Neurol* 2018;391:1574–5.

page 11 **affecting predominantly females**: Folsom DP, et al. *Dialogues Clin Neurosci* 2006;8:45–52.

page 12 **Emerging research is pointing**: Rahman A, et al. *Frontiers Res Topics* 2019;in press.

page 12 **The two major symptoms**: Feldman HA, et al. *J Clin Endocrinol Metab* 2002;87:589–98.

page 13 **It has been estimated**: Harlow SD, et al. *Menopause* 2012;19:387–95.

Chapter 2: Dispelling Myths Around Women's Brain Health

page 17 **than 1 to 2 percent of the population**: Clancy S. *Nat Educ* 2008;1:187.

page 17 **switching select genes on and off**: Jirtle RL, et al. *Nat Rev Genet* 2007; 8:253–62.

page 18 **medical and environmental factors**: Wong M, et al. *Nat Rev Neurosci* 2001;2:343–51.

page 18 **Medical conditions**: Jimenez-Sanchez G, et al. *Nat Genet* 2001;409:853–5.

page 18 **an unhealthy lifestyle**: Willett WC. *Science* 2002;296:695–8.

page 18 **medical and lifestyle shifts**: Norton S, et al. *Lancet Neurol* 2014;13: 788–94.

page 19 **less than five years**: www.cia.gov/library/publications/the-world -factbook/geos/us.html.

page 19 **less than two years**: Bennett JE, et al. *Lancet* 2015;386:163–70.

page 19 **rapidly narrowing gender gap**: Beltrán-Sánchez H, et al. *Proc Natl Acad Sci USA* 2015;201421942.

page 21 **Alzheimer's patients are women**: Throughout the book, I intentionally avoid characterizing women as being at higher "risk" of Alzheimer's than men. This is because, statistically, increased "prevalence" (i.e., the number of people affected) doesn't equal to increased "risk." In order to talk about increased risk, there has to be both increased prevalence and "incidence," which is the rate at which people develop a disease over time. While everybody agrees that Alzheimer's prevalence is higher in women than in men (two-thirds of Alzheimer's patients are indeed women), there is conflicting data over whether the incidence of Alzheimer's is also higher. This is mostly because very few studies have looked into it so far. So, statistically speaking, women aren't (yet) considered at higher "risk" of Alzheimer's than men. For an in-depth discussion about this topic, see Ferretti MT, et al. *Nat Rev Neurol* 2018; 14:457–69. Regardless of semantics, at the end of the day, more women than men end their lives battling dementia. Most importantly, the factors that put women at risk are not necessarily the same factors that put men at risk.

Our goal today is to identify what risk factors women need to watch out for and how to neutralize those risks.

page 21 **the same 2:1 ratio**: Vina J, Lloret A. *J Alzheimers Dis* 2010;20 Suppl 2:527–33.

page 21 **kills more men than women**: Gao S, et al. *Arch Gen Psychiatry* 1998; 55:809–15.

page 22 **99.6 percent drug failure rate**: Cummings JL, et al. *Alzheimers Res Ther* 2014;6:37–40.

page 22 **for men than for women**: Haywood WM, et al. *Am J Geriatr Pharmacother* 2006;4:273–86.

page 22 **every one of them has failed**: Andrieu S, et al. *Lancet Neurol* 2015; 14:926–44.

page 23 **brain plaques were gone**: Holmes C, et al. *Lancet* 2008;372:216–23.

page 23 **Recent clinical trials**: Kivipelto M, et al. *Nat Rev Neurol* 2018;14: 653–66.

Chapter 3: Unique Risks to Women's Brain Health

page 28 **than having an affected father**: Mosconi L, et al. *Proc Natl Acad Sci USA* 2010;107:5949–54.

page 28 **different effects on health**: Bertram L, et al. *Nat Rev Neurosci* 2008;9:768–78.

page 28 **than men with the gene**: Farrer LA, et al. *JAMA* 1997;278:1349–56.

page 29 **already in midlife**: Mosconi L, et al. *Neurology* 2017;89:1382–90.

page 29 **increased risk of Alzheimer's**: Scheltens P, et al. *Lancet* 2016; 388:505–17.

page 29 **other forms of dementia**: https://www.alz.org/national/documents /report_africanamericanssilentepidemic.pdf.

page 29 **than those who are white**: www.heart.org/HEARTORG/Conditions /More/MyHeartandStrokeNews/African-Americans-and-Heart -Disease_UCM_444863_Article.jsp#.WzaWkBJKhBy.

page 30 **"mini strokes"**: Morris MS. *Lancet Neurol* 2003;2:425–8.

page 31 **6 to 8 percent of all dementia patients**: Sims-Robinson C, et al. *Nat Rev Neurol* 2010;6:551–9.

page 31 **in a big way**: Biessels GJ, Reagan LP. *Nat Rev Neurosci* 2015;16:660–71.

page 31 **pre-diabetes or diabetes**: Menke A, et al. *JAMA* 2015;314:1021–9.

page 32 **later in life**: Nordstrom A, et al. *PLoS Med* 2018;15:e1002496

page 33 **longer to recover**: Harmon KG, et al. *Br J Sports Med* 2013;47:15–26.

page 33 **greater among women**: Stockl H, et al. *Lancet* 2013;382:859–65.

page 33 **in their lifetime**: www.cdc.gov/violenceprevention/pdf/cdc_nisvs_ipv _report_2013_v17_single_a.pdf.

page 34 **acting as a trigger**: Wyss-Coray T. *Nat Med* 2006;12:1005–15.

page 34 **worse in women**: Hall JR, et al. *J Alzheimers Dis* 2013;35:363–71.

page 35 **the jury is still out**: Breitner JC, et al. *Alzheimers Dement* 2011;7:402–11.

page 36 **triggering its appearance**: Perry V, et al. *Nat Rev Immunol* 2007; 7:161–7.

page 36 **cycles out of whack**: Klein SL, et al. *Lancet Infect Dis* 2010;10:338–49.

page 36 **12 million of whom are women**: National Institute of Mental Health: http://www.nimh.nih.gov/publicat/numbers.cfm.

page 36 **worsens during menopause**: Goldstein JM, et al. *Front Neurosci* 2014;8:247.

page 37 **later in life**: Goveas JS, et al. *J Am Geriatr Soc* 2011;59:57–66.

page 37 **in her lifetime**: www.womenshealth.gov/a-z-topics/thyroid-disease.

page 38 **her brain seem to remain**: Shadyab AH, et al. *Menopause* 2017; 24:35–44.

page 38 **higher risk of cognitive decline**: Gilsanz P, et al. *Neurology* 2019;92:in press.

page 40 **or widowed women**: Pankratz VS, et al. *Neurology* 2015;84:1433–42.

Chapter 4: The Brain's Journey from Pregnancy to Menopause

page 46 **2 million per second**: ed. Shonkoff JP, Phillips DA. *From Neurons to Neighborhoods*. Washington, DC: National Academies Press, 2000.

page 46 **to social signals**: Hoekzema E, et al. *Nat Neurosci* 2017;20:287–96.

page 47 **working memory**: Henry JD, et al. *J Clin Exp Neuropsych* 2007; 29:793–803.

page 47 **definitively unaltered**: Christensen H, et al. *Br J Psychiatry* 2010; 196:126–32.

page 48 **nearly twenty years**: Fraser Am, et al. *Circulation* 2012;125:1367–80.

page 49 **several weeks or more**: Wisner KL, et al. *New Engl J Med* 2002; 347:194–9.

page 52 **in recent years**: www.cdc.gov/nchs/data/databriefs/db309.pdf.

page 53 **reported in Europe**: van Keep PA, et al. *Maturitas* 1983;5:69–75.

page 53 **in China**: Han C, et al. *BMC Anesthesiology* 2103;17:103.

page 53 **memory decline and dementia**: Bove R, et al. *Neurology* 2014;82: 222–9.

page 53 **anxiety and depression**: Rocca WA, et al. *Menopause* 2018;25:1275–85.

page 57 **in part genetically linked**: Jiao X, et al. *Trends Endocrinol Metab* 2018;29:795–807.

page 58 **go through perimenopause**: Jacobs EG, et al. *J Neurosci* 2016;36:10163–73.

page 60 **future heart disease**: Thurston RC. *Climacteric* 2018;21:96–100.

page 63 **reproductive conflict**: Cant MA, et al. *Proc Natl Acad Sci USA* 2008; 105:5332–6.

Chapter 5: The Age of Precision Medicine

page 70 **may be inaccurate:** Dorschner MO, et al. *Am J Hum Genet* 2013; 93:631–40.

page 70 **40 percent of cases:** Tandy-Connor S, et al. *Genet Med* 2018;20:1515–21.

page 71 **presenilin 2 (PSEN2) genes:** Tanzi RE, et al. *Neuron* 2001;32:181–4.

page 71 **than many people fear:** Ritchie K, et al. *Lancet* 2002;360:1759–66.

page 79 **for clinical use:** www.genomicslawreport.com/index.php/2011/05/12/.

page 79 **by age eighty-five:** Qian J, et al. *PLoS Med* 2017;14:e1002254.

page 80 **psychological risks:** Green RC, et al. *N Engl J Med* 2009;361:245–54.

Chapter 6: Medical History and Laboratory Tests

page 85 **than their slimmer peers:** Shoberiri F, et al. *J Menopausal Med* 2016;22:14–9.

page 87 **the study of dementia prevention:** The SPRINT MIND investigators. *JAMA* 2019;321:553–61.

page 87 **blood pressure management:** Rodrigue KM, et al. *JAMA Neurol* 2013;70:600–6.

page 89 **with a regular metabolism:** Rettberg JR, et al. *Neurobiol Aging* 2016; 40:155–63.

page 89 **or sudden death:** Costello BT, et al. *Clin Cardiol* 2016;39:96–102.

page 89 **raising LDL cholesterol:** Ward H, et al. *Arch Intern Med* 2009; 169:1424–9.

page 90 **at or above 13:** Seshadri S, et al. *N Eng J Med* 2002;346:476–83.

page 91 **the symptoms of dementia:** Morris MS. *Lancet Neurol* 2003;2: 425–8.

page 91 **vitamin B12 deficiency:** Vidal-Alaball J, et al. *Cochrane Database Syst Rev* 2005;3:CD004655.

page 91 **dementia in late life:** Yurko-Mauro K, et al. *PLoS One* 2015;10:e0120391; Tan ZS, et al. *Neurology* 2012;78:658–64.

page 91 **the high-risk category:** Stark KD, et al. *Prog Lipid Res* 2016;63:132–52.

page 94 **in a variety of cognitive tasks:** Ferretti MT, et al. *Nat Rev Neurol* 2018;14:457–69.

page 94 **after menopause:** Rentz D, et al. *Menopause* 2017;24:400–8.

page 95 **diagnosed sooner:** Mielke M, et al. *Clin Epidemiol* 2014; 6:37–48.

page 96 **in women than in men:** Wiebers DO, et al. *Lancet.* 2003 Jul 12; 362(9378):103–10.

page 96 **interactions with our sex hormones:** https://seer.cancer.gov/statfacts /html/brain.html.

page 97 **those undergoing menopause:** Diaz JF, et al. *Arch Neurol* 1991; 48:1022–5.

page 97 **women in menopause:** Mosconi L, et al. *PLoS One* 2018;13: e0207885.

page 98 **via their PET scans:** Ossenkoppele R, et al. *JAMA* 2015;313:1939–49.

page 98 **25 percent of cases:** De Wilde A, et al. *JAMA Neurol* 2018;75:1062–70.

page 98 **symptoms of the disease:** Fantoni ER, et al. *J Alzheimers Dis* 2018; 63:783–96.

Chapter 8: Hormones, Antidepressants, and Other Meds: Do *You* Need Them?

page 120 **as well as overall mortality:** Lobo RA. *J Clin Endocrinol Metab* 2013;98:1771–80.

page 120 **who had never taken the hormones:** Grodstein F, et al. *Ann Intern Med* 2000;133:933–41.

page 121 **the opposite of what was intended:** Rossouw JE, et al. *JAMA* 2002; 288:321–33; Anderson GL, et al. *JAMA* 2004;291:1701–12.

page 121 **an increased risk of dementia:** Shumaker S, et al. *JAMA* 2003;289: 2651–62.

page 124 **than those who did not take MHT:** Manson JE, et al. *JAMA* 2017; 318:927–38.

page 124 **39 percent lower risk of death:** Salpeter SR, et al. *J Gen Intern Med* 2004;19:791–804.

page 124 **initiated soon after menopause:** Hodis HN, et al. *N Engl J Med* 2016; 374:1221–31.

page 124 **cardiac deaths:** Salpeter S, et al. *Am J Med* 2009;122:1016–22.

page 124 **cause of early menopause:** Doll KM, et al. *JAMA Surg* 2016;151:876–7.

page 124 **even premature death:** Shuster LT, et al. *Maturitas* 2009;65:161–6.

page 124 **they did not take estrogens:** Sarrel PM, et al. *Am J Pub Health* 2013;103:1583–8.

page 125 **than taking a placebo:** Chlebowski RT, et al. *N Engl J Med* 2009; 360:573–87.

page 125 **undergone a hysterectomy:** LaCroix AZ, et al. *JAMA* 2011;305:1305–14.

page 126 **cancer risk with MHT use:** North American Menopause Society. *Menopause* 2012;19:257–71.

page 126 **carry lower risk:** Ross RK, et al. *J Natl Cancer Inst* 2000;92:328–32.

page 128 **preexisting high risk of cancer:** Collaborative Group on Hormonal Factors in Breast Cancer. *Lancet* 1997;350:1047–59.

page 128 **doubling of the risk of dementia:** Shumaker S, et al. *JAMA* 2003;289: 2651–62.

page 128 **accelerating existing brain issues:** Wassertheil-Smoller S, et al. *JAMA* 2003;289:2673–84; Resnick SM, et al. *Neurology* 2009;72:135–42.

page 129 **compared with those who did not:** LeBlanc ES, et al. *JAMA* 2001;285: 1489–99.

page 129 **risk of future dementia:** Rocca WA, et al. *Neurology* 2007;69:1074–83.

page 129 **who did not take the drug:** Bove R, et al. *Neurology* 2014; 82:222–9.

page 129 **discontinued treatment**: Maki P. *Menopause* 2013;20:695–709.

page 129 **six years of menopause onset**: Henderson VW, et al. *Neurology* 2016;87:699–708; Gleason CE, et al. *PLoS Med* 2015;12:e1001833.

page 131 **with the APOE-4 gene**: Jacobs EG, et al. *PLoS One* 2013;8:e54713.

page 132 **40 percent of the patients**: Shilling V, et al. *Eur J Oncol Nurs* 2007; 11:6–15.

page 133 **increased Alzheimer's risk**: Benson JR. *J Natl Cancer Inst* 2002;94:1336; Espeland MA, et al. *J Womens Health* 2010;19:371–9.

page 133 **raise some concerns**: Eberling JL, et al. *Neuroimage* 2004;21:364–71; Yaffe K, et al. *Am J Psychiatry* 2005;162:683–90.

page 133 **for women over sixty-five**: Mehta L, et al. *Circulation* 2018;137:e30–66.

page 135 **those who used nothing**: Crandall C, et al. *Menopause* 2018;25:11–20.

page 137 **reduced mood swings**: North American Menopause Society. *Menopause practice. A clinician's guide.* 5th edition.

page 138 **with some IUDS**: Skovlund CW, et al. *JAMA Psych* 2016;73:1154–62.

page 138 **25 percent more likely**: Skovlund CW, et al. *JAMA Psych* 2016;73:1154–62.

page 139 **one or two incidences**: Orleans RJ, et al. *N Engl J Med* 2014;370:1777–9.

page 139 **after age forty**: https://www.cdc.gov/nchs/products/databriefs/db283 .htm.

page 140 **elsewhere in the body**: Banks WA. *Endocrinology* 2012;153:4111–9.

page 140 **its estrogen in-house**: Lu Y, et al. *J Neurosci* 2019;1970–18.

page 145 The diagrams incorporate the North American Menopause Society's Decision-Making Algorithm for Menopause Management, the American Association of Clinical Endocrinologists Guidelines for Management of Menopausal Symptoms as Related to Breast Cancer, the American College of Cardiology/American Heart Association ASCVD Risk Prediction Score, and the National Cancer Institute's Breast Cancer Risk Assessment Tool, as well as current data on dementia risk.

Chapter 9: Food Matters for Your Gray Matter

page 150 **from start to finish**: Gould E. *Nat Rev Neurosci* 2007;8:481–8.

page 150 **epigenetic lever**: Colvis CM, et al. *J Neurosci* 2005;25:10379–89.

page 151 **they respond to diets**: Lundsgaard AM, et al. *Front Endocrinol* 2014;5:e195.

page 153 **as her diet**: Heine PA, et al. *Proc Natl Acad Sci USA* 2000;97:12729–34.

page 153 **all observed after menopause**: Davis SR, et al. *Climacteric* 2012; 15:419–29.

page 155 **dietary interventions in women**: Kroenke CH, et al. *Menopause* 2012; 19:980–8.

page 155 **resistance against cancer**: Prentice RL, et al. *JAMA* 2006;295:629–42.

page 155 **or heart disease**: Howard BV, et al. *JAMA* 2006;295:655–66.

page 156 **with a fairly small sample:** https://blogs.plos.org/neuro/2016/07/16/ketones-to-combat-alzheimers-disease/.

page 158 **increased risk of heart disease:** Oh K, et al. *Am J Epidemiol* 2005; 161:672–9.

page 158 **by up to 67 percent:** Hu FB, et al. *N Eng J Med* 1997;337:1491–99.

page 158 **who ate fewer than 2 grams:** Morris MC, et al. *Neurobiol Aging* 2014; 35:S59–64.

page 159 **half that amount:** Okereke OI, et al. *Ann Neurol* 2012;72:124–34.

page 159 **than those who ate less:** Morris MC, et al. *Arch Neurol* 2003;60:194–200.

page 159 **in the long term:** Pottala JV, et al. *Neurology* 2015;82:435–42; Tan ZS, et al. *Neurology* 2012;78:658–64.

page 159 **lowest levels of Alzheimer's plaques:** Mosconi L, et al. *BMJ* 2014;4:e004850.

page 159 **replacing animal fats:** Rice MS, et al. *Am J Public Health* 2016;160:1592–8; Carruba G, et al. *Nutr Cancer* 2006;56:253–9.

page 159 **ovarian cancer:** Jones LW, et al. *Lancet Oncol* 2006;7:1017–26.

page 160 **higher amounts of vegetable oils:** Farvid MS, et al. *BMJ* 2014;348:3437.

page 160 **better cancer-survival rates:** Chlebowski RT, et al. *JAMA Oncol* 2016;e181212.

page 160 **"bad" estrogens in their bodies:** Wynder EL, et al. *JNCI* 2007;89:766–75.

page 160 **stroke later in life:** Hu FB, et al. *N Eng J Med* 1997; 337: 1491–9.

page 161 **type 2 diabetes:** Schulze MB, et al. *Am J Clin Nutr* 2004;80:348–56.

page 161 **cancer:** Monroe KR, et al. *Nutr Cancer* 2007;8:127–35.

page 161 **and dementia:** Knopman DS. *JAMA* 2009;302:686–7; Morris MC, et al. *Alzheimers Dement* 2015;11:1007–14.

page 161 **showed the best results:** Liu S, et al. *Am J Clin Nutr* 2000;71:1455–61.

page 161 **people without diabetes:** Crane PK, et al. *New Eng J Med* 2013;369: 540–8.

page 162 **suited to women's health:** Maki KC, et al. *J Nutr* 2015;145:S159–63.

page 162 **world's life-expectancy charts:** www.who.int/mediacentre/news/releases/2014/world-health-statistics-2014/en/.

page 163 **a positive sign for longevity:** Crous-Bou M, et al. *BMJ* 2014;349:g6674.

page 163 **sugary beverages:** Oh K, et al. *Am J Epidemiol* 2005;161:672–9.

page 163 **the largest trial to date:** Estruch T, et al. *Ann Intern Med* 2006; 145:1–11.

page 163 **much less cognitive decline:** Vallas-Pedret C, et al. *JAMA Intern Med* 2015;175:1094–103.

page 163 **eating a Western diet:** Mosconi L, et al. *J Prevent Alz Dis* 2014;1: 23–32; Walters M, et al. *BMJ Open* 2018;8:e023664.

page 163 **five additional years' worth of aging:** Berti V, et al. *Neurology* 2018; 90:e1789–98.

page 164 **for both genders**: Scarmeas N, et al. *JAMA* 2009;302:627–37.

page 164 **balancing estrogen in our favor**: Monroe KR, et al. *Nutr Cancer* 2007; 8:127–35.

page 164 **breast cancer occurrence in half**: Toledo E, et al. *JAMA Intern Med* 2015;175:1752–60.

page 164 **in as little as one year**: Gold EB, et al. *Menopause* 2006;13:423–33.

page 164 **hot flashes and night sweats**: Herber-Gast GC, et al. *Am J Clin Nutr* 2013;97:1092–9.

page 165 **chronic and mental illnesses**: Samieri C, et al. *Ann Intern Med* 2013; 159:584–91.

Chapter 10: Eight Steps to a Well-Nourished Brain

page 168 **health-packed greens**: Morris MC, et al. *Neurology* 2018; 90:e214–e222.

page 169 **didn't eat these berries**: Devore E, et al. *Ann Neurol* 2012;72:135–43.

page 169 **all those conditions**: Muga MA, et al. *BMC Geriatr* 2017 Nov 21;17:268.

page 169 **increased risk of colon cancer**: http://globocan.iarc.fr.

page 172 **for both women and men**: Knopman DS. *JAMA* 2009;302:686–7; Morris MC, et al. *Alzheimers Dement* 2015;11:1007–14.

page 172 **lowest risk of heart disease**: Liu S, et al. *Am J Clin Nutr* 1999;70: 412–9.

page 172 **lower risk of type 2 diabetes**: Schulze MB, et al. *Am J Clin Nutr* 2004; 80:348–56.

page 174 **as little as eight weeks**: Mastroiacovo D, et al. *Am J Clin Nutr* 2015;101:538–48.

page 175 **many fruits and vegetables**: Franke AA, et al. *Proc Soc Exp Biol Med* 1998;217:263–73.

page 175 **by up to 45 percent**: Franco O, et al. *JAMA* 2016;315:2554–63.

page 175 **their Western counterparts**: http://globocan.iarc.fr/Pages/fact _sheets_cancer.aspx.

page 176 **to develop breast cancer**: Hsieh CY, et al. *Cancer Res* 1998;58:3833–8.

page 176 **breast cancer risk in women**: Messina M, et al. *Oncology* 2013;27:430–7.

page 176 **can even reduce mortality**: Nechuta SJ, et al. *Am J Clin Nutr* 212;96: 123–32.

page 176 **circulating in your bloodstream**: Chen MN, et al. *Climacteric* 2015;18:260–9.

page 176 **isoflavone-rich soy foods**: www.aicr.org/cancer-research-update; Rock CL, et al. *Cancer J Clin* 2012;62:242–4.

page 177 **genetically modified soybeans**: www.ers.usda.gov/data-products /adoption-of-genetically-engineered-crops-in-the-us/recent -trends-in-ge-adoption.aspx.

page 177 **snacks and pastas**: Anderson JW, et al. *N Engl J Med* 1995;333:276–82.

page 179 **especially in women:** Mosconi L, et al. *BMJ* 2014;4:e004850.

page 179 **who consumed little to none:** Morris MC, et al. *JAMA* 2002;287: 3230–7.

page 179 **with vitamin C:** Engelhart MJ, et al. *JAMA* 2002;287:3223–9.

page 179 **helps regulate estrogen levels:** Ziaei S, et al. *Gynecol Obstet Invest* 2007;64:204–7.

page 182 **ORAC . . . units:** Carlsen MH, et al. *Nutr J* 2010;9:3–18.

page 182 **bacterial inhibition:** Tajkarimi MM, et al. *Food Control* 2010;21: 1199–218.

page 183 **for post-menopausal women:** Fiolet T, et al. *BMJ* 2018;360:k322.

page 183 **too much sodium:** Micha R, et al. *JAMA* 2017;317:912–24.

page 184 **balance to shoot for:** Simopoulos AP. *Am J Clin Nutr* 1991;54:438–63.

page 184 **risk of premature birth:** Saldeen P, et al. *Obstet Gynecol Surv* 2004;59:722–30.

page 185 **depression in both genders:** Gross G, et al. *PLoS One* 2014;9:e96905.

page 185 **more severe symptoms than men do:** Giles GE, et al. *Nutr Rev* 2013;71:727–41.

page 185 **by up to 70 percent:** Kalmijn S, et al. *Neurology* 2004;62:275–80.

page 185 **the later you enter menopause:** Dunneram Y, et al. *J Epidemiol Comm Health* 2018;72:733–40.

page 186 **better cognitive performance:** Okereke OI, et al. *Ann Neurol* 2012;72:124–34.

page 186 **patients with type 2 diabetes:** Devore EE, et al. *Diabetes Care* 2009;32:635–40.

page 186 **heart disease and stroke:** Hu FB, et al. *BMJ* 1998;317:1341.

page 187 **close to 30 percent:** Sacks FM, et al. *Circulation* 2017;136:e1–23.

page 188 **"we advise against the use of coconut oil":** Sacks FM, et al. *Circulation* 2017;136:e1–23.

page 188 **did not show this increase:** Khaw K, et al. *BMJ Open* 2018;8:e020167.

page 188 **substantial degree in butter:** Zong G, et al. *BMJ* 2016;355:i5796.

page 188 **diagnosed with Alzheimer's:** De la Rubia Orti JE, et al. *J Alzheimers Dis* 2018;65:577–87.

page 189 **who tolerate it well:** Chacarro JE, et al. *Hum Reproduct* 2007;22: 1340–7.

page 191 **heart disease and dementia:** Kivipelto M, et al. *Ann Int Med* 2002;137:149–55.

page 191 **doubling the risk of dementia:** Solomon A, et al. *Dement Geriatr Cog Dis* 2009;28:75–80.

page 191 **in healthy individuals:** Hu FB, et al. *JAMA* 1999;281:1387–94.

page 192 **heart failure later in life:** Djousse L, et al. *Circulation* 2008;117:512–6.

page 192 **an increased risk of stroke:** Bennet AM, et al. *JAMA* 2007;298: 1300–11.

page 192 **who consumed a comparable amount**: Kivipelto M, et al. *J Cell Mol Med* 2008;12:2762–71.

page 192 **a family history of Alzheimer's**: Mosconi L, et al. *BMJ* 2014;4:e004850.

page 192 **fat in the diet**: Shin JY, et al. *Am J Clin Nutr* 2013;98:146–59.

page 193 **cognitive performance in APOE-4 carriers**: Yassine HN, et al. *JAMA Neurol* 2018;74:339–47.

page 193 **people with the APOE-4 gene**: Van de Rest O, et al. *Neurology* 2016;86:2063–70.

page 193 **supporting brain longevity**: Chassaing B, et al. *Nature* 2015;519:92–6.

page 193 **the healthiest microbiomes**: Claesson MJ, et al. *Nature* 2012; 488:178–84.

page 193 **a poor-quality gut microbiome**: Chassaing B, et al. *Nature* 2015; 519:92–6.

page 194 **high complex-carbohydrate diets**: Caro H, et al. *J Clin Endocrinol Metabolism* 2016;101:233–42.

page 194 **many unpleasant problems**: Heitkemper MM, et al. *Gend Med* 2009;6:S152–67.

page 195 **risk of hot flashes**: Sievert LL, et al. *Ann Hum Biol* 2006;33:4–16.

page 195 **breast cancer**: Colditz GA, et al. *Nat Rev Cancer* 2005;5:388–96.

page 195 **alcohol consumption may pose even greater risks**: Livingston G, et al. *Lancet* 2017;390:2673–734.

page 196 **a potent antioxidant**: Price NL, et al. *Cell Metabolism* 2012;15:675–90.

page 196 **may promote a healthy brain**: Eskelinen MH, et al. *J Alzh Dis* 2009;16:85–91.

page 196 **among all beverages**: Streitburger DP, et al. *PLoS One* 2012;7:e44195.

page 198 **by up to 30 percent**: Edmonds CJ, et al. *Front Hum Neurosci* 2013;7:363; Benefer MD, et al. *Eur J Nutr* 2013;52:617–24.

page 198 **7 percent drink none at all**: Goodman AB, et al. *Prevent Chron Dis* 2013;10:E51.

page 198 **"purified" water and beer**: LaComb RP, et al. Food Surveys Research Group Dietary Data Brief No. 6, August 2011.

page 198 **risk of ovulatory infertility**: Caan B, et al. *Am J Public Health* 1998;88:270–4.

page 199 **thyroid function**: Diamanti-Kandarakis E, et al. *Endocr Rev* 2009; 30:293–342.

page 199 **raises serious concerns**: Korach KS., *Reproductive and Developmental Toxicology*, Marcel Dekker Ltd, 1998.

page 199 **increased risk of Alzheimer's**: Yan D, et al. *Sci Rep* 2016;6:32222.

page 199 **with the APOE-4 gene**: Livingston G, et al. *Lancet* 2017;390:2673–4.

page 202 **women in general**: www.niehs.nih.gov/health/topics/agents /pesticides/index.cfm.

page 204 **and promote longevity**: Mattson MP, et al. *J Nutr Biochem* 2005;16: 129–37.

page 204 **in as little as one year**: Kroenke CH, et al. *Menopause* 2012;19:980–8.

page 205 **to reduce this risk**: Michels KB, et al. *Cancer* 2007;109:2712–49.

page 205 **in as little as three months**: Witte AV, et al. *Proc Natl Acad Sci USA* 2009;106:1255–60.

page 205 **six months on the diet**: Harvie MN, et al. *Int J Obesity* 2011;35:714–27.

page 206 **burn fat more efficiently**: Mattson MP, Wan R. *J Nutr Biochem* 2005;16:129–37.

page 206 **against obesity and diabetes**: Chaix A, et al. *Cell Metab* 2014;20: 991–1005.

Chapter 11: Supplements for Women's Brains

page 209 **one supplement for brain-health reasons**: https://www.aarp.org /health/brain-health/global-council-on-brain-health/supplements/.

page 209 **from artificial supplements**: Hercberg S, et al. *Arch Intern Med* 2004;164:2335–42.

page 210 **the discomforts of menopause**: Franco O, et al. *J Am Med Assoc* 2016;315:2554–63

page 210 **validated clinical efficacy**: Franco O, et al. *J Am Med Assoc* 2016; 315:2554–63.

page 210 **patients with mild depression**: Larkin M. *Lancet* 2000;355:1619.

page 210 **mental clarity**: Scarmeas N, et al. *Lancet Neurol* 2018;17:1006-15.

page 210 **protective against Alzheimer's**: Mosconi L. *Brain Food: The Surprising Science of Eating for Cognitive Power.* Avery/Penguin Random House, 2018.

page 211 **balancing effects on homocysteine**: Tangney CC, et al. *Neurology* 2009;72:361–7.

page 211 **when measured via MRI scans**: Douaud G, et al. *Proc Natl Acad Sci USA* 2013;110:9523–8.

page 211 **together with omega-3s**: Jernerén F, et al. *Am J Clin Nutr* 2015;102: 215–21.

page 211 **particularly in APOE-4 carriers**: Yassine HN, et al. *JAMA Neurology* 2018;74:339–47.

page 212 **reduced risk of dementia**: Yurko-Mauro K, et al. *PLoS One* 2015;10:e0120391.

page 212 **overall cognitive function**: Tan MS, et al. *J Alzh Dis* 2015;43:589–603.

page 212 **following a TBI or stroke**: Raghavan A, et al. *Neural Regen Res* 2014;9:1104–7.

page 215 **hot flashes and night sweats**: Franco O, et al. *J Am Med Assoc* 2016;315:2554–63.

page 215 **a 46 percent reduction**: Cisafulli A, et al. *Menopause* 2004;11:400–4.

page 215 **good at easing night sweats**: Lipovac M, et al. *Gynecol Endocrinol* 2012;28:203–7.

page 215 **without any serious side effects**: www.aicr.org/cancer-research-update.

page 215 **at a dose of 400 IUs per day**: Ziaei S, et al. *Gynecol Obstet Invest* 2007;64:204–7.

page 216 **reduced hot flashes**: Franco O, et al. *JAMA* 2016;315:2554–63.

page 216 **it is superior to a placebo**: Franco O, et al. *JAMA* 2016;315:2554–63.

page 216 **ameliorate hot flashes**: Taku K, et al. *Menopause* 2012;19:776–90.

page 216 **at least in some women**: Ernst E. *Ann Int Med* 2002;136:42–53.

page 218 **short-term treatment of mild depression**: Larkin M. *Lancet* 2000; 355:1619.

page 218 **depressed mood**: Bae JH, et al. *Nutr Res* 2018;50:1–9.

page 218 **especially in women**: Yang JR, et al. *Neuropsychiatr Dis Treat* 2015;11:-2055–61.

page 218 **during perimenopause and post-menopause**: Franco O, et al. *JAMA* 2016;315:2554–63.

page 219 **help you fall asleep**: Brezinski A, et al. *Sleep Med Rev* 2005;9:41–50.

page 219 **insomnia, anxiety, and stress**: Cropley M, et al. *Phytother Res* 2002; 16:23–7.

page 219 **in as little as three months**: Henmi H, et al. *Fertil Steril* 2003;80:459–61.

page 220 **hot flashes and disturbed sleep**: Leonetti HB, et al. *Obstet Gynecol* 1999;94:225–8.

page 220 **the effects of supplementation are not very consistent**: Abbasi B, et al. *J Res Med Sci* 2012;17:1161–9.

page 221 **combat the effects of stress**: Stough C, et al. *Nutr J* 2014;13:122.

page 221 **blood sugar regulation**: Spasov AA, et al. *Phytomedicine* 2000;7:85–9; Darbinyan V, et al. *Phytomedicine* 2000;7:365–71.

page 222 **after taking ashwagandha**: Choudhary D, et al. *J Evid Based Compl Altern Med* 2017;22:96–106.

page 222 **after just sixty days**: Chandrasekhar K, et al. *Indian J Psychol Med* 2012;34:255–62.

page 222 **during times of stress**: Abdou AM, et al. *Biofactors* 2006;26:201–8.

page 223 **fat-burning properties**: Verpeut J, et al. *Nutr Res* 2013;33: doi:10.1016/j.nutres.2013.04.001.

page 223 **metformin or rosiglitazone**: Jun Y, et al. *Metabolism* 2008;57:712–7.

page 223 **markers of cardiovascular health**: Desideri G, et al. *Hypertension* 2012;11:1930–60.

Chapter 12: Women and Exercise: Could Less Be More?

page 225 **evident on multiple fronts**: Hillman CH, et al. *Nat Rev Neurosci* 2008;9:58–65.

page 226 **aging at the cellular level**: Tucker LA. *Prevent Med* 2017;100:145–51.

page 226 **enlargement of those areas**: Van Praag H. *Trends Neurosci* 2009;32: 283–90.

page 226 **higher number of Alzheimer's plaques**: Okonkwo OC, et al. *Neurology* 2014;83:1753–60.

page 226 **brain changes far ahead of time**: Walters M, et al. *BMJ* 2018;8:e023664.

page 227 **most convincing trials to date**: Erickson KI, et al. *Proc Natl Acad Sci USA* 2011;108:3017–22.

page 227 **exercised less or not at all**: Brown BM, et al. *Alzheimers Dement* 2017; 13:1197–1206.

page 227 **better off than those who don't**: Head D, et al. *Arch Neurology* 2012;69:636–43.

page 228 **obesity, or hypertension**: Norton S, et al. *Lancet Neurol* 2014;13:788–94.

page 228 **physical activity per week**: www.cdc.gov/nchs/data/nhis/earlyrelease /earlyrelease201605.pdf; accessed August 2018.

page 228 **once high school ends**: Armstrong S, et al. *JAMA Pediatr* 2018; 172:732–40.

page 228 **hampered from exercising**: Hull EE, et al. *J Phys Act Health* 2010; 7:577–83.

page 229 **more time to exercise**: Nomaguchi KM, et al. *J Marriage Fam* 2004;66:413–30.

page 229 **for women of all ages**: Middleton LE, et al. *J Am Geriatr Soc* 2010; 58:1322–6.

page 229 **later in life**: Hörder H, et al. *Neurology* 2018;90:e1298–35.

page 229 **women with a diagnosis of dementia**: Hogervorst E, et al. *J Alzheimers Dis Parkinsonism* 2012;2:e117.

page 230 **within just a few months**: Eggermont L, et al. *Neurosci Biobehav Rev* 2006;30:562–75.

page 230 **more in women than in men**: Middleton LE, et al. *J Am Geriatr Soc* 2010;58:1322–6.

page 230 **our sex hormones affect it**: Braun B, et al. *Exerc Sports Sci Rev* 2001;29:149–54.

page 231 **glucose more efficiently**: Ashley CD, et al. *Sports Med* 2000;29:221–7.

page 232 **the greater the benefits**: Cotman CW, et al. *Trends Neurosci* 2007;30: 464–72.

page 233 **strength and balance**: Lance C, et al. *J Sports Sci Med* 2006; 5: 662–71.

page 233 **for optimal ovulatory fertility**: Rich-Edwards JW, et al. *Epidemiology* 2002;13:184–90.

page 235 **heart disease, diabetes**: Earnest C, et al. *Am J Cardiol* 2013; 111:1805–11; Lucke J, et al. *Biol Res Nursing* 2010;12:162–70.

page 235 **diminished the returns**: Kyu H, et al. *BMJ* 2016;354:i3857.

page 236 **than those who exercised less**: Blumel JE, et al. *Menopause* 2016;23: 488–93.

page 238 **maintain bone density and mass**: Bonaiuti D, et al. *Cochrane Database Syst Rev* 2002;2:CD000333.

page 240 **by a good 35 percent**: Scarmeas N, et al. *JAMA* 2009;302:627-37.

Chapter 13: Be Mindful: De-Stress, Sleep, and Balance

page 242 **higher levels of stress than men**: www.apa.org/news/press/releases /stress/2010/national-report.pdf.

page 244 **before you even turn fifty**: Echouffo-Tcheugui JB, et al. *Neurology* 2018;91:e1961–70.

page 245 **"tend-and-befriend"**: Taylor SE, et al. *Psych Rev* 2000;107:411–29.

page 246 **the area in charge of reason**: Wang J, et al. *Soc Cogn Affect Neurosci* 2007;2:227–39.

page 246 **different areas of the brain**: Mather M, et al. *Neuroreport* 2010; 21:933–7.

page 246 **60 percent of these caregivers**: www.caregiving.org/data/Caregiving _in_the_US_2009_full_report.pdf.

page 246 **Hispanic and African American women**: Nebel RA, et al. *Alzheimers Dement* 2018;14:1171–83.

page 247 **chronic health conditions**: Navaie-Waliser M, et al. *Am J Pub Health* 2002;92:409–13.

page 247 **resting when necessary**: Schulz R, et al. *Ann Behav Med* 1997;19:110–6.

page 247 **heart disease, stroke**: www.apa.org/news/press/releases /stress/2010/national-report.pdf; Schulz R, et al. *JAMA* 1999;15:2215–9.

page 247 **developing Alzheimer's themselves**: Bottiggi Dassel K, et al. *Gerontologist* 2017; 57:319–28.

page 247 **than male caregivers**: https://www.caregiver.org/women-and -caregiving-facts-and-figures.

page 248 **an additional emotional toll**: Alzheimer's disease facts and figures. *Alzheimers Dement* 2016;12:459–509.

page 249 **a reduced risk of dementia**: Holt-Lunstad J, et al. *PLoS Medicine* 2010;7:e1000316.

page 249 **as often as possible**: Fratiglioni L et al. *Lancet* 2000;355:1315–9.

page 249 **employee recovery and health**: Park Y, et al. *J Occup Health Psychol* 2011;16:457–67.

page 249 **circadian rhythm**: Chang AM, et al. *Proc Natl Acad Sci USA* 2015;112:1232–7.

page 250 **for the mind and the body**: Bratman GN, et al. *Proc Natl Acad Sci USA* 2015;112:8567–72.

page 250 **liver disease, or endometriosis**: Rada G, et al. *Cochrane Database Syst Rev* 2010;9:CD004923.

page 251 **has a positive influence on neuroplasticity**: Tang YY, et al. *Nat Rev Neurosci* 2015;16:213–25.

page 252 **regularly practicing TM**: Schneider RH, et al. *Circulation* 2012;5: 750–8.

page 252 **Alzheimer's patients and their caregivers**: Paller KA, et al. *Am J Alzheimers Dis Other Demen* 2015;30:257–67.

page 252 **compared with a group that did not**: Carmody JF, et al. *Menopause* 2011;18:611–20.

page 253 **within eight weeks**: Khalsa DS. *J Alzheimers Dis* 2015;48:1–12.

page 253 **improvement in their overall cognitive function**: Khalsa DS, et al. Alzheimer's Association International Conference 2018.

page 254 **after just twelve weeks of treatment**: Eyre HA, et al. *Int Psychogeriatr* 2017;29:557–67.

page 254 **reduced symptoms of stress and insomnia**: Newton KM, et al. *Menopause* 2014;21:339–46.

page 254 **those on chemotherapies**: Cramer H, et al. *Cancer* 2015; 121:2175–84.

page 255 **achieved by MHT**: Avis NE, et al. *Menopause* 2016;23:626–37.

page 255 **experience more daytime sleepiness**: https://sleepfoundation.org /sleep-polls-data/sleep-in-america-poll/2007-women-and-sleep.

page 256 **dementia has made an appearance**: Yaffe K, et al. *Lancet Neurol* 2014;13:1017–28.

page 256 **relieving itself from harmful toxins**: Xie L, et al. *Science* 2013; 342:373–7.

page 256 **seemingly healthy people**: Spira AP, et al. *JAMA Neurology* 2013;70:1537–43.

page 256 **with poorer cognitive function**: Mander BA, et al. *Nat Neurosci* 2013;16:357–64.

page 257 **with a minimum of six for those sixty-five or older**: Isaacson RS, et al. *Alzheimers Dement* 2018;14:1663–73.

page 257 **a bit longer in women than in men**: Mourtazaev MS, et al. *Sleep* 1995;18:557–64.

page 257 **affecting over half of all post-menopausal women**: Jehan S, et al. *J Sleep Med Disord* 2016;3:1064–9.

page 257 **visit the National Sleep Foundation website**: www.sleepfoundation .org/sleep-disorders-problems/sleep-apnea-treatment.

Chapter 14: More Ways to Protect Your Brain

page 262 **lowering the risk of dementia later in life**: Fabrigoule C, et al. *Lancet Neurol* 2002;1:11.

page 263 **maintaining cognitive fitness over time**: Schneider AL, et al. *J Am Geriatr Soc* 2012;60:1847–53.

page 263 **as compared with those who did not**: Verghese J, et al. *Neurology* 2006;66:821–7.

page 263 **even prevent Alzheimer's plaques**: Landau SM, et al. *Arch Neurol* 2012;69:623–9.

page 263 **delayed onset of any cognitive decline**: Aguirre-Acevedo D, et al. *JAMA Neurol* 2016;73:431–8.

page 264 **formal education**: Vemuri P, et al. *Ann Neurol* 2012;72:730–8.

page 264 **higher, for women than for men**: www.census.gov/prod/2012pubs /p20-566.pdf.

page 265 **or cognitive performance**: Kable JW, et al. *J Neurosci* 2017; 37:7390–402.

page 265 **not in memory skills**: Rebok GW, et al. *J Am Geriatr Soc* 2014; 62:16–24; Wolinksy FD, et al. *PLoS One* 2013;8:e61624.

page 265 **limited or modest effects**: Lampit A, et al. *PLoS Medicine* 2014;11:e10001756.

page 267 **6 percent lead over female smokers**: www.lung.org/finding-cures /our-research/trend-reports/Tobacco-Trend-Report.pdf.

page 267 **smoke to relieve stress**: Smith PH, et al. *Prev Med* 2016;92:135–40.

page 267 **associated with habit formation**: Cosgrove K, et al. *J Neurosci* 2014; 34:16851–5.

page 268 **before they turned fifty**: http://dx.doi.org/10.1136/tobaccocontrol -2015-052510.

page 268 **persisted for over six years**: Gold EB, et al. *Am J Public Health* 2006;96:1226–35.

page 268 **Alzheimer's for both women and men**: Ott A, et al. *Lancet* 1998;351: 1840–3.

page 268 **diminishes this risk**: Hu FB, et al. *N Engl J Med* 2000;343:530–7.

page 268 **even steeper risks**: Livingston G, et al. *Lancet* 2017;390:2673–734.

page 269 **of all deaths worldwide**: Landrigan PJ, et al. *Lancet Comm* 2018;391: 462-512.

page 270 **contributing to cancer development**: www.breastcancer.org/risk /factors/cosmetics.

page 271 **who never took the medicines**: Gray SL, et al. *JAMA Intern Med* 2015;175:401–7.

page 271 **an increased Alzheimer's risk**: Billioti de Gage S, et al. *BMJ* 2014;349:g5205.

page 272 **often completely overlooked**: Teixeira FB, et al. *Front Aging Neurosci* 2017;9:327.

page 272 **brain inflammation and Alzheimer's plaques**: Kamer AR, et al. *Neurobiol Aging* 2015;36:627–33.

INDEX

Note: Page numbers in *italics* refer to diagrams. Page numbers followed by a *t* refer to tables.

Coconut-Lime Tofu with Mixed Vegetables, 294–95
coconut oil, 187–89
coffee, 196
cognitive decline/impairment
    and antioxidants, 179
    and APOE gene, 28
    and birth control pills, 137
    and blood pressure management, 87
    and brain shifts associated with menopause, 25
    and B vitamins, 90–91
    and cardiovascular disease, 30
    conditions that cause/mimic symptoms of, 82–83
    and dietary fats, 158–59
    drugs associated with, 270–72
    and exercise, 227, 229–30
    and fruits/vegetables, 168–69
    gender differences in, 94
    and grains, 172–73
    and hysterectomies, 124
    and inflammation, 34
    and intellectual engagement, 263
    and length of reproductive span, 38
    and loneliness, 266
    and Mediterranean diet, 163–64
    and menopause hormonal treatment, 129, 130
    risk factors for, 12, 26, 30–37
    and sleep deprivation, 255–56
    supplements for prevention of, 212
    See also Alzheimer's; dementia
cognitive health/function
    and B vitamins, 91
    and cognitive reserve, 263
    and diet, 150, 156, 173
    exercise's benefits for, 225–28, 229–30, 241
    and hydration, 197–99
    and intellectual engagement, 262–66
    and meditation, 253
    and menopause, 11, 58–59, 60
    and menopause hormonal treatment, 129
    and microbiome, 193, 194
    and pregnancy/baby brain, 47–48
    testing, 94–95
    and thyroid disease, 90
concussions, 30, 32, 214*t*
cortisol
    and alcohol, 195
    and high-intensity exercise, 231–32
    and penalties of prolonged stress, 61–62, 243, 244
    reference values for, 85*t*
    role of, in stress response, 246
    and supplements, 221, 222
C-reactive protein (CRP), 84*t*, 92, 212, 214*t*, 216, 216*t*
crying spells, 49
Cushing's syndrome, 93

dairy, 189–90, 288*t*, 289
death, leading causes of, 21
dementia
    and Ambien, xxiii
    and antioxidants, 179
    and birth control pills, 137
    and blood sugar, 161
    and cancer treatments, 133
    and carbohydrates, 161
    and cardiovascular disease, 30
    and cholesterol, 191
    clinical trials for, 80
    conditions that mimic symptoms of, 95–96
    and dietary fats, 158–59
    and exercise, 227, 229–30, 240
    and family-history questionnaire, 72–73, 74–75, 76
    gender differences in, 16, 26
    genetic risk of, 70–73
    and homocysteine levels, 90
    and hysterectomies, 129
    and length of reproductive span, 38
    and medications, 270–71
    and meditation, 253
    and Mediterranean diet, 164
    and menopause, 53, 59
    and menopause hormonal treatment, 121–22, 128–29, 130, 131
    and music-related memories, 266
    and omega-3s, 91
    and oophorectomies (removal of ovaries), 53
    and processed foods, 183
    and sleep deprivation, 256
    and systemic infections, 35
    and traumatic brain injury, 32
    and vitamins C and E, 212
    See also Alzheimer's
dental hygiene, 272
depression
    and Alzheimer's risks, 82
    and antidepressants, 61
    and birth control pills, 137–38
    drugs prescribed for, 271
    gender differences in, xviii, 36–37
    and hormonal fluctuations, 11–12
    impact on memory, 30
    and menopause, 11, 37, 60–61
    and omega-3s, 185, 210–11
    and ovaries removed prior to menopause, 53
    postpartum, 49–51
    prevalence of, 20, 36
    questionnaire on risk of, 108–9
    as risk factor for disease, 30, 36–37
    risk factors for, 18, 36
    and sleep, 60
    and social engagement, 266

and menopause, 11, 58–59
and number of children, 47
and omega-3s, 91
and oophorectomies (removal of ovaries), 53
and pregnancy/baby brain, 45–46, 47–48
and sleep, 60
and stress, 243–44
supplements for, 210–12, 213–14t
and traumatic brain injury, 32
men
    and body fat distribution, 151
    and declines in testosterone, 12
    life expectancies for, 19, 20
    and number of children, 47
    risk factors unique to, 40
    and testosterone, 43
meningiomas, xviii
menopause, 51–64
    age of onset, 54, 57–58
    and Alzheimer's risks, 9, 10–11, 21
    and birth control pills, 137
    cognitive changes associated with, 8–13, 9, 57, 58–59
    conditions that mimic symptoms of, 90
    and depression, 37
    diagnosis of, 93
    duration of, 54–55
    early/premature, 54, 185
    evolutionary function of, 63
    and exercise, 235–38
    and fruits/vegetables, 169
    genetic factors in, 57
    hormonal changes associated with, 7, 8, 9, 10–11, 55–56
    and insulin resistance, 32
    and menstruation cessation, 54–55, 143–44t
    and mental health issues, 11–12
    myths surrounding, 54–58
    number of women near or in, 12, 53
    ovaries removed prior to, 53, 54
    screener questionnaire for, 110–12
    and sex hormone levels, 85t, 93
    and supplements, 215–16, 216–17t
    symptoms of, 8, 9, 13, 51–52, 56, 58–63, 164, 169 (see also specific symptoms, including hot flashes)
    taboos surrounding, 52
    triggered by surgeries/treatments, 53, 124
    as turning point for medical risks, 26
    See also perimenopause
menopause hormonal treatment (MHT), 119–48
    and Alzheimer's risks, 128–29
    antidepressants in lieu of, 138–40
    benefits of, 124–25
    bio-identical hormones, 135–36
    and birth control pills, 136–38
    and cancer-risk concerns, 120, 121, 125–28, 131, 141, 144
    contraindications to, 141–42t

and dementia risk, 130, 131
and diet plan, 207
and heart disease risk, 120–21, 124, 126, 130, 141, 144
history of, 120–23
and hysterectomies, 126, 129, 130, 146, 146t
making informed decisions about, 140–48, 141–42t, 143–44t, 145t, 146t
managing symptoms without, 147–48
new generation of hormones for, 134–38
and oophorectomies (removal of ovaries), 53
oral versus topical, 134–35
primary indications for, 142
soy isoflavones in lieu of, 215
"window of opportunity" for, 123–24, 147
See also Women's Health Initiative study
menstrual cycle
    and alcohol/caffeine metabolism, 196
    cessation of, 54–55, 143–44t, 191
    difficult, 43
    hormones associated with, 42, 42–43, 93
    pain in, 184
    and PMS, 43
mental health issues, xviii, 11–12. See also specific conditions, including depression
metabolic disorders, 31–32
metabolism, 153, 223, 224t
microbiome, 193–95
migraines, xviii, 43
mild cognitive impairment, 79, 87, 211, 252, 254, 271
milk, 189–90
mind-body techniques, 250–55, 258
mindfulness meditation, 252
misdiagnosis of women's conditions, xxiii–xxiv
"momnesia," 47–48
monounsaturated fats, 158, 186–87, 192
moods and mood swings
    and birth control pills, 137
    and B vitamins, 91
    exercise's impact on, 225
    and menopause, 11, 60–61
    and menstrual cycle, 43
    and postpartum depression, 49
    and sleep, 60
    and supplements, 217–18, 218–19t, 222, 222t
motherhood, 46–51, 255
muscles, 152, 230–31
music, 266
Must-Have Green Salad recipe, 298
myths around women's brain health, 15–24
    on disease due to longer life spans, 19–22
    on genes as destiny, 16–19
    on impending cures, 22–23

nature, restorative power of, 250
neuroendocrine system of women, 43–45, 44, 56

tests for Alzheimer's prevention *(cont.)*
   fasting glucose and insulin tests, 84*t*, 88–89
   homocysteine, 84*t*, 90
   omega-3s, 84*t*, 90–92
   thyroid, 84*t*, 90
   waist-to-height ratio, 83*t*, 86
thalidomide, xx
thyroid, 44, 84*t*, 90
thyroid disease, 30, 37, 90
time-restricted feeding, 206–7
Transcendental Meditation (TM), 252
trans fats, 158–59, 160, 182–83, 191, 192–93
transgender women, 14
transient ischemic attacks (TIA), 30
traumatic brain injury (TBI), 30, 32–33, 214*t*
triglycerides, 32, 84*t*, 89, 142*t*, 205
tryptophan, 259
23andMe, 68, 69, 70, 80

urinary tract infections (UTIs), 35, 36

vaginal bleeding, 141*t*
vaginal dryness, 142
valerian root, 219, 220*t*
vegetable oils, refined, 187
vegetables
   antioxidants in, 180, 181–82*t*
   and fiber, 170, 171*t*
   guidelines for, 167, 168–69
   and Mediterranean diet, 165
   organic, 203
   serving sizes for, 288*t*, 289
   and vitamin D, 190
vegetarians and vegans, 186, 191, 211, 212, 213*t*, 219*t*, 221
Veggie Burgers recipe, 306–7
Vellutata di Broccoli recipe, 307–8
vitamin B5, 221
vitamin B6, 210, 213*t*, 260
vitamin B12, 82, 84*t*, 90–91, 210, 211, 213*t*, 221, 260
vitamin C, 179, 210, 212, 214*t*, 219, 220*t*
vitamin D, 190
vitamin E, 179, 180, 210, 212, 214*t*, 215–16, 216*t*

waist-to-height ratio, 83*t*, 86
walking, 227, 237
water and hydration, 196–99, 197*t*
weight gain
   estrogen's role in, 32, 152–53
   gender differences in, 151–53
   and metabolism support, 223, 224*t*
   during pregnancy, 49
   and testosterone levels, 43
   and thyroid disease symptoms, 90
weight loss, 35, 204
whales, 63
white matter disease, 96–97
wine, 195–96
Women's Alzheimer's Movement (WAM), x, xi
Women's Brain Initiative (WBI), 281
women's equality, xv, 7
Women's Health Initiative study
   about, 121–22
   ages of participants, 155
   and Alzheimer's risks, 128
   and cancer-risk concerns, 121, 125–27
   and dietary fats, 160
   dietary modification arm of, 154–56
   and heart-disease related deaths, 124
   memory study (WHIMS), 128
   and smoking, 268
   systemic therapy used by, 134
   and "window of opportunity" for MHT, 123
Women's Healthy Eating and Living Study, 164
Wyeth Pharmaceuticals, 120

X chromosome, relative size of, 4
xenoestrogens, 199, 200–201*t*, 270

Y chromosome, relative size of, 4
Yentl syndrome, xxiv
yoga and Pilates, 237–38, 239*t*, 254

Zucchini Infornati (In the Oven) recipe, 308
Zulresso (brexanolone), 50